NOVEL INFECTIOUS AGENTS AND THE CENTRAL NERVOUS SYSTEM

The Ciba Foundation is an international scientific and educational charity. It was established in 1947 by the Swiss chemical and pharmaceutical company of CIBA Limited—now CIBA-GEIGY Limited. The Foundation operates independently in London under English trust law.

The Ciba Foundation exists to promote international cooperation in biological, medical and chemical research. It organizes about eight international multidisciplinary symposia each year on topics that seem ready for discussion by a small group of research workers. The papers and discussions are published in the Ciba Foundation symposium series. The Foundation also holds many shorter meetings (not published), organized by the Foundation itself or by outside scientific organizations. The staff always welcome suggestions for future meetings.

The Foundation's house at 41 Portland Place, London, W1N 4BN, provides facilities for meetings of all kinds. Its Media Resource Service supplies information to journalists on all scientific and technological topics. The library, open seven days a week to any graduate in science or medicine, also provides information on scientific meetings throughout the world and answers general enquiries on biomedical and chemical subjects. Scientists from any part of the world may stay in the house during working visits to London.

Ciba Foundation Symposium 135

NOVEL INFECTIOUS AGENTS AND THE CENTRAL NERVOUS SYSTEM

A Wiley – Interscience Publication

1988

JOHN WILEY & SONS

Chichester · New York · Brisbane · Toronto · Singapore

Published in 1988 by John Wiley & Sons Ltd, Chichester, UK.

Suggested series entry for library catalogues:
Ciba Foundation Symposia

Ciba Foundation Symposium 135
x + 278 pages, 44 figures, 29 tables

Library of Congress Cataloging-in-Publication Data

Novel infectious agents and the central nervous system.
    p. cm. — (Ciba Foundation symposium ; 135)
    'A Wiley–Interscience publication.'
    Papers and discussions from the Symposium on Novel Infectious
Agents and the Central Nervous System, held at the Ciba Foundation,
London, June 30–July 2, 1987.
    Includes indexes.
    ISBN 0 471 91512 2
    1. Central nervous system—Diseases—Etiology—Congresses.
2. Scrapie—Congresses. 3. Prions—Congresses. I. Symposium on
Novel Infectious Agents and the Central Nervous System (1987 : Ciba
Foundation) II. Ciba Foundation. III. Series.
RC385.N68   1988
616.8'3—dc19   87–31740
                                                          CIP

British Library Cataloguing in Publication Data

Novel infectious agents and the central
    nervous system. — (Ciba Foundation
    symposium ; 135).
    1. Central nervous system — Diseases
    I. Series
    616.8   RC360
    ISBN 0 471 91512 2

Typeset by Inforum Ltd, Portsmouth
Printed and bound in Great Britain.

Contents

Participants

J.W. Almond Department of Microbiology, University of Reading, London Road, Reading, Berks RG1 5AQ, UK

K. Beyreuther ZMBH – Zentrum für Molekulare Biologie, Universität Heidelberg, Im Neuenheimer Feld 282, D-6900 Heidelberg, Federal Republic of Germany

D.C. Bolton Laboratory of Molecular Structure & Function, Institute for Basic Research in Developmental Disabilities, 1050 Forest Hill Road, Staten Island, New York 10314, USA

F. Brown Wellcome Biotechnology Ltd, Langley Court, Beckenham, Kent BR3 3BS, UK

P. Brown Nervous System Studies Laboratory, NINCDS, Building 36, Room 5B 21, National Institutes of Health, Bethesda, Maryland 20892, USA

G.A. Carlson The Jackson Laboratory, Bar Harbor, Maine 04609, USA

R.I. Carp Department of Virology, Institute for Basic Research in Developmental Disabilities, 1050 Forest Hill Road, Staten Island, New York 10314, USA

B. Chesebro Laboratory of Persistent Viral Diseases, National Institutes of Health, Rocky Mountain Laboratories, Hamilton, Montana 59840, USA

S. DeArmond Department of Pathology (Neuropathology), Box 0506, University of California, School of Medicine, San Francisco, California 94143, USA

A.G. Dickinson AFRC & MRC Neuropathogenesis Unit, Ogston Building, West Mains Road, Edinburgh EH9 3JF, UK

H. Diringer Department of Biochemistry, Robert Koch Institut des Bundesgesundheitsamtes, Nordufer 20, D-1000 Berlin 65, Federal Republic of Germany

D. Dormont   Division of Radiobiology & Radioprotection, Centre de Recherches du Service de Santé des Armées, 1 Bis rue Raoul Batany, F-92140 Clamart, France

H. Fraser   AFRC & MRC Neuropathogenesis Unit, Ogston Building, West Mains Road, Edinburgh EH9 3JF, UK

R. Gabizon   Department of Neurology, University of California, School of Medicine, San Francisco, California 94143, USA

A.T. Haase   Department of Microbiology, University of Minnesota Medical School, 1460 Mayo Memorial Building, Box 196 UMHC, 420 Delaware St SE, Minneapolis, Minnesota 55455, USA

J. Hope   AFRC & MRC Neuropathogenesis Unit, Ogston Building, West Mains Road, Edinburgh EH9 3JF, UK

R.H. Kimberlin   AFRC & MRC Neuropathogenesis Unit, Ogston Building, West Mains Road, Edinburgh EH9 3JF, UK

M.P. McKinley   Department of Neurology, University of California, School of Medicine, San Francisco, California 94143, USA

L. Manuelidis   Neuropathology Section, Yale University, School of Medicine, PO Box 3333, 333 Cedar Street, New Haven, Connecticut 06510, USA

C.L. Masters   Department of Neuropathology, Royal Perth Hospital, Box X 2213, GPO, Perth, Western Australia 6001

P.A. Merz   Departments of Virology & Pathological Neurobiology, Institute for Basic Research in Developmental Disabilities, 1050 Forest Hill Road, Staten Island, New York 10314, USA

B. Oesch   Institut für Molekularbiologie I, Universität Zürich, Hönggerberg, CH-8093 Zürich, Switzerland

S.B. Prusiner   Department of Neurology, HSE-781, University of California, School of Medicine, San Francisco, California 94143-0518, USA

G.W. Roberts (*Ciba Foundation Bursar*)   Division of Psychiatry, Clinical Research Centre, Watford Road, Harrow, Middlesex HA1 3UJ, UK

N. Stahl   Department of Neurology, HSE-781, University of California, School of Medicine, San Francisco, California 94143-0518, USA

J. Tateishi   Department of Neuropathology, Neurological Institute, Kyushu University 60, Maidashi, Fukuoka 812, Japan

H.M. Wisniewski   Institute for Basic Research in Developmental Disabilities, 1050 Forest Hill Road, Staten Island, New York 10314, USA

Introduction

Wellcome Biotechnology Ltd, Langley Court, Beckenham, Kent BR3 3BS

1988 Novel infectious agents and the central nervous system. Wiley, Chichester (Ciba Foundation Symposium 135) p 1–2

The increasing awareness that progressive degeneration of the central nervous system, as occurs in Alzheimer's disease, may be caused by a transmissible agent has focused attention on conditions such as Creutzfeld-Jakob disease and kuru in man and scrapie in sheep and goats, which are known to be caused by such agents. These transmissible diseases are linked by a similar pathology and the agents causing them are usually referred to as unconventional viruses. However, one of the more intriguing features of the agents is the uncertainty about their composition and physical organization.

The brilliant work on the epidemiology of kuru and the accumulating evidence that scrapie, kuru and Creutzfeld-Jakob disease have a similar aetiology have thrown into relief the opportunity for understanding these diseases. Those working on scrapie have had the advantage since 1961 of a cheap and readily available animal model. They have the additional advantage that the agent is present in large amounts in the brain of the moribund mouse. These factors have made scrapie the model for the study of this group of agents.

Why then are we still uncertain about the nature of the scrapie agent? One of the main reasons is that the only way to assay it is by measuring its infectivity. Since this can only be performed in animals, with its inherent inaccuracy, the interpretation of purification studies is difficult. Moreover, the assays take upwards of six months. Another reason is the nature of the infectious material, because brain tissue is a particularly difficult starting point for chemical studies. Nevertheless, over the last few years several proposals have been made about the nature of the scrapie agent. Some of these have been controversial and, to those engaged on work with conventional viruses, sometimes scarcely credible. Thus, the idea of an infectious membrane, carbohydrate or protein is difficult to grasp after 30 years of Crick and Watson. More recently, attention has been focused on three hypotheses. The first of these is that the scrapie agent is a virus after all, being identical with the fibrils seen on electron microscopical examination of preparations from infected animals. The second hypothesis postulates the existence of a virino, which is proposed to consist of a low molecular weight scrapie-specific nucleic acid and a protein derived from the host. The third and clearly most provocative hypothesis is that the agent is a self-replicating protein. This last hypothesis was originally based on the observation that the infectivity of scrapie is not affected by several agents which should inactivate nucleic acids, whereas it is inactivated by several protein-specific reagents. More important, however, is the fact that a scrapie-specific nucleic acid has not been detected. During the past few years, application of the methods of molecular biology has started to make considerable impact on the study of scrapie and the related agents and the general feeling in the field is one of optimism that this intriguing problem may soon be solved.

The clinical neurology and epidemiology of Creutzfeldt-Jakob disease, with special reference to iatrogenic cases

Paul Brown

Laboratory of Central Nervous System Studies, NINCDS, National Institutes of Health, Bethesda, Maryland 20892, USA

Abstract. The clinical characteristics of Creutzfeldt-Jakob disease (CJD) in a newly analysed group of 223 cases transmitted to primates at the NIH are compared to a recent large series of neuropathologically verified cases in France, and the limited conclusions from worldwide epidemiological studies are briefly summarized. Discussion then focuses on iatrogenic CJD, with special attention to the interplay of clinical, laboratory and epidemiological features of the current outbreak of CJD in hypopituitary dwarfs treated with growth hormone extracted from pools of human pituitary glands.

1988 Novel infectious agents and the central nervous system. Wiley, Chichester (Ciba Foundation Symposium 135) p 3–23

For nearly 50 years after Alfons Jakob reported on a group of patients that included the first unequivocal case of the disease that now bears his name (Jakob 1921) interest languished in this arcane footnote to neurology, and, in part engendered by Jakob's own descriptions, confusion surrounded its very definition as a disease entity.

As the years passed, the pernicious medical instinct for renaming things led to a profusion of terms for a heterogeneous collection of subacute and chronic neurological disorders that paraded under the rubric of Creutzfeldt-Jakob disease (CJD). At the core of this collection there was nevertheless a growing number of patients with neuropathologically characteristic spongiform encephalopathy, which was slowly gaining appreciation as a critical diagnostic feature.

When the transmissible nature of CJD was finally revealed (Gibbs et al 1968), two things happened: first, a burgeoning interest in the disease pushed the publication rate through a series of swings around an exponential progression that is currently approaching 100 publications per year (Fig. 1); second, the clinical and pathological definition of CJD as a disease entity could at last

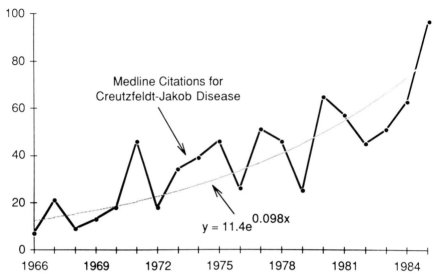

FIG. 1.   Medline citations of Creutzfeldt-Jakob disease 1966–1985. Solid line connects actual number of citations each year; shaded line represents a 'best fit' curve by the method of least squares, which is exponential in form.

be securely anchored to a single, unimpeachable criterion: transmission of disease to experimental animals inoculated with homogenates of brain tissue from suspected patients (Roos et al 1973, Traub et al 1977, Bernoulli et al 1979).

Sporadic CJD: clinical features

After 20 years of diagnostic refinement based on this criterion of transmission, a final evaluation of its performance is appropriate. For this purpose, the clinical features of a series of 223 transmitted cases of CJD referred to the Laboratory of Central Nervous System Studies at the NIH between 1968 and 1982 may be compared to a series of 230 pathologically verified cases identified in France during the same period of time (Brown et al 1986). As shown in Tables 1 and 2, and in Figs. 2 and 3, there is not much to choose between the two series. Another large series of pathologically verified cases from England and Wales (Will & Matthews 1984) is not suitable for a similarly detailed comparison because of a somewhat different analytical format, but it conforms in all essential respects to the French and NIH series.

In the transmitted series, spongiform change was clearly evident by light microscopy in the brains of all but three patients, in whom neuropathological changes were stated to be absent, but whose slides were unobtainable for review. Thus, the criterion of transmissibility has both validated the pathological benchmark of spongiform change and refined a spectrum of diverse

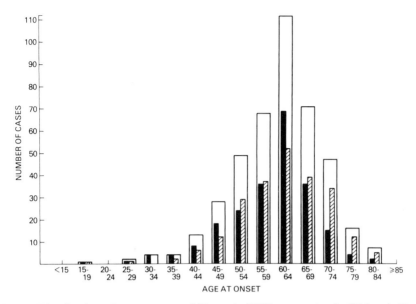

FIG. 2.   Distribution of age at onset of illness in NIH case series (solid bars), French case series (cross-hatched bars), and combined series (open bars). In some age groups, the combined series total does not equal the sums of the individual series, because 29 transmitted patients in the French series were included in the NIH transmitted series, and so have been included only once in the combined totals.

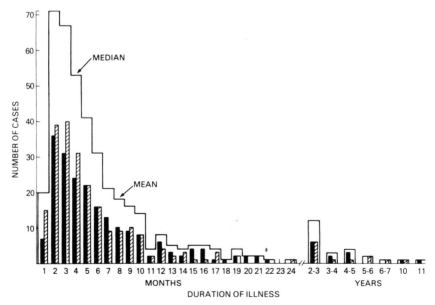

FIG. 3.   Distribution of durations of illness in NIH case series (solid bars), French case series (cross-hatched bars), and combined series (open bars). The individual and combined series case totals are subject to the same proviso noted in Fig. 2.

TABLE 1 **Percentage frequencies of symptoms and signs at the onset of Creutzfeldt-Jakob disease in two large consecutive case series, based either on the criterion of disease transmission (NIH) or neuropathology (French)**

Symptoms/signs	Clinical presentation			
	NIH (n = 223)		French (n = 230)	
Mental deterioration	67		64	
Dementia		48		31
Behavioural abnormalities		25		29
Higher cortical function		12		15
Cerebellar	33		34	
Visual/oculomotor	16		17	
Visual		13		14
Oculomotor		4		6
Vertigo	10		7	
Headache	10		7	
Sensory	6		5	
Movement disorder	5		0.4	
Myoclonus		1		0
Other		4		0.4
Extra-pyramidal	1		2	
Pyramidal	0.5		2	
Lower motor neuron	0		0.4	
Seizures	0		0.4	
Periodic EEG activity	0		0	
Triphasic 1 cycle/second		0		0
Slow wave burst/suppression		0		0

clinical disorders into the single nosological entity of CJD.

Typically, the disease affects individuals between 50 and 75 years of age, and is slightly more prevalent in females. In about 40% of patients, the illness begins as a gradually progressive mental deterioration, usually manifested as memory loss, errors in judgement, mood change, or uncharacteristic behaviour; less often, mental deterioration takes the form of higher cortical function defects such as aphasia or apraxia. In another 25% of patients, the onset of mental deterioration coincides with the appearance of physical neurological symptoms, and in the remaining 35% of patients, the onset consists exclusively of physical symptoms. In this latter group, cerebellar or visual/oculomotor signs may dominate the clinical presentation, and often evolve rapidly. In fact, the sudden onset of vertigo, diplopia, ataxia, paralysis or paresthesias can lead to a mistaken initial diagnosis of cerebrovascular accident or multiple sclerosis.

TABLE 2 **Percentage frequencies of symptoms and signs during the clinical course of Creutzfeldt-Jakob disease in two large consecutive case series, based either on the criterion of disease transmission (NIH) or neuropathology (French)**

Symptoms/signs	Clinical course	
	NIH (n = 223)	French (n = 230)
Mental deterioration	100	100
Dementia	100	96
Behavioural abnormalities	77	49
Higher cortical function	51	47
Movement disorder	86	91
Myoclonus	80	88
Other	37	26
Cerebellar	70	61
Pyramidal	67	43
Extra-pyramidal	57	67
Visual/oculomotor	40	42
Visual	23	31
Oculomotor	18	16
Seizures	18	8
Headache	16	14
Vertigo	16	10
Lower motor neuron	13	11
Sensory	5	11
Periodic EEG activity	59	80
Triphasic 1 cycle/second	46	56
Slow wave burst/suppression	14	32

In relentless progression, mental deterioration and mood alteration evolve into a state of dementia, confusion and mutism; visual deterioration continues to cortical blindness (often with hallucinations); and motor impairments progress to increasingly severe incoordination, marked oppositional rigidity, and involuntary movements (usually myoclonic, but often trembling and sometimes choreo-athetoid or complex movements). Most patients die within six months of the onset of illness and there are no verified cases of recovery.

Although this consistent and characteristic clinical picture is seen in the majority of patients, the existence of a small proportion of clinically atypical patients has also been confirmed by the criterion of transmissibility, including some cases of the Gerstmann-Sträussler-Scheinker syndrome (Masters et al 1981, Tateishi et al 1984), a few cases with prominent amyotrophic signs (Salazar et al 1983), and some otherwise typical cases of unusually long duration (Brown et al 1984).

Sporadic CJD: epidemiology

The epidemiology of CJD was extensively discussed in 1980 (Brown 1980). It has been further elaborated in a series of studies carried out in several countries over the past decade, recently reviewed (Brown et al 1987), and summarized in Table 3.

The major results that have emerged from the composite of these studies can be briefly stated: CJD occurs worldwide in a consistent pattern of disease frequency and distribution, with a currently stable incidence of about one new case per million people per year in large metropolitan centres and about half that incidence in the general population; case clustering appears to be founded less in geography than in genetic predisposition, whether as high-incidence foci in ethnic or comparatively inbred local populations, or as familial disease, which accounts for 5–10% of all cases. Symptomatic patients are not important in directly spreading disease; evidence for environmental sources of CJD infection is either anecdotal or statistically tenuous. Direct inoculation of the agent remains the only proven mechanism for spreading CJD but documented cases of iatrogenic CJD are rare.

Therefore, although epidemiological investigation of CJD has provided a good description of its occurrence in the world population, the question of how, or even if, the sporadic disease is acquired has not been resolved. For help, we may have to turn from epidemiology to molecular biology, where by virtue of a series of recent discoveries, the old self-replicating membrane hypothesis (Hunter et al 1968) has, like the fabled Phoenix, risen from its own ashes to be reborn as a modern alternative for nucleic acid-directed replication mechanisms.

The identification of a ubiquitous gene encoding a membrane protein with an amyloid configuration that is somehow uniquely modified in individuals with CJD (or animals with scrapie) and which influences the length of the incubation period in these diseases has led to several interesting new hypotheses (German & Marsh 1983, Prusiner 1984, Wills 1986). These all share the idea of a self-regulating mechanism for the production of a 'pathological' protein without having recourse to DNA-directed replication. Such a protein could account for the occurrence of sporadic (i.e., 'spontaneous') CJD in the majority of human cases, and also explain iatrogenic (or experimental) CJD, where direct introduction of the pathological protein molecule would provide the seed for its own replication.

However, such explanations for the origin of CJD evolved in the rarified air of pure molecular biology and must eventually submit themselves to a broader, if more mundane, biological perspective, that includes the phenomena of strain variation and apparent spontaneous mutation of infectious isolates, infectious-like pathogenesis in host species, and the contagious character of natural scrapie in sheep and goats. It must also be pointed out that the peculiarities of

TABLE 3 Summary of regional and national surveys of Creutzfeldt-Jakob disease

Country	Survey years	Total no. of cases	Male: female ratio	Familial cases (%)	National annual mortality rate (cases/million)	Regional case concentration (no. of cases)	Regional annual mortality rate (cases/million)
Chile	1955–1972	19	1.04[a]	27[a]	0.10	Santiago (14)	0.25
	1973–1977	16			0.31	Santiago (11)	0.73
	1978–1983	46			0.69	Santiago (16)	0.77
	1980–1982					rural (4)	8.33
Czechoslovakia	1972–1986	46	0.92	22	0.66	rural (17)[b]	3.20
						rural (5)	2.96
England and Wales	1964–1973	46[a]	0.53	7	0.09	2 rural (3,5)	
	1970–1979	158	0.60	4–6	0.31		
	1980–1984	120	0.69	6	0.47		
France	1968–1977	178	0.81	6–9	0.34	Paris (28)	1.22
	1978–1982	151			0.58	Paris (13)	1.19
Hungary	1960–1986	65[a]	0.55	11	0.39	Budapest (33)	0.64
						rural (10)	
Israel	1963–1972	23	1.90	4	1.07 (0.47)[c]	Libyan-born (13)	42.22
	1963–1977					Libyan-born (20)[d]	44.41
Italy	1958–1971	32	1.00	8	0.05	Rome (21)	0.50
	1974–1979					Genoa (6)	0.93
	1975–1979					Parma rural (10)	1.38
	1972–1985	87	0.53	0	0.11		
Japan	1975–1977	75[e]	0.79	6	0.15 (0.45)[f]	Fukuoka (5)	1.10[g]
United States	1973–1977	265	0.95		0.26	Boston (22)	0.43
	1979	148[h]	0.84		0.66		
	1980	142[h]			0.63		

[a] Histopathologically-confirmed cases only
[b] 35% familial cases
[c] Excluding Libyan-born cases
[d] 35% familial cases
[e] Questionnaire survey of neurology services
[f] Estimated period prevalence rate
[g] Point prevalence rate (1978)
[h] U.S. mortality statistics (death certificates)

sporadic CJD in the human population could all be plausibly explained by the transfer of an infectious agent by inefficient routes of infection during the early preclinical stage of a disease that had a 'natural' incubation period of several decades. Whichever of these various explanations proves correct, the outcome promises to be both novel and exciting.

Iatrogenic CJD

The few proven or highly likely cases of iatrogenically acquired CJD are summarized in Table 4. Until recently, iatrogenic CJD was only recognized as a consequence of surgical procedures involving the eye (Duffy et al 1974) or brain (Bernoulli et al 1977, Foncin 1980, Will & Matthews 1982). To this small group of well known cases has been added a patient who underwent resection of a mastoidal cholesteatoma with replacement of a damaged section of underlying dura by a dura mater graft (Prichard et al 1987). The onset of CJD occurred 18 months after the operation. As no other patient with a dementing or otherwise suspect illness had undergone surgery in the hospital during the preceding several months, cross-contamination by instruments appeared a far less likely explanation than infection from the graft, which had been obtained from a commercial source of pooled dural patches from unidentified human cadavers.

TABLE 4   Summary of all proven or probable cases of iatrogenic Creutzfeldt-Jakob disease

Source of infection	Route of inoculation	Incubation period	Clinical duration
Corneal transplant	intraocular	18 months	8 months
Deep EEG electrodes	intracerebral	16 months	8 months
		20 months	23 months
Surgical instruments	intracerebral	18 months	2 months
		18 months	3 months
		19 months	3 months
		28 months	6 months
Dura mater graft	intracerebral	19 months	4 months
Human growth hormone	subcutaneous/ intramuscular	?–10 years	–[a]
		4–18 years	6 months
		6–13 years	19 months
		8–12 years	11 months
		12–15 years	14 months
		15–21 years	10 months
		19–23 years	3 months

[a] Patient died of pneumonia in the preclinical incubation phase of CJD

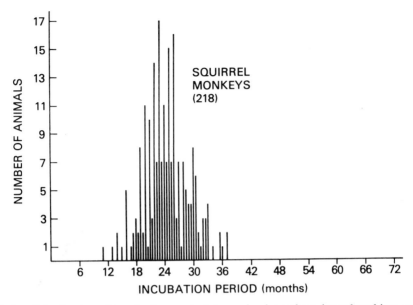

FIG. 4. Distribution of incubation periods in squirrel monkeys inoculated intracerebrally with 1–10% brain homogenates from patients with Creutzfeldt-Jakob disease.

TABLE 5 Results of primate experiments in which identical inocula (either 1% or 10% human CJD brain homogenates) were given by intracerebral or peripheral routes to different animals

Human case	Inoculated species	Duration of incubation period (months)	
		Intracerebral inoculation	Peripheral inoculation
Coc.	Squirrel monkey	11, 20	i.m.: non-CJD death (26)
Dow.	Spider monkey	25, 28, 34, 37	i.p.: non-CJD death (39, 41)
Gra.	Chimpanzee	13	i.m.: alive, no sx (156)
	Spider monkey	4 (sacrificed)	i.v.: non-CJD death (31)
Mat.	Chimpanzee	26	i.m.: 11
	Squirrel monkey	20	i.m.: non-CJD death (35)
Tuc.	Squirrel monkey	19, 24	s.c.: alive, no sx (136)
			i.v.: alive, no sx (136)
Woo.	Squirrel monkey	22, 22, 28, 30	s.c.: alive, no sx (116)
	Chimpanzee	12	s.c.: alive, no sx (116)
			i.d.: 19
			i.v., i.p., i.m.: 16

i.m., intramuscular; i.p., intraperitoneal; i.v., intravenous; s.c., subcutaneous; i.d., intradermal; sx, symptoms

TABLE 6   The effect of inoculum dose and route of inoculation on the incubation period in primates inoculated with primate-passaged, human strains of Creutzfeldt-Jakob disease or kuru

Human case	Inoculated species	Inoculation route	Inoculum dose (LD_{50})	Incubation period (months)
Eir. (kuru)	Chimpanzee	i.c.	10 000	10
			10 000	11
			20 000	12
		i.p., i.m., s.c.	75 000	18
Mat. (CJD)	Squirrel monkey	i.c.	20 000	16
		i.c.	20 000	18
		i.c.	10 000	20
		i.c.	20 000	30
		i.d., s.c.	80 000	24
Sep. (kuru)	Capuchin monkey	i.c.	20	17
		i.v., i.p., i.m., s.c.	80	81
Eir. (kuru)	Chimpanzee	i.c.	30	15
		i.v., i.p., i.m., s.c.	50	142
Mat.	Squirrel monkey	i.c.	200	18
(CJD)		i.d., s.c.	800	no transmission

i.c., intracerebral; i.v., intravenous; i.p., intraperitoneal; i.m., intramuscular, s.c., subcutaneous; i.d., intradermal

The other, more ominous, recent event has been the discovery of a small but growing number of cases of CJD developing in hypopituitary dwarfs treated with growth hormone derived from pools of human cadaver pituitary glands (Brown et al 1985, Brown 1988). The long incubation periods of 4–19 years between the last dose of hormone and the onset of CJD symptoms made the connection much more difficult to establish than in those patients undergoing surgical procedures, in whom incubation periods ranged from 16 to 28 months.

Primate transmission experiments in our NIH laboratory provide an excellent approximation to these human accidents. When CJD human brain homogenates are inoculated intracerebrally into a sensitive primate host such as the squirrel monkey, CJD is regularly transmissible after incubation periods that range from 12 to 36 months in a bell-shaped distribution curve around a mean value of 24 months (Fig. 4). When the same brain homogenates are inoculated by a peripheral rather than intracerebral route, however, transmission occurs only irregularly (Table 5). These experiments were conducted using 10% homogenates of untitred brain tissue from different CJD patients and, depending on the individual patient, the inoculum could have contained from 10 to 10 000 mean lethal doses.

A more precise relationship between inoculum dose and route of inoculation can be derived from experiments using primate-passaged, titred strains of virus (Table 6). When a high dose of virus is used, the incubation period is not very different after intracerebral or peripheral inoculation. When a low dose of virus is used, the incubation period is similarly short after intracerebral inoculation but after peripheral inoculation the incubation period stretches out from months to years, or the disease may not be transmitted at all. This probably applies to the human growth hormone recipients, explaining the very long incubation periods observed in these patients, and also contributing to the rarity of disease transmission. Indeed, the arithmetical probability of including an infected gland in a pituitary pool and the dilution factor during its processing suggest that the level of hormone contamination was probably so low that only an occasional ampoule from a contaminated batch contained even a single infectious particle.

Even more interesting than these extremely long incubation periods has been the unusual, almost stereotyped clinical picture of CJD in this group of patients. In all but one (who died in a preclinical stage of disease), the presenting symptom was cerebellar ataxia. Although the clinical presentation in sporadic CJD includes cerebellar signs in about one-third of patients, most of these have the coincidental appearance of mental deterioration or other neurological signs. In only about 10% of sporadic patients is the onset limited exclusively to cerebellar signs.

The evolution of illness in the growth hormone-treated patients was also unusual in that cerebellar and basal ganglion signs continued to dominate the clinical picture. Mental deterioration was a comparatively minor and often late-appearing feature, and none of the patients has shown the characteristic periodic electroencephalographic (EEG) activity that occurs in the majority of patients with sporadic CJD.

Thus, the illness in these iatrogenic growth hormone-treated patients shows a greater resemblance to kuru than to typical sporadic CJD cases in adults. Since all the iatrogenic cases were in young adults, one obvious explanation could be that the clinical form of illness is a function of the age at which it occurs. Kuru, for example, is typically a disease of young adults who were infected in childhood and adolescence. What about the small subset of non-iatrogenic CJD patients who die before the age of 40? Table 7 compares the clinical picture in a group of 15 young non-iatrogenic patients to the six iatrogenic growth hormone cases.

It is evident that young growth hormone-treated patients present a picture of CJD that is as different from sporadic CJD in young adults as it is from the disease in older adults. Almost all the young non-iatrogenic patients presented

TABLE 7 Clinical features of CJD in six growth hormone recipients (left side of table) and in 15 non-iatrogenic cases dying before the age of 40 years (right side of table)

Patient	JRo	ALa	PGr	DMc	WTa	TSt	MNa	DSo	MPr	EKe	SYa	BDe	YMa	JDe	LSi	MMa	RCo	MLe	STu	SFe	AFl
Age	20	22	23	31	32	37	16	18	19	20	26	26	27	31	31	34	35	35	35	35	39
Sex	M	F	M	F	M	M	M	M	F	F	M	F	F	F	F	F	M	M	M	F	F
Duration (months)	6	11	19	14	10	3	26	24	4	37	18	32	54	12	132	5	3	10	18	7	19
Mental deterioration																					
Dementia	+	000	000	000	000	000	000	000	+	000	000	0	+	0	000	000	+	0	000	0	+
Behavioural	000	+	0	+	0	000	+		000	000		000	+	000	000	000	000	000	000	000	000
Higher cortical	+		+	+		+	+			+	+	+	+		+	+	+				
Cerebellar																					
Ataxia	000	000	000	000	000	000	+		0	0	+	+	000	000	0	+	000	+		+	+
Nystagmus	000		0	0	+	000				+		+	+								+
Dysarthria	0	+	+	+	+	+	+	+		+	+	+	0	+	+	+		+		+	
Tremor			+	0	+							+	+	+		+					
Dysphagia	+		+		+	+						+	+		+						
Visual/oculomotor																					
Visual	+		+	+			+			0	0										
Oculomotor					+	+				+		+							0	0	
Movement disorder																					
Myoclonus	+	+	+	+	+	+	+	+	+	+	+	+	+	+	+	+	+	+	+	+	+
Other		+	+		+	+	+	+	0	+	000	+	+	+	+	+	+	000	+	+	+
Pyramidal							+	+		0	0	+	+	+			+			+	
Extra-pyramidial	+	+	+	+	+	+	+		+	+	+	+	+	+			+			+	+
Sensory	0						+									0					
Headache								000	000	0										0	
EEG Periodicity	+	0	+	+	+	+	+	+	+	+	+	+	+	+	+	+	+	+			+

Evolution of illness is indicated by the symbols: 000, present at onset; 0, present early in course; +, present later in course

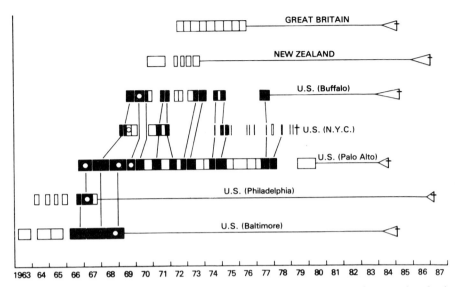

FIG. 5. Schematic representation of the time course of hormone therapy, incubation period, and illness and death in each of the seven neuropathologically verified cases of Creutzfeldt-Jakob disease in human growth hormone recipients. For each patient, the boxes indicate successive lots of hormone used during the course of therapy. Lots that were shared by more than one patient are shown in black, with inter-connecting lines. Boxes containing circles are lots that contained hormone extracted from a single batch of pituitary glands. △, period of illness; †, time of death.

with some form of mental deterioration and, although three had cerebellar signs, in only one of them (an unusual familial Japanese case with plaques and white matter involvement) was the onset exclusively cerebellar. Moreover, in contrast to the growth hormone-treated patients, CJD in the young non-iatrogenic group progressed with a characteristic accumulation of neurological signs and, more often than not, the appearance of periodic EEG activity. Thus, the youth of iatrogenic growth hormone-treated patients does not explain their distinctive clinical picture.

A second possible explanation could be that infection in the growth hormone-treated patients was due to a single strain of CJD virus with distinctive biological characteristics. The phenomenon of strain variation among the unconventional viruses has been particularly well documented in experimental scrapie infections (Bruce & Dickinson 1987), but has also been shown to apply to naturally occurring CJD (Gibbs et al 1979). For this explanation to have merit, however, there must be strong evidence for a common source of infection, and it was obvious from the start that no common lot of growth hormone had been shared by the three original U.S. patients. With the identification of two new cases during the past year, a minimum of three contaminated lots is now required to account for the five U.S. cases (Fig. 5).

In retrospect, however, our focus on lots of hormone that were distributed to patients was too narrow; we should have also been looking at the batches of pituitary glands from which the hormone lots were prepared, because there was no one-to-one relationship between lots of hormone and batches of pituitary glands. The constituents of a given lot of hormone always originated from several different batches of pituitary glands; and conversely, various fractions and remainders from a given batch of glands always found their way into several different lots of hormone. By going back to the original protocols it was possible to follow an individual batch of pituitary glands through its various processing steps into multiple lots of hormone. We have been able to identify one batch, processed in 1967, from which extracts found their way into at least one lot of hormone taken by each of the five U.S. patients at some point between 1967 and 1970.

However, even assuming this batch to have been the single source of infection for the U.S. patients, the two foreign patients (from England and New Zealand) remained unaccounted for. We subsequently learned that hormone received by the New Zealand patient was processed in the same laboratory that made hormone for distribution in the U.S., using pools of pituitary glands collected in the U.S. and New Zealand. Although the New Zealand patient did not share any hormone lot with the U.S. cases, the possibility that extracts from the same batch of pituitary glands mentioned above might have been included in New Zealand lots of hormone has not been excluded with equal certainty.

This still left the English case to explain, since the hormone given to this patient was reported to have been made exclusively from glands collected in the United Kingdom and processed in England. When we discovered that the physician who processed the hormone had apprenticed in the laboratory producing hormone for U.S. patients, we inquired whether some early lots might have in fact been prepared there, or whether any (potentially contaminated) equipment might have been brought to England. Neither conjecture proved correct, so the English case remains undeniably separate from all other cases, and closes discussion of the statistically improbable proposal that the outbreak of CJD in growth hormone recipients may have resulted from a single infected pituitary gland.

The most intriguing explanation for the distinctive clinical picture of CJD in growth hormone recipients is that the subcutaneous route of infection, with viraemic entry into the brain, produces a different sequence of pathology than is seen in the patient with sporadic CJD. It is true that when infected brain tissue is inoculated subcutaneously into primates, the disease does not differ clinically or pathologically from that following any other route of infection. However, in the milieu of infected pituitary tissue, it is reasonable to suppose that the biologically 'sticky' infectious particle of CJD might bind to the growth hormone protein during the course of purification. Were this to occur, the virus could be introduced into the central nervous system as an unwanted passenger on growth hormone molecules bound to receptor sites in the hypothalamus, then spread to nearby basal ganglion structures and their cerebellar projections.

A final thought about CJD in growth hormone recipients concerns the question of host susceptibility. If humans are uniformly susceptible to the infectious agent of CJD, then iatrogenic introduction of the agent will inevitably lead to illness and death, and no further explanation is required other than having been exposed to a contaminated ampoule of hormone. However, it appears more likely that human genetic factors may also influence susceptibility to infection and/or illness, as is true of experimental CJD and scrapie in animals. Genotypic analysis of future cases occurring under this extraordinary circumstance of iatrogenic infection acquired via a common exposure could reveal the existence of such human host determinants.

References

Bernoulli C, Siegfried J, Baumgartner G et al 1977 Danger of accidental person-to-person transmission of Creutzfeldt-Jakob disease by surgery. Lancet 1:478–479

Bernoulli CC, Masters CL, Gajdusek DC et al 1979 Early clinical features of Creutzfeldt-Jakob disease (subacute spongiform encephalopathy). In: Prusiner SB, Hadlow WJ (eds) Slow transmissible diseases of the nervous system. Academic Press, New York, vol 1:229–251

Brown P 1980 An epidemiologic critique of Creutzfeldt-Jakob disease. Epidemiol Rev 2:113–135

Brown P 1988 Human growth hormone therapy and Creutzfeldt-Jakob disease: a drama in three acts. Pediatrics, in press

Brown P, Rodgers-Johnson P, Cathala F et al 1984 Creutzfeldt-Jakob disease of long duration: clinicopathological characteristics, transmissibility, and differential diagnosis. Ann Neurol 16:295–304

Brown P, Gajdusek DC, Gibbs CJ Jr, Asher DM 1985 Potential epidemic of Creutzfeldt-Jakob disease from human growth hormone therapy. N Engl J Med 313:728–731

Brown P, Cathala F, Castaigne P, Gajdusek DC 1986 Creutzfeldt-Jakob disease: clinical analysis of a consecutive series of 230 neuropathologically-verified cases. Ann Neurol 20:597–602

Brown P, Cathala F, Raubertas RF et al 1987 The epidemiology of Creutzfeldt-Jakob disease: conclusion of a 15-year investigation in France and review of the world literature. Neurology 37:895–904

Bruce EM, Dickinson AG 1987 Biological evidence that scrapie agent has an independent genome. J Gen Virol 68:79–89

Duffy P, Wolf J, Collins G et al 1974 Possible person-to-person transmission of Creutzfeldt-Jakob disease. N Engl J Med: 290:692–693

Foncin J, Gaches J, Cathala F, et al 1980 Transmission iatrogène interhumaine possible de maladie de Creutzfeldt-Jakob avec atteinte des grains du cervelet. Rev Neurol (Paris) 136:280

German TL, Marsh RF 1983 The scrapie agent: a unique self-replicating pathogen. Prog Mol Subcell Biol 8:111–121

Gibbs CJ Jr, Gajdusek DC, Asher DM et al 1968 Creutzfeldt-Jakob disease (subacute spongiform encephalopathy): transmission to the chimpanzee. Science (Wash DC) 161:388–389

Gibbs CJ Jr, Gajdusek DC, Amyx H 1979 Strain variation in the viruses of Creutzfeldt-Jakob disease and kuru. In: Prusiner SB, Hadlow WJ (eds) Slow transmissible diseases of the nervous system. Academic Press, New York, vol 2:87–110

Hunter GD, Kimberlin RH, Gibbons RA 1968 Scrapie: a modified membrane hypothesis. J Theor Biol 20:355–357

Jakob A 1921 Uber eigenartige erkrankung des zentralnervensystems mit bemerkenswertem anatomischen befunde (spastische pseudosklerose-encephalomyelopathie mit disseminierten degenerationsherden). Dtsch Z Nervenheilkd 70:132–146

Masters CL, Gajdusek DC, Gibbs CJ Jr 1981 Creutzfeldt-Jakob disease virus isolations from the Gerstmann-Sträussler syndrome, with an analysis of the various forms of amyloid plaque deposition in the virus-induced spongiform encephalopathies. Brain 104:559–588

Prichard J, Thadani V, Kalb R, Manuelidis E 1987 Rapidly progressive dementia in a patient who received a cadaveric dura mater graft. Morb Mortal Wkly Rep 36:49–55

Prusiner SB 1984 Prions. Sci Am 251:50–59

Roos R, Gajdusek DC, Gibbs CJ Jr 1973 The clinical characteristics of transmissible Creutzfeldt-Jakob disease. Brain 96:1–20

Salazar AM, Masters CL, Gajdusek DC, Gibbs CJ Jr 1983 Syndromes of amyotrophic lateral sclerosis and dementia: relation to transmissible Creutzfeldt-Jakob disease. Ann Neurol 14:17–26

Tateishi J, Sato Y, Nagara H, Boellard JW 1984 Experimental transmission of human spongiform encephalopathy to small rodents. IV. Positive transmission from a typical case of Gerstmann-Sträussler-Scheinker disease. Acta Neuropathol 64:85–88

Traub R, Gajdusek DC, Gibbs CJ Jr 1977 Transmissible virus dementia: the relation of transmissible spongiform encephalopathy to Creutzfeldt-Jakob disease. In: Smith NL, Kinsbourne M (eds) Aging and dementia. Spectrum, New York, p 91–154

Will RG, Matthews WB 1982 Evidence for case-to-case transmission of Creutzfeldt-Jakob disease. J Neurol Neurosurg Psychiatry 45:235–238

Will RG, Matthews WB 1984 A retrospective study of Creutzfeldt-Jakob disease in England and Wales 1970–79. I: clinical features. J Neurol Neurosurg Psychiatry 47:134–140

Wills PR 1986 Scrapie, ribosomal proteins and biological information. J Theor Biol 122:157–178

DISCUSSION

Hope: Has anyone found PrP protein in normal pituitary or in the pituitaries of affected animals?

P. Brown: We have never looked.

Hope: Have you looked for scrapie-associated fibrils?

P. Brown: No, it's a good idea. We have recently inoculated pituitaries from CJD patients into chimps to verify that pituitary tissue is infectious. It is already known that pituitaries from scrapie-infected animals can be infectious.

Kimberlin: I find the incubation period differences that you showed between i.c. and peripheral routes very impressive. One of the differences between very long incubation scrapie models and short ones is this problem of neuroinvasion, and I think the same applies to peripherally injected CJD.

P. Brown: You all know the excellent data that are available for scrapie. The data I have shown come from 20 years of primate experiments on CJD, and, for identical inocula given into the brain or the periphery, these represent the total available information.

Merz: Paul, do you have any plans to see if the spleens have CJD infectivity? Richard Kimberlin's work has shown that this is a major source from which scrapie agent can get into the central nervous sytem after peripheral inoculation. If I remember correctly, human CJD spleen isolations are very rare in your laboratory.

P. Brown: Yes, they are rare to vanishing, only a single isolation in 24 attempts. We will certainly now study the spleen from growth hormone-treated cases of CJD as they arise. Only two patients, neither of whom has yet been published, have been diagnosed while still alive. None of the other patients' organs has been available for examination. One of these two patients had a full autopsy and material is available. I have looked for PrP and SAF, and they were present in the brains of these patients.

We thought that since the inoculation with growth hormone and the agent might constitute a kind of immunization, with patients being given multiple doses of the infectious agent it would be interesting to look for an antibody against these proteins in this group of young patients. They do not have antibody to the protein and probably were not immunized. I suspect that each of these patients was infected with only one contaminated vial and therefore had only a single exposure.

Masters: I would propose an alternate hypothesis to your idea of 'piggy-backing' into the hypothalamus. I have always thought that the cerebellar propensity of kuru was best explained on the basis of low dose entry through the gastrointestinal tract or skin by some pathway which involves retrograde transport into the cerebellum. This could take the form of retrograde spread through the fifth nerve to the brainstem or from the autonomic nervous system which innervates the gastrointestinal tract or spleen.

Of the cases that you looked at, how many have had electroencephalogram (EEG) examinations in the final stages?

P. Brown: EEGs were done repeatedly in every patient: all have been abnormal but not periodic.

Chesebro: With regard to these low dose transmissions in the animals, I was struck by the inability to get the virus to multiply at all. Have you looked at any of the animals which received those peripheral inoculations to see if they had infection in the spleen, for instance? Have you made a secondary pass from the splenic tissue?

P. Brown: It would be very nice to do, but these experiments were not designed to yield this sort of information. This work was done between 5 and 20 years ago and none of the tissues that we would have liked to use was kept.

Chesebro: Does anybody have any evidence for transmission of the agent and replication in the periphery of the host without any agent reaching the CNS? Does it depend on dose?

Kimberlin: There is very good evidence for this and it is dose related to some extent. In my paper I refer to the persistent high level of 87V infectivity in the spleen, which scarcely, if ever, penetrates the CNS within the lifespan of IM mice.

Dickinson: We published a paper on incubation period longer than lifespan (Dickinson et al 1975). If you take all the strains of scrapie that exist, that title may be more typical of the range of naturally occurring strains than are the quick incubation models.

Chesebro: Are these data applicable to humans?

Kimberlin: I don't see why not. I am sure that the mechanisms and rules that we are learning with scrapie will be useful for human diseases.

Chesebro: But if you can't isolate CJD infectivity easily from human spleen, maybe it doesn't replicate there.

Manuelidis: You can isolate infectivity from human blood and blood contains spleen-derived cells. We have transmitted CJD from human buffy coat (Manuelidis et al 1985) and have extended these findings in several additional cases. In rodents with CJD there is both viraemia (Manuelidis et al 1978a) and splenic infectivity (Manuelidis & Manuelidis 1979), although the level of infectivity can be quite low in the spleen of some rodent models of CJD. Low infectivity of human spleen might easily be missed in cross-species transmissions. The human disease probably entails a splenic phase of infectivity.

I would question an exclusively neuronal pathway for infection to and within the CNS. Specific neurons with special metabolic profiles or activity states might be peculiarly susceptible to an agent, even if generally seeded by viraemia. It is well known that in conventional virus infections, for example poliomyelitis, general viraemia occurs, but only selected neurons are affected by the virus; several routes of spread to the CNS can occur with conventional viruses (Johnson & Mims 1968). With respect to the cerebellar signs in growth hormone-treated patients, one has to consider the age of the patients, their hormonal state (and the potential differential sensitivity of selected neurons), as well as the extended incubation time.

The cerebellar signs in growth hormone-treated patients that you presented are quite interesting. It is possible that the agent may develop unique properties (as a consequence of its peculiar isolation, or inoculation at very low dilution). The extended incubation times in these growth hormone-treated patients with cerebellar signs is intriguing when one considers the cerebellar signs in long incubation Gerstmann-Sträussler Scheinker (GSS) disease. Only one of our numerous human CJD isolates clearly affects the cerebellum in rodents (Manuelidis et al 1978b), therefore unique properties of the agent or 'strains' of the agent in these cases deserve further attention.

P. Brown: One of the problems with a simple viraemic explanation is that in experimentally induced disease in a primate such as the Capuchin monkey, which has a clinical phase that lasts for some months (comparable to the duration in a human), there is absolutely no difference in the clinical disease after intracerebral or peripheral routes of inoculation.

Manuelidis: How many different strains or different isolates have been used?

P. Brown: The same isolate in different monkeys or different isolates in different monkeys.

Diringer: It is interesting to follow routes into the central nervous system via the pituitary, because little is known about this gland as a route of entry of viruses into the central nervous system. We did a kinetic experiment to investigate whether entry of the scrapie virus was via the pineal body. This seems not to be the case because infectivity in the pineal gland develops at the same time as in the central nervous system. We have not yet looked at the pituitary.

Carp: We do see a difference in clinical symptoms, if we go to an extreme case and inject directly into the central nervous system. We put the 22L strain of scrapie directly into the cerebellum: ataxia appeared two or three weeks before the classical symptoms of scrapie (Kim et al 1987). We place these mice on a grid work and they behave as though they are drunk! This is quite distinctive for that particular agent injected directly into the cerebellum – we don't see it if we inject into the cortex, caudate nucleus, thalamus or substantia nigra, nor do we see this early change with other strains of scrapie, for example 139A, ME7 or 87V.

Wisniewski: We have made a split cerebellum preparation by injecting 22L scrapie agent into one half of the cerebellum—all the lesions were on the side of the injection. The two hemispheres were separated by scar tissue. Therefore, it appears that transport through axons and dendrites is of critical importance in the spread of scrapie agent from one side of the cerebellum to the other side.

Fraser: If you inject scrapie (for example strains ME7, 87V) into one eye, you get asymmetrical targeting to the visual central targets on the contralateral side of the brain (Fraser & Dickinson 1985).

P. Brown: In the case of CJD that was diagnosed after death but died before symptoms developed, there was only a single lesion, a single focus of pathology, and that was in the corpus striatum. Unfortunately, the slides of the hypothalamus were lost before they could be reviewed so we don't know for certain if there were any pathological changes in the hypothalamus, but there was none anywhere else in the brain.

Dickinson: I don't believe the growth hormone-treated cases of CJD come from minute amounts of infectivity let through into the final product by inadequacy of the chemical protocol. What I think happens, is that human inadequacies and lack of understanding lead to occasional rather large cross-contaminations between steps of the protocol. Even so, that might end up as only relatively small amounts of operational infectivity. The infective dose by an i.c. route is quite different from the infective dose by a peripheral route, so a relatively large focus of contamination passing into occasional vials as a 'lump' of infectivity, which could be thousands of i.c. infective doses, could still be only a very small number of peripheral infective doses.

Gabizon: Dr Brown, did you consider the possibility that in these growth hormone cases, it is not only contamination of the growth hormone but that individuals who lack growth hormone also have some genetic susceptibiity to CJD?

P. Brown: I think if that were the correct explanation, we should by now have seen a case of CJD in a growth hormone-deficient patient who was not treated, and we haven't. In some three thousand known cases of CJD there is not a single case of this sort.

Gabizon: I meant that this specific disease, when inoculated into people who don't have growth hormone, acts differently to when inoculated into 'normal' individuals.

P. Brown: I would be disinclined to think so, because in many cases the growth hormone has been fully replaced. You would then have to ask whether in a group of patients who were growth hormone-deficient but have now been treated, there could be something special. It is theoretically possible. However, most of this growth hormone deficiency is not known to be genetically influenced: about one third of the cases are caused by a tumour pathology and indeed the British case with CJD had a craniopharyngeoma as the reason for growth hormone deficiency.

Dormont: Do you have data on the sleep patterns of these patients?

P. Brown: No.

Dormont: These patients were all treated with growth hormone extracted by the 'old-fashioned procedures'. Perhaps we should refer to them as brain extract-treated patients, because the extraction of growth hormone ten years ago was very basic.

P. Brown: It was a fairly harsh procedure; the most important modern revision is the inclusion of a Sephadex 100 column adsorption step, which may non-specifically adsorb the infectious agent. The old-fashioned method of extraction included a series of organic solvent extracts, and treatments at pH 2 and pH 10.

There are also two possible cases of CJD—not yet verified—who only began treatment in 1982. That is modern therapy, post 1977.

Prusiner: Do you think that the form of the infectious particle (prion) is important? It can exist in a lot of different forms, a membrane form, a rod form, or a liposome form. The processing of the prion after subcutaneous inoculation may be similar to the processing of the infectious particle as it comes down the gastrointestinal tract in kuru: it crosses the epithelium of presumably the small intestine, enters the blood stream and then finds its way to the brain. One might study this by labelling the scrapie prion proteins in purified preparations, inoculating them peripherally and then determining where they go. There are small regions of the brain in which the blood-brain barrier is defective or doesn't exist, they may act as routes by which the scrapie agent is taken up selectively, and that uptake may depend on the physical form of the particle.

P. Brown: It is possible, however I continue to be attracted by the notion of entry in this particular circumstance via receptors, since this hormone does have a population of specific receptors in the hypothalamus. The only pre-clinical case we know of had lesions in the corpus striatum. I think that in the future we are going to see another dozen or so cases of CJD caused by growth hormone therapy, so we will have the opportunity to detect a case very early and do more focused studies. Experimentally, of course, we might also do it in primates.

References

Dickinson AG, Fraser H, Outram GW 1975 Scrapie incubation time can exceed natural lifespan. Nature (Lond) 256:732–733

Fraser H, Dickinson AG 1985 Targeting of scrapie lesions and spread of agent via the retino-tectal projection. Brain Res 346:32–41

Johnson RT, Mims CA 1968 Pathogenesis of viral infections of the nervous system. N Engl J Med 278:23–30, 84–92

Kim YS, Carp RI, Callahan SM, Wisniewski HM 1987 Incubation periods and survival times for mice injected stereotaxically with three scrapie strains in different brain regions. J Gen Virol 68:695–702

Manuelidis EE, Manuelidis L 1979 Observations on Creutzfeldt-Jakob disease propagated in small rodents. In: Prusiner S, Hadlow WJ (eds) Slow transmissible diseases of the nervous system. Academic Press, New York, 2:147–173

Manuelidis EE, Gorgacz EJ, Manuelidis L 1978a Viremia in experimental Creutzfeldt-Jakob disease. Science (Wash DC) 200:1069–1071

Manuelidis EE, Manuelidis L, Pincus JH, Collins WF 1978b Transmission from man to hamster of Creutzfeldt-Jakob disease with clinical recovery. Lancet 2:40–42

Manuelidis EE, Kim JH, Mericangas JR, Manuelidis L 1985 Transmission of Creutzfeldt-Jakob disease from human blood. Lancet 2:896–897

Neuropathology of unconventional virus infections: molecular pathology of spongiform change and amyloid plaque deposition

Colin L. Masters[a] and Konrad Beyreuther[b]

[a]Department of Pathology, University of Western Australia; [a]Department of Neuropathology, Royal Perth Hospital, Perth, Western Australia; [b]Center for Molecular Biology, University of Heidelberg, Im Neuenheimer Feld 282, D-6900 Heidelberg, Federal Republic of Germany

Abstract. To the triad of neuronal loss, gliosis and spongiform change as characteristic morphological changes associated with infection of the central nervous system, one can now add the presence of scrapie-associated filaments (SAF)/PrP rods. While the host's immune response is conspicuous by its absence, the vigorous astrocytic response is presumptive evidence of the host's ability to recognize and respond to the primary neuronal insult.

We assume that the spongiform change and vacuolation of neurons are of fundamental importance in the pathogenesis of the disease, realizing that neither is specific or essential for the replication of the infectious agent. The topographical distribution of lesions is partly explained by the portal of entry and retrograde spread of the virus. The temporal progression of the lesions is more clearly determined by the host genes, best illustrated by studies of the incubation period. The molecular basis of the spongiform change is unknown but it is presumed to involve some disturbance of membrane metabolism. The recognition of PrP as a membrane glycoprotein invites proposals for its role in the development of these spongiform lesions.

Extracellular amyloid occurs as plaques or congophilic angiopathy in some instances, and provides the best evidence that Alzheimer's disease (AD) is in some way related to the unconventional virus diseases. However, the protein subunit (A4) of the amyloid fibril in AD and its precursor are quite distinct from the PrP subunit which constitutes the amyloid fibril in these infectious diseases. It is still unclear whether the PrP subunit in the SAF has exactly the same composition as in the extracellular amyloid fibril. Our results suggest that only a fragment of the PrP molecule is the major constituent of the extracellular fibril. Since both PrP and A4 are derived from membrane glycoproteins, the elucidation of their normal function is likely to lead to a better understanding of the spongiform and amyloidogenic lesions in these diseases.

1988 Novel infectious agents and the central nervous system. Wiley, Chichester (Ciba Foundation Symposium 135) p 24–36

One of the more remarkable features of the unconventional virus diseases is the absence of any cytopathic changes in non-neuronal tissues in spite of demonstrable agent replication in such unaffected organs as spleen, lung, liver, kidney and gastrointestinal tract. Since the lesions in the brain are clearly not mediated by the immune system, we must conclude that the spongiform change and amyloidogenesis are crucial elements in the replication cycle of the virus, but these lesions are not essential for its replication strategy. It is only within the last few years that we have been able to consider the pathogenesis of the neuropathological lesions in molecular terms and in this paper we briefly summarize some current studies in this area.

Pathology of spongiform change

Most observers agree that the vacuolation of the neuropil is the result of membranous dilations occurring mainly in the dendrites of neurons, suggesting that the primary lesion in some way disturbs the integrity of the post-synaptic/ dendritic compartment. Vacuolation has also been described in the soma of neurons, in astrocytes, and within the myelin sheaths of oligodendroglia, the latter apparently of importance to the white matter lesions seen occasionally in both natural and experimental infections.

At present, the spongiform lesion is the major morphological criterion discernible by light microscopy for the diagnosis of Creutzfeldt-Jakob disease (CJD), kuru and scrapie. This criterion may now be supplemented by the immunocytochemical demonstration of PrP in those cases of CJD, kuru and the Gerstmann-Sträussler syndrome (GSS) that develop amyloid plaques, but these form only a small proportion of all cases. The specificity of the spongiform change has long been debated. There are many conditions in which vacuolation in the brain can occur – some artifactual, others clearly related to a variety of metabolic disturbances. The neuropathologist relies mainly on the topography of the lesions and the distinction drawn between *spongiform change* and *status spongiosus* (Masters & Richardson 1978).

The topographical distribution of spongiform change in the human brain is rather characteristic: in most cases the lesions are widespread in the cerebral cortex, striatum, thalamus, upper brain stem and the molecular layer of the cerebellum. Within the cerebral cortex, the spongiform change often gives the appearance of a laminar distribution but it is never confined to the more superficial layers (layers I and II). This may be an important point for differential diagnosis, since many unrelated anoxic and metabolic disturbances will cause a superficial vacuolation of the cerebral cortex. Another characteristic feature is the peculiar distribution of spongiform change within the hippocampal region, where it is often absent from the subiculum and parahippocampal gyrus. There are exceptions in which the topography of the spongiform change is different from that in the standard case (for example, where the cerebral cortex is spared).

The distinction between *spongiform change* and *status spongiosus* is important. The latter term carries no connotation of specificity and may be used for a variety of conditions in which there is disruption and rarefaction of the neuropil. In the context of the unconventional virus diseases, status spongiosus correctly describes the end-stage gliotic cerebrum seen in cases of CJD of long clinical duration (Masters & Richardson 1978). Such gliotic rarefaction of the brain is rarely seen in either natural or experimental infections of animals, probably a reflection of the shorter duration of clinical disease when compared to humans.

As a marker of infectivity, the spongiform lesion has proven of great value in the development of virus-strain 'typing' techniques and in demonstrating and monitoring the spread of infectivity through neuronal pathways (see Kimberlin & Walker, Dickinson & Outram, this volume). It has become clear from these studies that the principal determinants of spongiform change lie not only at the level of genes controlling virus-host interaction, but also in the temporal progression of virus replication within the nervous system. The linkage of genes controlling the incubation period of scrapie with the PrP gene (Carlson et al 1986) suggests a role for PrP in the replication cycle of the virus.

The molecular basis of spongiform change is unknown. There are several ideas which might be usefully developed, all pointing to an involvement of membrane glycoproteins. Spongiform lesions occur in conventional virus infections and may be related to the abnormal processing of Pr 80^{env} of murine leukaemia viruses (Wong et al 1985, Rassart et al 1986) or the G antigen of vesicular stomatitis virus (Robain et al 1986). The recognition of PrP as a neuronal glycoprotein (Bolton et al 1982, 1985, Oesch et al 1985, Kretzschmar et al 1986), which is post-translationally modified during the course of infection, also suggests that it may have an important role in the development of the spongiform lesion. It will be necessary to determine whether these virus-associated glycoproteins are released from membranes and then play a direct role in the development of post-synaptic vacuoles. It is also possible that the abnormal processing of the PrP glycoprotein leads to vacuole formation after insertion of the molecule into the membrane. In either event, the accumulation of the glycoprotein (or a degradation product) may result in its aggregation into amyloid filaments (see below). The close association of the PrP glycoprotein with infectivity (Bolton et al 1982) and the linkage of its gene with a locus that influences the incubation period (Carlson et al 1986) provide the basis for its proposed central role in the development of the spongiform change.

In Alzheimer's disease (AD), spongiform change is occasionally seen in the region of the hippocampus and inferior temporal gyrus. The overall topography of lesions in AD is, of course, quite different from that in the unconventional virus diseases. In AD there is strong evidence for an olfactory/limbic origin of the disease process, which then spreads to corticocortical association areas. One must remember that the time course of illness in AD is different, at least one order of magnitude longer than in the unconventional virus diseases. If both AD and CJD have a similar pathogenesis, it is conceivable that vacuolation and spongiform change do not usually occur in AD because of the slower time course of events.

Amyloid fibrils in unconventional virus infections

Approximately 10 per cent of all cases of CJD and more than 70 per cent of cases of kuru show amyloid plaque deposition, as revealed by routine light microscopy (Masters et al 1981a,b). A variable proportion of experimentally infected animals also develop amyloid plaques (Bruce & Dickinson 1985). Most, if not all, cases of unconventional virus disease show the presence of scrapie-associated filaments (SAF) (Merz et al 1984, Diringer et al 1983), which are composed of aggregates of the PrP molecule. Using negative staining techniques, it is now apparent that the SAF are indistinguishable from the PrP rods. The SAF, however, are quite distinct from extracellular amyloid fibrils. Recent observations suggest that the SAF may be associated with intracellular tubulofilaments (Narang et al 1987). Immunocytochemical and biochemical studies of the extracellular amyloid deposits in the unconventional virus diseases show that these are also composed of aggregates of PrP (Prusiner et al 1983, Barry et al 1985, Kitamoto et al 1986, Beyreuther & Masters, unpublished observations).

In AD, in which cerebral amyloidogenesis is pathognomonic, the amyloid protein is composed of a small 4 kDa subunit (A4 protein) (Masters et al 1985a,b), which is derived from a much larger precusor cell-surface glycoprotein (Kang et al 1987). There are clearly two different forms of amyloid fibril: intracellular filaments, which form the neurofibrillary tangle composed of paired helical and straight filaments, and the extracellular filaments, which form plaque cores and congophilic angiopathy. Our studies (Masters et al 1985a,b) show that both types of amyloid are built from the same A4 subunit. It is highly probable that the precursor for A4 is cleaved and/or processed by different mechanisms giving rise to either the intracellular or extracellular filament. One such processing mechanism may be ubiquitination (Mori et al 1987, Perry et al 1987). In different disease states there are unknown factors which drive the amyloidogenic pathway preferentially in one of the two directions (Guiroy et al 1987). One aspect needs to be emphasized: there is no evidence, and indeed it would be highly unlikely, that once the A4 has polymerized into a fibril it can interchange between the intracellular and extracellular compartments.

The precursor-product relationships are schematically summarized in Fig. 1, comparing the pathways of fibril formation in both the conventional virus diseases and AD. The intracellular forms of SAF are speculative and con-

I   Unconventional virus disease

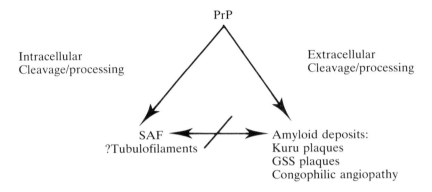

**II   Alzheimer's disease and
    related conditions**

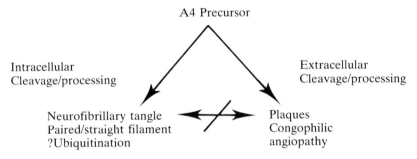

FIG. 1.   Schematic interrelationships between intracellular and extracellular amyloidogenesis from neuronal membrane glycoproteins.

troversial. It has been argued that the SAF are artifacts of detergent solubilization (Meyer et al 1986); however, the identification of SAF structures *in
situ* would suggest that they do represent genuine products of some *in vivo*
metabolic process (Narang et al 1987). When AD brains are subjected to an
SAF purification protocol, structures resembling paired helical filaments are
readily identifiable (Rubenstein et al 1986). The similarities between SAF
and paired helical filament fragments are quite striking at an ultrastructural
level, whereas the extracellular amyloid filaments in both AD and the unconventional virus diseases are virtually indistinguishable by morphological
criteria. If the pathways proposed in this schematic outline prove to be
correct, then the central questions will concern the nature of the cleavage/
processing mechanisms, and their relationship to the infectious unit.

Acknowledgements

This research was supported in part by grants from the National Health & Medical Research Council of Australia (CLM), and the Deutsche Forschungsgemeinshaft, Bundesministerium für Forschung and Technologie, and Fonds der Chemischen Industrie (KB).

References

Barry RA, McKinley MP, Bendheim PE et al 1985 Antibodies to the scrapie protein decorate prion rods. J Immunol 135:603–613

Bolton DC, McKinley MP, Prusiner SB 1982 Identification of a protein that purifies with the scrapie prion. Science (Wash DC) 218:1309–1311

Bolton DC, Meyer RK, Prusiner SB 1985 Scrapie PrP 27–30 is a sialoglycoprotein. J Virol 63:596–606

Bruce ME, Dickinson AG 1985 Genetic control of amyloid plaque production and incubation period in scrapie-infected mice. J Neuropath & Exp Neurol 44:285–294

Carlson GA, Kingsbury DT, Goodman PA et al 1986 Linkage of prion protein and scrapie incubation time genes. Cell 46:503–511

Dickinson AG, Outram GW 1988 Genetic aspects of unconventional virus infections: the basis of the virino hypothesis. In: Novel infectious agents and the central nervous system. Wiley, Chichester (Ciba Found Symp 135) p 63–84

Diringer H, Gelderblom H, Hilmert H, Ozel, M, Edelbluth C, Kimberlin RH 1983 Scrapie infectivity, fibrils and low molecular weight protein. Nature (Lond) 306:476–478

Guiroy DC, Miyazaki M, Multhaup G et al 1987 Amyloid of neurofibrillary tangles of Guamanian parkinsonism-dementia and Alzheimer disease share identical amino acid sequence. Proc Natl Acad Sci USA 84:2073–2077

Kang J, Lemaire H-G, Unterbeck A et al 1987 The precursor of Alzheimer's disease amyloid A4 protein resembles a cell-surface receptor. Nature (Lond) 325:733–736

Kimberlin RH, Walker CA 1988 Pathogenesis of experimental scrapie. In: Novel infectious agents and the central nervous system. Wiley, Chichester (Ciba Found Symp 135) p 37–62

Kitamoto T, Tateishi J, Tashima T et al 1986 Amyloid plaques in Creutzfeldt-Jakob disease stain with prion protein antibodies. Ann Neurol 20:204–208.

Kretzschmar HA, Prusiner SB, Stowring LE, De Armond SJ 1986 Scrapie prion proteins are synthesized in neurons. Am J Pathol 122:1–5

Masters CL, Richardson EP Jr 1978 Subacute spongiform encephalopathy (Creutzfeldt-Jakob disease). The nature and progression of spongiform change. Brain 101:333–344

Masters CL, Gajdusek DC, Gibbs CJ Jr 1981a The familial occurrence of Creutzfeldt-Jakob and Alzheimer's disease. Brain 104:535–558

Masters CL, Gajdusek DC, Gibbs CJ, Jr 1981b Creutzfeldt-Jakob disease virus isolation from the Gerstmann-Sträussler syndrome. With an analysis of the various forms of amyloid plaque deposition in the virus-induced spongiform encephalopathies. Brain 104:559–587

Masters CL, Simms G, Weinman NA, Multhaup G, McDonald BL, Beyreuther K 1985a Amyloid plaque core protein in Alzheimer disease and Down syndrome. Proc Natl Acad Sci USA 82:4245–4249

Masters CL, Multhaup G, Simms G, Pottgiesser J, Martins RN, Beyreuther K 1985b

Neuronal origin of a cerebral amyloid: neurofibrillary tangles of Alzheimer's disease contain the same protein as the amyloid of plaque cores and blood vessels. EMBO (Eur Mol Biol Organ) J 4:2757–2763

Merz PA, Rohwer RG, Kascsak R et al 1984 Infection-specific particle from the unconventional slow virus diseases. Science (Wash DC) 225:437–440

Meyer RK, McKinley MP, Bowman KA, Braunfeld MB, Barry RA, Prusiner SB 1986 Separation and properties of cellular and scrapie prion proteins. Proc Natl Acad Sci USA 83:2310–2314

Mori H, Kondo J, Ihara Y 1987 Ubiquitin is a component of paired helical filaments in Alzheimer's disease. Science (Wash DC) 235:1641–1644

Narang HK, Asher DM, Gajdusek DC 1987 Tubulofilaments in negatively stained scrapie-infected brains: relationship to scrapie-associated fibrils. Proc Natl Acad Sci USA 84:7730–7735

Oesch B, Westaway D, Wälchli M et al 1985 A cellular gene encodes scrapie PrP 27–30 protein. Cell 40:735–746

Perry G, Friedman R, Shaw G, Chau V 1987 Ubiquitin is detected in neurofibrillary tangles and senile plaque neurites of Alzheimer disease brains. Proc Natl Acad Sci USA 84:3033–3036

Prusiner SB, McKinley MP, Bowman KA et al 1983 Scrapie prions aggregate to form amyloid-like birefringent rods. Cell 35:349–358

Rassart E, Nelbach L, Jolicoeur P 1986 Cas-Br-E murine leukemia virus: sequencing of the paralytogenic region of its genome and derivation of specific probes to study its origin and the structure of its recombinant genomes in leukemic tissues. J Virol 60:910–919

Robain O, Chany-Fournier F, Cerutti I, Màzlo M, Chany C 1986 Role of VSV G antigen in the development of experimental spongiform encephalopathy in mice. Acta Neuropathol 70:220–226

Rubenstein R, Kascsak RJ, Merz PA, Wisniewski HM, Carp RI, Iqbal K 1986 Paired helical filaments associated with Alzheimer disease are readily soluble structures. Brain Res 372:80–88

Wong PKY, Knupp C, Yuen PH, Soong MM, Zachary JF, Tompkins WAF 1985 tsl, a paralytogenic mutant of Moloney murine leukemia virus TB, has enhanced ability to replicate in the central nervous system and primary nerve cell culture. J Virol 55:760–767

DISCUSSION

Dickinson: In your histological series there was no picture of fully developed scrapie in a sheep with no vacuolation. Paul Brown said earlier that vacuolation is pretty well a *sine qua non* of this set of clinical diseases in humans. We don't use that criterion in sheep. We only know that vacuolation can be absent from advanced scrapie because we know when we injected the sheep, what we injected it with and we can predict the course of the disease. If such a sheep had presented itself as a natural case, we would have no way of knowing why the sheep died without doing a transmission from it. This extends to the human situation; when somebody dies with a variety of neurological signs but showing no vacuolation we do not know whether the cause was one of this set of degenerative conditions which have an infective basis.

Masters: You are drawing attention to the spectrum of pathological change. We still don't understand the molecular basis of spongiform change. What you say is absolutely correct. Vacuolation is not a reliable marker of infectivity in the natural infection in sheep, but it does seem more reliable in the human diseases.

Dickinson: We have differed before about the regression relationship between the amount of vacuolation and the duration of the disease – it would seem to me that a simpler explanation is more consistent with all the experimental findings. No one has done the serial killing experiment and found vacuolation regressing, therefore a simpler explanation of this regression you describe is that those individuals in whom vacuolation is a less dominant feature are able to survive for longer.

Masters: It is not possible to do that sort of experiment in humans!

Dickinson: In the experimental systems that are available nothing correlating with your explanation is present.

Masters: That may be because the duration of clinical disease in animals is much less than in the human.

P. Brown: You and Dr Tateishi have done probably the only more or less quantitative assessements of spongiform change related to the length of the disease. How does that compare with 'anecdotal' observations, for example those verified cases in our long duration of CJD series, cases of 10 and 13 years, which were riddled with spongiform change. The brain of the chimp that had CJD for ten years was also riddled with spongiform change. These are contrasting elements and we need to study a whole series to know whether this spongiform change is common or not.

Masters: I agree that it is a difficult point. One explanation for these long duration cases is that there is a pre-existing neurological disease of undefined nature, which predisposes to infection. CJD is then superimposed for the last 2–3 years before death.

P. Brown: We have considered that as an alternative. Firstly, it does not apply to the experimental case. Secondly, I don't think that it applies to humans, because some of the long duration cases were not 75-year-old people who were gradually failing and then 10 years later failed very quickly. One individual was only 35 years old at onset and he definitely had a slowly progressive dementing disease – if it wasn't CJD, it would be extraordinary for two rare diseases to occur in a 35-year-old person, who died of verified transmitted CJD.

Masters: I don't believe that these vacuoles are static phenomena. There must be a constant and rapid turnover of membranes within these fluid-filled vacuoles. In the average case of CJD, these vacuoles diminish after a certain stage of neuronal loss. This relationship is not usually apparent in animals, only in humans.

P. Brown: With the exceptions we just mentioned!

Tateishi: I would like to report on the immunostaining of amyloid plaques in human patient and mouse brains infected with CJD (Tateishi et al 1984). We have obtained a high titre rabbit antiserum raised against the CJD-infected mouse PrP or against the amyloid core protein of a GSS patient. Species-specific antisera and formic acid pre-treatment (Kitamoto et al 1987) increased the specificity and sensitivity of the immunostaining of amyloid plaques in formalin-fixed and paraffin-embedded tissue sections. Small and ill-defined plaques, not stained by routine stains, could be detected by the immunostaining. In aged mice, spongiform changes due to ageing occur often, as reported by Fraser & McBride (1985). In such a mouse it is difficult to differentiate spongiform change from CJD changes, and amyloid plaques become a good marker for the pathology of CJD infection. We looked at amyloid plaques in mice comparing routine staining methods, such as Congo red, and immunostaining with anti-mouse CJD antiserum. By routine staining only a few mice in 14 transmission cases show the amyloid plaques after a long incubation period (more than 403 days after i.c. inoculation), but by immunostaining all of 33 transmission cases show amyloid plaques after a shorter incubation period (more than 245 days).

The detection rate of amyloid plaques in CJD and GSS patients was compared between Congo red and anti-human GSS antiserum stainings. By Congo red staining, only three cases out of 26 CJD patients were positive, but by immunostaining 16 cases were positive. Eleven GSS cases were all positive by both methods. If all CJD and GSS patients are grouped according to the duration of their clinical illness, scoring for amyloid plaques is negative before six months of clinical course but 100% positive after one year clinical course. Therefore the incidence of amyloid plaques is determined by the length of the clinical course and there is no difference between CJD and GSS.

Masters: Dr Tateishi's data are in good agreement with our findings.

Fraser: I would like to emphasize that although Colin has described great variety in the pathology of these diseases, the extent to which we can regulate this variety by using controlled biological systems has not been defined and needs to be emphasized. With specified host genotypes and strains of scrapie, there is very precise control over the details of the neuropathology (Fraser 1979).

There seems to be an extraordinary lack of association between the two main lesions that we have been discussing. We don't know why plaques occur sometimes to excess and why sometimes degeneration in the absence of plaques occurs to excess. We have done a lot of work infecting mice with 'wild-type' strains isolated from natural sheep scrapie, in which the prominent lesion is numerous cerebral plaques in the cerebral cortex and elsewhere, whereas the spongiform change is restricted to sub-cortical parts of the brain. Under controlled circumstances these strains can mutate to strains with a very different pathology. In one wild-type strain of scrapie (87V), which has a very long incubation period, both spongiform degeneration and plaques occur. If you map these two lesions in brain sections following intraocular injection, there is initial targeting of spongiform degeneration into the contralateral superior colliculus, but there is no such targeting of amyloid plaques in the visual system. The plaques occur in quite unrelated areas. Similarly, with intracerebral infection with this agent the spongiform change occurs in the raphé, the medulla, the thalamus, the mid-line, the forebrain and the basal forebrain, but the plaques occur in unrelated areas such as the cortex (Fraser et al 1986). We need to resolve the neuroanatomical basis of this disassociation.

In some models, ME7 agent in VM mice, or 22A in LM mice for example, there is total destruction of the pyramidal layer hippocampal neurons. In the same part of the brain in other scrapie models you get a different pathology, in this case with severe spongiosis but without the neuronal destruction (Scott & Fraser 1984). So in the mouse you can control experimentally the variety of pathology that you can see in field or natural disease situations where you have no experimental control (Fraser & Bruce 1983).

DeArmond: One possibility is that when the protein is released from neurons after necrosis or by secretion, it is then subject to extracellular bulk flow of fluids in the CNS. The distribution of amyloid plaques that we find in the hamster is precisely what would be expected if one injected indian ink into the brain. They develop around blood vessels and beneath both the ventricular surface and the pial surface.

Masters: What we now see in Alzheimer's disease fits exactly with your concept of the distribution of plaques. In Alzheimer's disease, the accumulation of this amyloidogenic material around the blood vessels in the subarachnoid space can only be explained by the flow of this protein or its precursor. It is difficult to understand how a polymerized amyloid fibril can flow anywhere, so the precursor must be able to translocate in some fashion.

DeArmond: We find that the protein accumulates in these areas and doesn't form plaques immediately. Most of the prion protein immunoreactive material which occurs in perivascular, sub-pial and sub-ventricular regions does not show Congo red staining or green birefringence. Something else has to happen to the extracellular prion protein once it reaches those locations.

Dickinson: Concerning the scrapie-associated fibrils (SAF), I think most people agree that all the fibrils that have been talked about, which have a major component or a sole component of PrP, are essentially the same. The only statement which has ever made me doubt whether the things are the same is Stanley Prusiner's first reference to 'prion rods', where he said 'while these rods are frequently found in scrapie preparations, they do not appear to be unique since a few rods of similar size and shape have been found in control fractions' (Prusiner et al 1982).

Merz: At an EMBO meeting in Edinburgh, Scotland in 1984 this question arose as to whether or not the SAF were the same as the prion rods or the amyloid rods (Merz et al 1981, Prusiner et al 1982, 1983). Experiments were set up to answer that question, using antibodies to identify whether or not the SAF and prion or amyloid rods, as isolated in purified preparations, were identical. SAF antisera were raised against scrapie strain ME7 SAF purified by Heino Diringer's method (Kascsak et al 1986). We also used Paul Bendheim and Stan Prusiner's scrapie 263K PrP antisera (Bendheim et al 1984) and scrapie 263K antisera from Heino Diringer (Diringer et al 1984). These were used on isolated SAF which had not been treated with proteinase K and on fibrils that had been purified with proteinase K. Both types of preparation of SAF from infections with three strains of scrapie decorated with the three antisera.

The PrP proteins were also shown to be in both types of fibril by Western blotting with similar preparations; I personally consider this issue closed (Merz et al 1987).

Masters: But there is a difference between SAF and amyloid filaments. The issue now is to identify the molecular basis for the differences between the amyloid filament and the SAF structure.

Merz: The question is, which amyloid? GSS, CJD or scrapie in mice?

Masters: Is there a structural difference between the mouse amyloid and the GSS amyloid?

Merz: Yes, ultrastructurally there is a difference between the 87V amyloid isolated from mice and that from the human GSS. 87V amyloid seems to be composed of two fibrils in a parallel array. Each of the two fibrils is 4–8 nm in diameter with a twist every 15–25 nm. The GSS amyloid fibrils are 7–9 nm in diameter twisting every 70 nm. The amyloids were isolated from affected brains and observed ultrastructurally after negative staining (Merz et al 1983a,b).

Diringer: Colin, were all the SAF that you showed from scrapie cases?

Masters: One was CJD. The amyloid was from a GSS case.

Merz: The SAF from GSS was published, it is not the same as amyloid from GSS (Merz et al 1983b).

DeArmond: Prion rods and SAF are more or less artifacts created in an *in vitro* system—that is, protein has been dissolved chemically and then reconstituted *in vitro* and a rod-like structure appears. Colin, do you equate SAF to the amyloid filaments that appear in scrapie?

Masters: I drew a distinction between SAF and the extracellular amyloid. There are possibly two different pathways involved, one leading to SAF and the other to the extracellular amyloid. The basic question is, if SAF exist *in vivo* and are not just a preparative artifact, then in which compartment of the brain do they exist?

Prusiner: I think there are clear differences between prion rods and SAF and I think it's a lack of precision on the part of the people who say that all this is the same (Diener 1987, Prusiner et al 1987). Let me quote Pat Merz' original description of SAF (Merz et al 1981): "SAF of type 1 is a fibril comprised of two filaments. The fibrils are 12–16 nm in width with a space of 2–4 nm between the filaments. At their narrowest, the fibrils are 4–6 nm in width with no observable space between the two filaments. The fibrils narrow to 4–6 nm usually every 40–60 nm, although in some of the fibrils the narrowing is found every 80–110 nm. Within the fibril the space between the individual filaments can be observed for 40–60 nm along the length of the fibril between each narrow portion. . . . Type 2 is composed of four filaments with a space between each filament of 3–4 nm at its widest. The fibril measures 27–34 nm at its widest and 9–12 nm at its narrowest. The fibril narrows every 100–120 nm."

I agree with Colin Masters that what he called SAF look like our preparations of prion rods (Prusiner et al 1982, 1983). They do not look like the SAF that Pat Merz described (Merz et al 1981). Subsequently, electron micrographs of SAF from a CJD case were published in which the filaments intersect at regular intervals (Merz et al 1983c).

SAF have a regular morphology, both for type 1 and type 2. There are two or four sub-filaments helically wound and they intersect with regular perodicity. The morphology has been used to differentiate these from intermediate filaments and amyloids (Merz et al 1984). Prion rods, on the other hand, have a non-uniform morphology; they are heterogeneous, they have no regular substructure and they are indistinguishable from many purified amyloids (Prusiner et al 1983).

Masters: Do you therefore agree that there is a difference between the amyloid and the prion rods, or would you say that amyloid filaments are identical morphologically with prion rods?

Prusiner: In scrapie they are identical except for the length (DeArmond et al 1985). In the hamster, where we isolate the prion rods, in thin sections we find the amyloid filaments to be indistinguishable morphologically.

Wisniewski: What about negative staining?

Prusiner: We have not done negative staining of the amyloid filaments. We have not been able to isolate the amyloid filaments from the extracellular space.

Wisniewski: I think you are comparing amyloid fibres assembled under different conditions. One has to remember that amyloidogenic proteins under different conditions of polymerization show different morphologies. Small changes in conditions produce morphologically different assemblies of the same protein.

References

Bendheim PE, Barry RA, DeArmond SJ, Stites DP, Prusiner SB 1984 Antibodies to a scrapie prion protein. Nature (Lond) 310:418–421
DeArmond SJ, McKinley MP, Barry RA, Braunfeld MB, McColloch JR, Prusiner SB

1985 Identification of prion amyloid filaments in scapie-infected brain. Cell 41:221–235

Diener TO 1987 PrP and the nature of the scrapie agent. Cell 49:719–721

Diringer H, Rahn HC, Bode L 1984 Antibodies to protein of scrapie associated fibrils. Lancet 2:345

Fraser H 1979 Neuropathology of scrapie. The precision of the lesions and their diversity. In: Prusiner SB, Hadlow WJ (eds) Slow transmissible diseases of the nervous system. Academic Press, New York, vol 1:387–405

Fraser H, Bruce ME 1983 Experimental control of cerebral amyloid in scrapie in mice. In: Behan PO et al (eds) Immunology of nervous system infections. Elsevier, Amsterdam (Prog Brain Res 59) p 281–290

Fraser H, McBride, PA 1985 Parallels and contrasts between scrapie and dementia of the Alzheimer type and ageing: strategies and problems for experiments involving lifespan studies. In: Traber J, Gispen W (eds) Senile dementia of the Alzheimer type. Springer-Verlag, Berlin, p 250–268

Fraser H, McBride PA, Scott JR, Bruce ME 1986 Infectious degeneration of the nervous system. In: Triger DR (ed) Advanced medicine. Ballière Tindall, London, vol 22:371–383

Kascsak RK, Rubenstein R, Merz PA et al 1986 Immunological analysis of scrapie associated fibrils isolated from four different scrapie agents. J Virol 59:676–683

Kitamoto T, Ogomori K, Tateishi J, Prusiner SB 1987 Formic acid pretreatment enhances immunostaining of cerebral and systemic amyloids. Lab Invest, 57:230–236

Merz PA, Somerville RA, Wisniewski HM, Iqbal K 1981 Abnormal fibrils from scrapie-infected brain. Acta Neuropathol 54:63–74

Merz PA, Wisniewski HM, Somerville RA, Bobin SA, Iqbal K, Masters CL 1983a Ultrastructure of amyloid fibrils from neuritic and amyloid plaques. Acta Neuropathol 60:113–124

Merz PA, Somerville RA, Wisniewski HM 1983b Abnormal fibrils in scrapie and senile dementia of the Alzheimer type. In: Court LA, Cathala F (eds) Virus non conventionnels et affections du systeme nerveux central. Masson, Paris, p 259–281

Merz PA, Somerville RA, Wisniewski HM, Manuelidis L, Manuelidis EE 1983c Scrapie-associated fibrils in Creutzfeldt-Jakob disease. Nature (Lond) 306:474–476

Merz PA, Rohwer RG, Kascsak R, Wisniewski HM, Somerville RA, Gibbs CJ, Jr, Gajdusek DC 1984 Infection-specific particles from the unconventional slow virus diseases. Science (Wash DC) 225:437–440

Merz PA, Kascsak RJ, Rubenstein R, Fama CL, Carp RI, Wisniewski HM 1987 Antisera to SAF protein and 'prion' protein decorate scrapie associated fibrils. J Virol 61:42–49

Prusiner SB, Bolton DC, Groth DF, Bowman KA, Cochran SP, McKinley MP 1982 Further purification and characterization of scrapie prions. Biochemistry 21:6942–6950

Prusiner SB, McKinley MP, Bowman KA et al 1983 Scrapie prions aggregate to form amyloid-like birefringent rods. Cell 35:349–358

Prusiner SB, Gabizon R, McKinley MP 1987 On the biology of prions. Acta Neuropathol 72:299–314

Scott JR, Fraser H 1984 Degenerative hippocampal pathology in mice infected with scrapie. Acta Neuropathol 65:62–68

Tateishi J, Nagara H, Hikita K, Sato Y 1984 Amyloid plaques in the brains of mice with Creutzfeldt-Jakob disease. Ann Neurol 15:278–280

Pathogenesis of experimental scrapie

Richard H. Kimberlin and Carol A. Walker*

*AFRC & MRC Neuropathogenesis Unit, West Mains Road, Edinburgh, EH9 3JF and
MRC Radiobiology Unit, Chilton, Didcot, OX11 0RD, UK

Abstract. Most of our understanding of the pathogenesis of the unconventional slow infections comes from studies of experimental scrapie in mice and hamsters. After injection by non-neural peripheral routes, pathogenesis necessarily involves the lymphoreticular system (LRS) before the central nervous system (CNS). Available evidence indicates haematogenous spread from the site of injection to the scrapie replication sites in the LRS; later, infection spreads along visceral autonomic nerves from the LRS to the thoracic spinal cord, and thence to brain. The cells in the LRS which are important to scrapie pathogenesis are long lived. Neuroinvasion and spread of infection within the CNS probably involve neuronal pathways. We suggest that disease develops after infection has reached certain clinical target areas in the CNS but only when scrapie replication there has caused sufficient functional damage. Restriction of the replication process in both LRS and CNS is indicated by the occurrence of plateau concentrations of infectivity, especially in some long incubation scrapie models. A remarkable feature of these is that both neuroinvasion and clinical disease occur long after infectivity plateaux have been reached in the LRS and CNS, respectively. We propose that the slowness of scrapie is related to (1) limitations of cell-to-cell spread of infection from LRS to CNS, and (2) limitations on spread between neurons, coupled with restrictions on replication in brain.

1988 Novel infectious agents and the central nervous system. Wiley, Chichester (Ciba Foundation Symposium 135) p 37–62

The list of diseases caused by 'unconventional' slow viruses includes transmissible mink encephalopathy, kuru, Creutzfeldt-Jakob disease (CJD), a variant of CJD called Gerstmann-Sträussler syndrome, and chronic wasting disease of mule deer and elk. Our understanding of the pathogenesis of these diseases is based almost entirely on scrapie. The most important single step forward occurred over 25 years ago when the first successful transmissions of scrapie to mice were reported. This development led to large scale bioassays (still the only method for measuring infectivity) and a much greater experimental sophistication than was possible in sheep and goats. Subsequently many mouse scrapie models have been obtained with different ranges of incubation period. These models vary mainly in the strain of agent and the *Sinc* genotype of mouse (*Sinc* is the major murine gene controlling incubation period; see Dickinson, this volume). Not surprisingly, most studies have focused on the shorter incubation models involving passages of the original 'Chandler' isolate from which the 139A strain was derived, and also the ME7 strain which has a different origin. About 10 years ago the high speed scrapie strain, 263K, was isolated in golden hamsters. This model has been widely used in scrapie research because of its exceptionally short incubation period (minimum of about 60 days) and high infectivity titres in brain (about 10^{10} i.c. ID_{50} units/g).

The intracerebral (i.c.) route of injection is used universally for bioassays of infectivity because it is the most efficient and sensitive (see later). However, this route bypasses the need for the extraneural events of pathogenesis established by Eklund et al (1967) in a major study of 'Chandler' scrapie injected subcutaneously (s.c.). Spleen is usually the first tissue to become infected. Scrapie replication proceeds in many tissues of the lymphoreticular system (LRS) including spleen, lymph nodes, thymus and submaxillary salivary gland. Later, replication occurs in spinal cord and brain, and titres here eventually become much higher than those in the LRS. At all times the level of viraemia is very low or undetectable. Many subsequent studies have confirmed this pattern and Hadlow et al (1982) have shown that infection of the LRS precedes the neural events of pathogenesis in the natural disease of sheep.

The importance of spleen in mouse scrapie was demonstrated by splenectomy or genetic asplenia, which lengthened the incubation period of intraperitoneally (i.p.) injected 139A or ME7 scrapie (Fraser & Dickinson 1970, 1978, Clarke & Haig 1971, Dickinson & Fraser 1972). No effect was seen with i.c. injected scrapie, showing that the infection of spleen by 'escaped' inoculum and the subsequent replication there do not contribute to pathogenesis. Neonatal or adult thymectomy (McFarlin et al 1971, Fraser & Dickinson 1978) did not affect the incubation period of i.p. injected scrapie, suggesting that only some tissues or cell types of the LRS are important in pathogenesis.

Many other studies have been carried out to fill in the details of scrapie pathogenesis in the LRS and CNS. In this paper we attempt to synthesize the salient findings into a coherent picture, at the risk of oversimplification. We also speculate on the nature of the constraints which make scrapie a slow disease.

Establishment of infection

We have compared the effective titres of standard scrapie brain inocula adminstered by a variety of routes to give a measure of their relative efficiencies of infection (Kimberlin & Walker 1978). Intraspinal (i.s.) and i.c. are the most efficient routes (Kimberlin et al 1987) but several hundred i.c. ID_{50} units are required to give one ID_{50} by the intrasciatic route (Kimberlin et al 1983b). Table 1 shows that among the non-neural routes intravenous (i.v.) injection is much more efficient than s.c., although the efficiency of the latter depends

TABLE 1   Relative efficiency of infection of different routes as measured by titration of standard scrapie brain inocula

Route of infection	No. of titrations	Effective titre[a] ($\log_{10} ID_{50} \pm SEM$)	i.c. units per ID_{50}
139A scrapie in adult female CW mice (Sinc[s7]*)*			
i.c.	14	7.03 ± .13	1
i.v.	16	6.06 ± .11	9
i.p.	50	4.40 ± .06	430
s.c.[b]	11	2.64 ± .11	24 500
263K scrapie in adult female golden hamsters			
i.c.	26	8.50 ± 0.10	1
i.p.	2	3.90 ± 0.10	40 000

[a] Titres are expressed per 30mg of mouse brain and 50mg of hamster brain
[b] Subcutaneous injection in the 'scruff' of the neck
139A data taken from Kimberlin & Walker (1983), 263K data from Kimberlin & Walker (1977, 1988)

considerably on the site of injection (Kimberlin & Walker 1979a).

To understand the basis of these differences, we studied the distribution of scrapie infectivity and of radioactively labelled liposomes after injection by the i.c., i.v., i.p. and s.c. routes (Millson et al 1979). In all cases, inoculum was widely distributed in blood and many tissues after only 30 minutes (see also Hotchin et al 1983). There was substantial uptake by organs such as liver, in which scrapie does not replicate (Eklund et al 1967, Millson et al 1979), suggesting that much of the inoculum may be ineffective in establishing scrapie infection. With the i.c. route, it is the inoculum remaining locally at the site of injection which is important in scrapie pathogenesis (see Kimberlin & Walker 1983). The opposite is true for the peripheral routes. The initial uptake of scrapie inoculum by liver, lung and spleen was in the order i.v.> i.p.> s.c. This pattern corresponds to the relative efficiencies of infection shown in Table 1 and is inversely related to the localization of inoculum at the injection site (Millson et al 1979). We suggest that experimental scrapie infection may be established very rapidly by blood-borne inoculum, a proportion of which is taken up by spleen and lymph nodes.

It is interesting that the dose–incubation curves for the i.v., i.p. and s.c. routes are virtually identical after correcting for the differences in the relative efficiency of infection (Kimberlin & Walker 1978, 1983). This means that the subsequent pathogenesis of scrapie given by these routes of infection follows common pathways.

Multiplication in the lymphoreticular system

The pattern of 139A replication in spleen after i.p. and i.c. infection is shown in Fig. 1a and 1b, respectively. Reducing the dose injected shifts the replica-

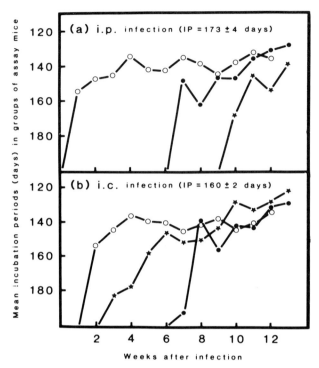

FIG. 1.   Replication curves of 139A in spleen (○), spinal cord (●) and brain (★) of CW mice infected with (a) about 1800 i.p. ID_{50} units or (b) about 250 i.c. ID_{50} units. From Fig. 1a, 2a in Kimberlin & Walker (1979a). Replication is indicated by the progressive shortening of incubation period in successive groups of assay mice. IP, incubation period (days ± SEM).

tion curves to the right; injecting the same effective dose by different peripheral routes causes replication to start at the same time after infection. In all cases, titres in spleen increase quite rapidly and then reach a plateau concentration which is maintained for the remainder of the incubation period. Infectivity plateaux in spleen have been observed in many studies (Table 2; see later).

The identity of the cells in the LRS which support replication of scrapie is not known. However, three studies have defined some properties of the cell types which are important in scrapie pathogenesis. First, Fraser & Dickinson (1978) increased the interval between splenectomy and i.p. injection of scrapie by up to 70 days and showed that the cells lost to scrapie pathogenesis by removal of spleen are not replaced. Secondly, Fraser & Farquhar (1987) found that exposing mice to ionizing radiation, under a wide variety of conditions, had no effect on the incubation period of peripherally injected scrapie. These observations rule out any role of lymphocytes in scrapie pathogenesis and suggest that the important cells are long lived. Thirdly,

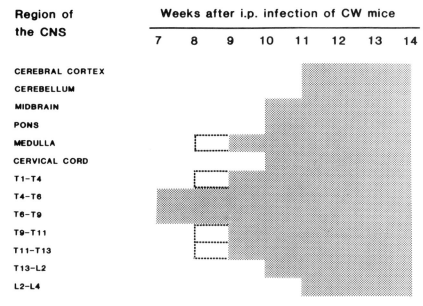

FIG. 2.   Comparison of the onset of 139A replication in 13 regions of the CNS. Neuroinvasion occurs in the spinal cord between thoracic vertebrae 4–9. The mean incubation period in the donor mice was 24 weeks. The stippled areas indicate the period when replication was taking place in each region of the CNS. The open areas denote uncertainties in the times of onset of replication because some of the assay groups at eight weeks were lost. From Table 1 in Kimberlin & Walker (1982).

Clarke & Kimberlin (1984) took spleens at a stage when the concentration of infectivity was at a plateau and separated each of them into a pulp fraction (containing about 80% of the spleen weight and most of the readily isolated cells) and a residual, stromal fraction from the trabecular framework of the spleen. The concentration of infectivity in the stroma was, on average 10 times that in the pulp fractions, indicating the potential importance in pathogenesis of some structurally stable cell populations in spleen. The likely presence of nerve endings in the stromal fraction is interesting in view of the evidence that neuroinvasion occurs via peripheral nerves (next section).

Invasion of the central nervous system

The invasion of the CNS by 139A scrapie is a controlled event; with each non-neural route of infection tested, replication in brain was detected after 40–50% of the incubation period had elapsed (Kimberlin & Walker 1979a). Fig. 1a illustrates that it is always preceded by replication in the spinal cord. It is interesting that 'spillover' of i.c. injected inoculum initiated replication in spleen, which was followed by replication in the spinal cord at about the same time as with peripherally injected scrapie (Fig. 1b).

In later studies we adjusted the doses of 139A injected i.v., i.p. and s.c. to give similar incubation periods. This gave almost identical patterns showing that replication in thoracic spinal cord precedes that in lumbar cord and brain (Kimberlin & Walker 1980). Fig. 2 illustrates that the pattern of replication curves indicated neuroinvasion in the region of the spinal cord between thoracic vertebrae 4 and 9 (Kimberlin & Walker 1982). We concluded that 139A scrapie infection spreads from spleen and visceral lymph nodes along autonomic (probably sympathetic) nerve fibres to mid-thoracic cord. Direct evidence for the centripetal invasion of the CNS along peripheral nerves was obtained by studies of the sciatic nerve (Kimberlin et al 1983b).

Viraemia is barely detectable four days after infection with 139A scrapie (Millson et al 1979). Once in the CNS, infection spreads slowly to the rest of the spinal cord, and to major regions of the brain in a caudal-rostral sequence (Kimberlin & Walker 1982, Cole & Kimberlin 1985). Widespread infection of the spinal cord and brain leads to a centrifugal spread of infection to peripheral nerves (Kimberlin et al 1983a, Buyukmihci et al 1980, 1985).

Studies of 263K scrapie in hamsters also suggest a neural pathway to thoracic cord following i.p. infection (Kimberlin & Walker 1986a). This is interesting because Diringer (1984) detected a persistent, low level viraemia by the use of extraction methods to concentrate 263K scrapie from blood and thereby increase the sensitivity of its detection. Using the same methods, he demonstrated infection of brain after only five days, which persisted for at least another 35 days with no evidence of replication as would have occurred with i.c. injected 263K. We have argued that Diringer's observation is an example of limited infection (possibly of capillary endothelial cells), which is not relevant to pathogenesis (Kimberlin & Walker 1986a, see later). However, it would be worth studying other experimental models, in particular the K.Fu strain of CJD in mice, which appears to maintain a relatively high level of viraemia throughout incubation (Kuroda et al 1983).

Spread and multiplication in the central nervous system

Two studies, one of which is illustrated in Fig. 2, enabled us to calculate the overall rate of spread of scrapie within the CNS to be about 0.5–2.0 mm/day (Kimberlin & Walker 1982, Kimberlin et al 1983b). This is much slower than the rate of spread of conventional neurotropic viruses and is comparable to the rate of slow intra-axonal transport of cytoskeletal proteins. Infection of the eye shows that infectivity first occurs in brain in the contralateral superior colliculus, to which the majority of retinal ganglion cells project (Fraser 1982, Fraser & Dickinson 1985, Kimberlin & Walker 1986a). This is strong evidence for intraneuronal (presumably intra-axonal) transport of scrapie and we suggest that neurons may be the most important cells for the spread of scrapie in the peripheral nervous system and the CNS.

We believe that infection can spread more easily along some neuronal

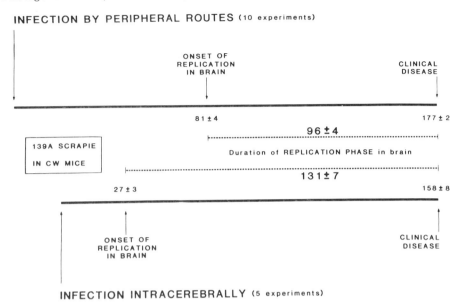

INFECTION BY PERIPHERAL ROUTES (10 experiments)

ONSET OF
REPLICATION
IN BRAIN

CLINICAL
DISEASE

81 ± 4 177 ± 2

96 ± 4

139A SCRAPIE

IN CW MICE

Duration of REPLICATION PHASE in brain

131 ± 7

27 ± 3 158 ± 8

ONSET OF
REPLICATION
IN BRAIN

CLINICAL
DISEASE

INFECTION INTRACEREBRALLY (5 experiments)

FIG. 3. The duration of the replication phase in brain is shorter using non-neural peripheral routes of infection than after intracerebral infection of anterior brain. Data presented in days as mean values ± SEM and taken from Table 5 in Kimberlin & Walker (1983). The peripheral routes used are: i.p. (4 experiments); i.v. (2); s.c., scruff of neck (2) and hind foot pad (2).

pathways than others. The origin of this idea was an analysis of 10 experiments using the i.v., i.p. or s.c. routes, which produced three findings (Kimberlin & Walker 1983). First, the interval between infection and the onset of replication in brain varied in direct proportion to the incubation period. In contrast, the duration of the replication phase in brain, from the time of onset to clinical disease, was constant. However, the most remarkable finding was that the duration of the replication phase was *longer* after i.c. infection than after infection by the non-neural peripheral routes, despite the *shorter* average i.c. incubation periods in these experiments (Fig. 3). This means that the neuropathogenesis of scrapie is faster when infection enters brain from spinal cord after peripheral infection than when injected i.c. into anterior brain. This conclusion is supported by the shorter incubation periods after intra-sciatic infection than after i.c. infection, once corrections have been made for the differences in the effective scrapie dose injected (Kimberlin et al 1983b). We then used intraspinal infection to bypass the lymphoreticular phase of pathogenesis after i.v., i.p. or s.c. infection and produce just the neural phase. As expected, the duration of the replication phase in brain was shorter after intraspinal than after i.c. infection and, consequently, so were the incubation periods of all three scrapie models tested (Kimberlin et al 1987, see Fig. 4).

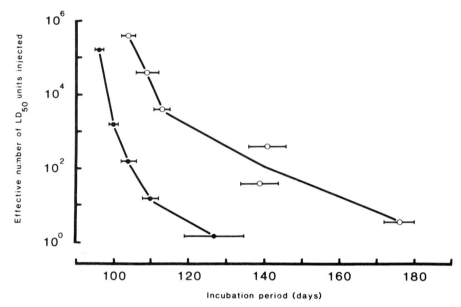

FIG. 4.   Dose–incubation curves of 139A scrapie in CW mice. Intraspinal infection
(●) gives shorter incubation periods than intracerebral infection (○). Data from Fig.
1a in Kimberlin et al (1987).

We have also studied 263K scrapie in golden hamsters and again found that
the duration of the replication phase after i.p. infection was shorter than after
i.c. infection. In addition, the duration of the replication phase after infection
of the eye (which provides an alternative pathway to the brain) was even
longer than with the i.c. route (Kimberlin & Walker 1986a).

Previously, we have suggested that the development of the fatal clinical
disease depends on scrapie agent replicating and causing cell dysfunction
(perhaps cell death) in a small number of so called 'clinical target areas'
(CTA: see Kimberlin & Walker 1983). The major conclusion from all of the
above studies is that the site of invasion (or injection) of the CNS affects the
duration of the replication phase in brain by determining the neural pathways
by which the CTA are reached (Kimberlin & Walker 1986a, Kimberlin et al
1987). If we assume that scrapie infection is transported mainly within
neurons, then it is easy to see how the rate of spread of infection to the CTA
would be related to (1) the anatomical complexity of neuronal pathways from
the site of invasion, and (2) the ease or difficulty with which infection can
spread between different types of connecting neurons (see examples in Fig.
5). Infection spreading from the spinal cord (after injection i.v., i.p., s.c., i.s.
or into the sciatic nerve) would gain relatively easy access to the CTA in
contrast to the more complex pathways (eg. Fig. 5d) applicable to i.c. infection or infection of the eye. We envisage that the CTA constitute a very small

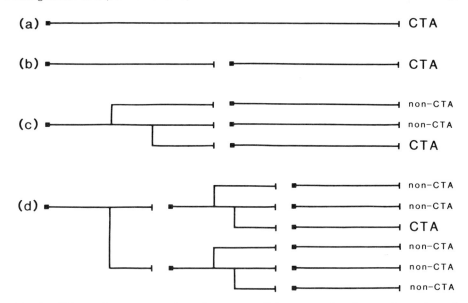

FIG. 5. Schematic representation of some possible neuronal pathways from sites of scrapie invasion of the CNS (a-d) to clinical target areas (CTA) and the rest of the CNS (non-CTA). From Fig. 3 in Kimberlin & Walker (1988).

portion of the CNS so that, even with the i.c. route, the pathways to the CTA would vary according to the precise site of injection with consequent effects on incubation period. Studies of four scrapie models using stereotactic i.c. injection techniques support this view (Gorde et al 1982, Kim et al 1987).

Elsewhere (Kimberlin & Walker 1988), we have discussed in detail how the differential targeting of scrapie infection to the CTA and non-CTA determines the major disease parameters of each scrapie model. For example, targeting to the CTA is a major factor in determining the length of incubation and we have suggested that the CTA may be among the last areas of the CNS to be reached by scrapie agent in some of the very long incubation models. In contrast, the overall rate of scrapie replication in brain largely reflects events in the non-CTA: it is a function of the intrinsic replication rate in cells to which infection has spread, and the efficiency of spread to other potential replication sites. As Fig. 1 indicates, the replication rate of 139A in brain is considerably faster after infection i.p. than i.c., and the same difference has been found with 263K in hamsters (Kimberlin & Walker 1986a, Czub et al 1986). We suggest the reason is that i.p. infection leads to more efficient targeting of scrapie to non-CTA, as well as to CTA, than does i.c. infection.

Evidence for restrictions on the replication of scrapie

Table 2 lists the published studies of different scrapie models, in all of which

TABLE 2 Occurrence of plateau concentrations of scrapie infectivity in various tissues other than brain

Scrapie model	Tissues with an infectivity plateau	References
263K/golden hamster	Spleen, lymph nodes	Kimberlin & Walker (1986a)
'Chandler'/$Sinc^{s7}$ mice	Spleen, lymph nodes, thymus, salivary gland	Eklund et al (1967)[a]
139A/$Sinc^{s7}$	Spleen	Clarke & Haig (1971), Hunter et al (1972), Kimberlin & Walker (1979a)
	Salivary gland	Millson et al (1979)[a]
	Spinal cord, spinal nerves, dorsal root ganglia	Kimberlin et al (1983a)
ME7/$Sinc^{s7}$ mice	Spleen	Dickinson et al (1969)[a], Mould et al (1970)
ME7/$Sinc^{p7}$ mice	Spleen	Dickinson et al (1969)[a]
87V/$Sinc^{p7}$	Spleen	Collis & Kimberlin (1985), Bruce (1985)

[a] Coincident viraemia not detected

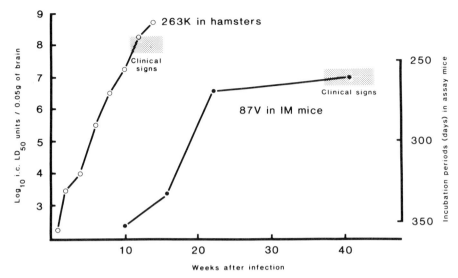

FIG. 6.   Differences in the shape of the scrapie replication curves in brain in relation to incubation period, after i.c. infection. The concentration of 263K scrapie increased up to the time of clinical disease but the replication of 87V virtually stopped several months beforehand. From Fig. 2 in Kimberlin & Walker (1986a) and from Collis & Kimberlin (1985). (N.B. Differences in the assay procedures used do not permit comparisons of absolute replication rate.)

the concentration of infectivity in lymphoreticular tissues reached stable plateau levels. With 87V scrapie in IM mice, the plateau in spleen lasted over a year. Clarke & Haig (1971) demonstrated a remarkably close correlation between total 139A infectivity and spleen weight, later confirmed by Clarke & Kimberlin (1984).

The occurrence of plateau titres is not limited to lymphoreticular tissues: they occur in the CNS, in both thoracic and lumbar spinal cords, and in the spinal nerves and dorsal root ganglia of the peripheral nervous system (Kimberlin et al 1983a and b). Plateau titres in the CNS are at least tenfold higher than those in the peripheral nervous system, which are comparable to those in the LRS. It would be interesting to know the cellular basis of these titre patterns.

In brain, no infectivity plateau was apparent with 263K scrapie injected i.c. (Fig. 6) but this model is exceptional in having the shortest incubation range of any so far described. However, the replication curves for i.c. injected (Kimberlin & Walker 1988) and i.p. injected 139A in CW mice (Kimberlin et al 1983a) tend towards a plateau in brain, as do those for i.c. injected ME7 in C57BL mice (Dickinson et al 1969, Kimberlin & Walker, unpublished). Plateaux of ME7 in the optic nerve and superior colliculus occur after infection of the eye (Fraser & Dickinson 1985). Two studies of 87V scrapie in IM

TABLE 3 Onset of agent replication in relation to incubation period

Scrapie model	Dilution of scrapie brain inoculum	Onset of replication (weeks)		Incubation period (weeks)	Reference
		Spleen	Brain		
263K/golden hamster	1%	1	9	16	Kimberlin & Walker (1986a)
139A/$Sinc^{s7}$ mice	0.1–1%	1–3	10–11	24–27	Kimberlin & Walker (1979a)
'Chandler'/$Sinc^{s7}$ mice[a]	1%	4	16	23–30	Eklund et al (1967)
ME7/$Sinc^{s7}$ mice	1%	1	ND	38	Dickinson & Fraser (1969)
ME7/$Sinc^{p7}$ mice	1%	~ 4	ND	77	Dickinson & Fraser (1969)
87V/$Sinc^{p7}$ mice	10%	4	>55	>70	Bruce (1985)
87V/$Sinc^{p7}$ mice	1%	4	(>80)	(>80)	Collis & Kimberlin (1985)

[a] Subcutaneous infection; i.p. infection was used in all other cases
ND, not determined. Brackets indicate that replication or clinical disease had not occurred at the time shown

mice, a much slower scrapie model, reveal striking evidence for plateaux in brain, as illustrated in Fig. 6 (Bruce 1985, Collis & Kimberlin 1985).

The occurrence of infectivity plateaux clearly indicates a restriction on the scrapie replication process. It can be argued that replication takes place in stable, long-lived cell populations in both the LRS (radiation resistant cells) and the nervous system (possibly in neurons). The restriction can therefore be seen in terms of a finite number of cells that can support replication, and a limitation on the net replication process in individual cells. Infectivity plateaux may be due to either a complete cessation of agent synthesis in these stable cells or to a dynamic equilibrium between synthesis and loss of infectivity. The loss could arise through destruction or 'export' of infection, but if the latter occurs, it does not lead to the accumulation or maintenance of an appreciable level of viraemia (Table 2).

A limited number of scrapie replication sites has been suggested as the most likely explanation of competition between strains of scrapie (Dickinson & Outram 1979). This occurs when two scrapie strains of different incubation period in a given strain of mouse are injected at different times. Under certain conditions, the 'slower' strain can completely prevent the second, 'faster' strain from producing scrapie. Competition occurs when either the i.c. (Dickinson et al 1972) or the i.p. route of infection is used (Dickinson et al 1975a, Kimberlin & Walker 1985), indicating that strains can compete for cell sites in both the LRS and the CNS.

Evidence for limitations on the cell-to-cell spread of scrapie agent

Not enough comparative studies have been done to determine whether or not the rate of scrapie replication in the LRS varies in different tissues and in different scrapie models. However, for all the scrapie models listed in Table 3 replication in spleen starts within about four weeks of i.p. infection, regardless of incubation period and with only a small difference attributable to *Sinc* gene. It is interesting that the timing of invasion of the brain cannot be predicted from the onset of replication in spleen. For example, neuroinvasion occurred three weeks before the titre of 263K had reached a plateau in hamster spleen (Kimberlin & Walker 1986a), and 5–6 weeks after 139A scrapie plateaued in CW mice (Fig. 1a, Kimberlin & Walker 1979a). However, with low doses of 87V scrapie in IM mice neuroinvasion had still not occurred 60 weeks after the spleen plateau had been reached (Collis & Kimberlin 1985). This remarkable situation suggests that cell-to-cell spread of scrapie may be restricted in some way. The restriction could be at the cellular interface between the LRS and the nervous system. Alternatively, at least two cellular compartments in the LRS may be involved in scrapie pathogenesis, with rapid uptake and replication of scrapie taking place in one but with restricted spread of infection to a second compartment from which neuroinvasion could occur.

In the CNS, there are indications that scrapie replication is faster in the short incubation models than in the larger ones, but better comparative studies are needed. *Sinc* gene clearly has a substantial effect on the onset of replication of ME7 in brain (Dickinson et al 1969). There are dramatic differences in the shape of the replication curve according to the scrapie model. For example, Fig. 6 shows a constant exponential rate of 263K replication in hamster brain which is interrupted only by the fatal disease. In contrast, 87V reaches a virtual plateau concentration of infectivity in brain long before the clinical disease develops. This clearly indicates a limitation on cell-to-cell spread of infectivity, which, for convenience, we can think of in terms of neurons. We have discussed (Kimberlin & Walker 1988) that the ease with which infection by a given strain of scrapie can spread along various pathways depends on the physiological and neurochemical properties of different types of connecting neurons. This would effectively create a hierarchy of cells that can support scrapie replication, according to their accessibility. We suggest that the gradual slowing down of 87V replication occurs as only the replication sites in the less accessible cells in the non-CTA remain. The cells in the CTA would be among the last to be reached with the consequence of a much longer incubation period.

Conclusions and qualifications

One of the great paradoxes of scrapie and the related diseases is why they are so slow when no known host responses are induced to slow them down; neither the immune system nor interferon production seems to be involved. Studies of experimental scrapie have revealed that slowness is coupled to remarkable predictability and that both features are predetermined by the combination of host genotype, strain of agent and the route of infection.

The route of injection is one determinant of the effective scrapie titre that establishes infection in the LRS, but the efficiency of a given route can be modified in either direction by treatment of the host with drugs at around the time of scrapie injection. For example, phytohaemagglutinin can increase the effective dose by up to 100 times (A.G. Dickinson, personal communication, R.H. Kimberlin, unpublished) and certain polyanions can reduce it by 100 to 1000 times (Kimberlin & Walker 1986b). The extent of these modifications is equivalent to a major part of a dose–incubation range. The efficiency of infection can also be reduced when scrapie inoculum prepared from one strain of mice is injected into mice of the same *Sinc* genotype but different strain (Kimberlin & Walker 1978). We therefore suggest that an altered efficiency of infection may underly the influence on incubation period of the gene called 'PID-1', which is located within the D subregion of the major histocompatibility (H-2) complex in mice (Kingsbury et al 1983).

Subsequent pathogenesis is subject to constraints on the cell-to-cell spread of infection and on the intrinsic rate of replication in infected cells. These two factors may be closely related if replication is needed before infection can spread to other cells (Kimberlin & Walker 1988). The length of incubation period in different scrapie models is determined by at least two major factors, (1) the rate of spread of infection from LRS to CNS (neuroinvasion), and (2) dynamics of replication in the CNS and of the spread of infection to the CTA. The controlling effect of *Sinc* gene on the incubation period of mouse scrapie is clearly exerted at the neural stage of pathogenesis (and possibly on the access of scrapie to the nervous system) but its effect in the LRS seems to be much less.

The events of pathogenesis we have described are based entirely on studies of animals that were infected as adults. Neonatal mice are much less susceptible to scrapie infection: incubation periods after peripheral injection can be much longer (Outram et al 1973, Hotchin & Buckley, 1977) and infection by i.c., i.p. and s.c. routes is less efficient (Kimberlin & Walker 1978). This raises many questions about the differential maturation of cell populations which can either be infected by scrapie, or actively degrade it or sequester it without inactivation. Studies on neonates (Hotchin & Buckley 1977), adults (Dickinson et al 1975b) and interspecies transmission from hamsters to mice (Kimberlin & Walker 1979b), have all provided examples of long term persistence of infection at a low level, perhaps accompanied by very slow replication. But it is not clear whether disease can develop from these situations, or whether they represent 'dead-end' infections of the wrong cells for pathogenesis to occur.

There are many other uncertainties of scrapie pathogenesis concerning the relevance of experimental routes of infection to natural infection, the identity of the cells in the LRS which support replication, whether or not neuroinvasion invariably occurs via peripheral nerves, the extent to which cells other than neurons are important in pathogenesis, the locations of the CTA in different scrapie models, and the nature of the molecular lesions underlying the development of disease.

Looking to the future, the short incubation models can be exploited to yield further information about some of the mechanisms of scrapie pathogenesis but more studies of the slow scrapie models are needed to learn about the controls. Infection of the eye (Fraser & Dickinson 1985) provides a relatively simple neuroanatomical system to study the spread of infection within and between neurons, and stereotactic injection techniques will help to locate the clinical target areas (Kim et al 1987). Much interest is currently centred on a glycoprotein, PrP, which is the major constituent of scrapie-associated fibrils (SAF). The occurrence of SAF in brain extracts has become a pathological hallmark of scrapie and the related diseases. Studies of the pathogenesis of SAF from normal PrP could reveal much about the type of molecular lesions underlying the clinical disease. Even greater revelations would occur if it turns out that PrP is also a functional component of the infectious agent and/ or the protein product of *Sinc* gene.

References

Bruce ME 1985 Agent replication dynamics in a long incubation period model of mouse scrapie. J Gen Virol 66:2517–2522

Buyukmihci N, Rorvik M, Marsh RF 1980 Replication of the scrapie agent in ocular neural tissues. Proc Nat Acad Sci USA 77:1169–1171

Buyukmihci N, Goehring-Harmon F, Marsh RF 1985 Asymmetry of retinal lesions in experimental scrapie after intracerebral inoculation of hamsters. Exp Neurol 87:172–176

Clarke MC, Haig DA 1971 Multiplication of scrapie agent in mouse spleen. Res Vet Sci 12:195–197

Clarke MC, Kimberlin RH 1984 Pathogenesis of mouse scrapie: distribution of agent in the pulp and stroma of infected spleens. Vet Microbiol 9:215–225

Cole S, Kimberlin RH 1985 Pathogenesis of mouse scrapie: dynamics of vacuolation in brain and spinal cord after intraperitoneal infection. Neuropathol Appl Neurobiol 11:213–227

Collis SC, Kimberlin RH 1985 Long-term persistence of scrapie infection in mouse spleens in the absence of clinical disease. FEMS (Fed Eur Microbiol Soc) Microbiol Lett 29:111–114

Czub M, Braig HR, Diringer H 1986 Pathogenesis of scrapie: study of the temporal development of clinical symptoms, of infectivity titres and scrapie-associated fibrils in brains of hamsters infected intraperitoneally. J Gen Virol 67:2005–2009

Dickinson AG, Fraser H 1969 Genetical control of the concentration of ME7 scrapie agent in mouse spleen. J Comp Pathol 79:363–366

Dickinson AG, Fraser H 1972 Scrapie: effect of Dh gene on incubation period of extraneurally injected agent. Heredity 29:91–93

Dickinson AG, Outram GW 1979 The scrapie replication-site hypothesis and its implications for pathogenesis. In: Prusiner SB, Hadlow WJ (eds) Slow transmissible diseases of the nervous system. Academic Press, New York vol 2:13–31

Dickinson AG, Outram GW 1988 Genetic aspects of unconventional virus infections: the basis of the virino hypothesis. In: Novel infectious agents and the central nervous system. Wiley, Chichester (Ciba Found Symp 135) p 63–84

Dickinson AG, Meikle VMH, Fraser H 1969 Genetical control of the concentration of ME7 scrapie agent in the brain of mice. J Comp Pathol 79:15–22

Dickinson AG, Fraser H, Meikle VMH, Outram GW 1972 Competition between different scrapie agents in mice. Nature (Lond) 237:244–245

Dickinson AG, Fraser H, McConnell I, Outram GW, Sales DI, Taylor DM 1975a Extraneural competition between different scrapie agents leading to loss of infectivity. Nature (Lond) 253:556

Dickinson AG, Fraser H, Outram GW 1975b Scrapie incubation time can exceed natural lifespan. Nature (Lond) 256:732–733

Diringer H 1984 Sustained viremia in experimental hamster scrapie. Arch Virol 82:105–109

Eklund CM, Kennedy RC, Hadlow WJ 1967 Pathogenesis of scrapie virus infection in the mouse. J Infect Dis 117:15–22

Fraser H 1982 Neuronal spread of scrapie agent and targeting of lesions within the retino-tectal pathway. Nature (Lond) 295:149–150

Fraser H, Dickinson AG 1970 Pathogenesis of scrapie in the mouse: the role of the spleen. Nature (Lond) 226:462–463

Fraser H, Dickinson AG 1978 Studies of the lymphoreticular system in the pathogenesis of scrapie: the role of spleen and thymus. J Comp Pathol 88:563–573

Fraser H, Dickinson AG 1985 Targeting of scrapie lesions and spread of agent via the retino-tectal projection. Brain Res 346:32–41

Fraser H, Farquhar CF 1987 Ionising radiation has no influence on scrapie incubation period in mice. Vet Microbiol 13:211–223

Gorde JM, Tamalet J, Toga M, Bert J 1982 Changes in the nigrostriatal system following microinjection of an unconventional agent. Brain Res 240:87–93

Hadlow WJ, Kennedy RC, Race RE 1982 Natural infection of Suffolk sheep with scrapie virus. J Infect Dis 146:657–664

Hotchin J, Buckley R 1977 Latent form of scrapie virus: a new factor in slow-virus disease. Science (Wash DC) 196:668–671

Hotchin J, Sikora E, Baker F 1983 Disappearance of scrapie virus from tissues of the mouse. Intervirology 19:205–212

Hunter GD, Kimberlin RH, Millson GC 1972 Absence of eclipse phase in scrapie mice. Nature (Lond) 235:31–32

Kim YS, Carp RI, Callahan SM, Wisniewski HM 1987 Incubation period and survival times for mice injected stereotaxically with three scrapie strains in different brain regions. J Gen Virol 68:695–702

Kimberlin RH, Walker CA 1977 Characteristics of a short incubation model of scrapie in the golden hamster. J Gen Virol 34:295–304

Kimberlin RH, Walker CA 1978 Pathogenesis of mouse scrapie: effect of route of inoculation on infectivity titres and dose-response curves. J Comp Pathol 88:39–47

Kimberlin RH, Walker CA 1979a Pathogenesis of mouse scrapie: Dynamics of agent replication in spleen, spinal cord and brain after infection by different routes. J Comp Pathol 89:551–562

Kimberlin RH, Walker CA 1979b Pathogenesis of scrapie: agent multiplication in brain at the first and second passage of hamster scrapie in mice. J Gen Virol 42:107–117

Kimberlin RH, Walker CA 1980 Pathogenesis of mouse scrapie: evidence for neural spread of infection to the CNS. J Gen Virol 51:183–187

Kimberlin RH, Walker CA 1982 Pathogenesis of mouse scrapie: patterns of agent replication in different parts of the CNS following intraperitoneal infection. J R Soc Med 75:618–624

Kimberlin RH, Walker CA 1983 Invasion of the CNS by scrapie agent and its spread to different parts of the brain. In: Court LA, Cathala F (eds) Virus non-conventionnels et affections du système nerveux central. Masson, Paris, p 17–33

Kimberlin RH, Walker CA 1985 Competition between strains of scrapie depends on the blocking agent being infectious. Intervirology 23:74–81

Kimberlin RH, Walker CA 1986a Pathogenesis of scrapie (strain 263K) in hamsters infected intracerebrally, intraperitoneally or intraocularly. J Gen Virol 67:255–263

Kimberlin RH, Walker CA 1986b Suppression of scrapie infection in mice by hetero-polyanion 23, dextran sulfate, and some other polyanions. Antimicrob Agents Chemother 30:409–413

Kimberlin RH, Walker CA 1988 Transport, targeting and replication of scrapie in the CNS. In: Court LA et al (eds) Unconventional viruses and central nervous system diseases. Atelier d'Arts Graphiques, Abbaye de Melleray, in press

Kimberlin RH, Field HJ, Walker CA 1983a Pathogenesis of mouse scrapie: evidence for spread of infection from central to peripheral nervous system. J Gen Virol 64:713–716

Kimberlin RH, Hall SM, Walker CA 1983b Pathogenesis of mouse scrapie: evidence for direct neural spread of infection to the CNS after injection of sciatic nerve. J Neurol Sci 61:315–325

Kimberlin RH, Cole S, Walker CA 1987 Pathogenesis of scrapie is faster when infection is intraspinal instead of intracerebral. Microb Pathogen 2:405–415

Kingsbury DT, Kasper KC, Stites DP, Watson JD, Hogan RN, Prusiner SB 1983 Genetic control of scrapie and Creutzfeldt-Jakob disease in mice. J Immunol 131:491–496

Kuroda Y, Gibbs CJ Jr, Amyx HL, Gajdusek DC 1983 Creutzfeldt-Jakob disease in mice: persistent viremia and preferential replication of virus in low-density lymphocytes. Infect Immun 41:154–161

McFarlin DE, Raff MC, Simpson E, Nehlsen SH 1971 Scrapie in immunologically deficient mice. Nature (Lond) 233:336

Millson GC, Kimberlin RH, Manning EJ, Collis SC 1979 Early distribution of radioactive liposomes and scrapie infectivity in mouse tissues following administration by different routes. Vet Microbiol 4:89–99

Mould DL, Dawson A McL, Rennie JC 1970 Very early replication of scrapie in lymphocytic tissue. Nature (Lond) 228:779–780

Outram GW, Dickinson AG, Fraser H 1973 Developmental maturation of susceptibility to scrapie in mice. Nature (Lond) 241:536–537

DISCUSSION

Merz: If I understand correctly, you support Bob Rohwer's finding of a continual accumulation of 263K scrapie in hamster brain.

Kimberlin: Yes. His results were published in a paper that was mainly about scrapie-induced cell fusion (Moreau-Dubois et al 1982).

Merz: At that time, there was disagreement as to whether the scrapie 263K replication curve plateaued or whether it was a continual log increase.

Kimberlin: Yes. Both curves were obtained after i.c. infection and they are very similar. However, as I explained, this was with 263K scrapie in hamsters. Other scrapie models do not give a continual log increase in titre.

Prusiner: In your Fig. 6, one single point creates the plateau of 87V scrapie in IM mice. How many times did you measure that point?

Kimberlin: That is one curve done by Dr Susan Collis and myself, but there are other data using the same model which show the same thing (Bruce 1985). I am not trying to be final about this—more data are needed on the replication dynamics of long incubation models. But we have enough information for me to show some major differences between the replication curves of 263K in hamsters and 87V scrapie in IM mice.

Carlson: I would like to emphasize that we are talking about plateaux of replication. By this type of an assay it is not possible to distinguish between the rate of replication in an organ and a balance between replication, accumulation and catabolism.

Kimberlin: I agree, we have no idea whether we are dealing with a static or a dynamic plateau. In some ways, competition experiments with two different strains of scrapie injected into the same mice might indicate that plateaux in the lymphoreticular system are functionally static. Competition is one of the classic predictions that you can make to test the idea of a limitation of the replication and spread of scrapie infectivity. However, we cannot really answer your question at the moment. One approach might be to do a competition experiment and measure the replication dynamics of each scrapie strain in, for example, spleen.

Carlson: Was the competition based on clinical disease, rather than on increase in titre of scrapie infectivity?

Kimberlin: Competition is measured by changes in the incubation period but there is enough information to interpret competition in terms of the net replication and spread of the competing strains.

Carp: I agree that breakdown of scrapie could be a factor in the production of a plateau. We have shown that peritoneal macrophages *in vitro* can inactivate scrapie (Carp & Callahan 1981, 1982). We also have evidence that if we induce macrophages in the peritoneal cavity, we get a longer incubation period following intraperitoneal injection of scrapie (Carp & Callahan 1985). Both of these results suggest that catabolic events can affect the level of infectivity.

Merz: The sites of replication for the scrapie agents are not really known, because there are no tissue culture systems or accepted agent markers to identify these sites. The assay measures accumulation of infectivity, not replication in a given area. Replication could occur elsewhere, followed by movement of the agent.

Kimberlin: It is very difficult to distinguish between accumulation and replication *in vivo*. There is always the argument that infectivity may accumulate in one tissue because it is being transported from sites of replication in another. Perhaps the only place where you can argue that replication really occurs is the very first place where an increase in infectivity is found. However, these arguments are difficult to resolve. It is reasonable to draw on some of the lessons from virology and argue that where you do get a substantial increase in titre it is either because the infectious agent is replicating there or because it is being targeted to that place.

Merz: A meeting like this is helpful to clarify definitions, such as the term 'replication'.

Kimberlin: All our data on the spread of infectivity to and within the CNS are based on measurement of relative times of onset of replication in different regions. My interpretation of those data is not substantially affected by whether we are measuring accumulation or replication. If it is accumulation, infectivity still has to replicate and then spread to a given region to accumulate.

Bolton: The proper term when you are measuring the agent in certain sites is accumulation, not replication, which has very definite molecular implications. We still do not know at what sites the agent is being replicated.

Kimberlin: Bearing in mind that *in vivo* it is almost impossible to prove replication at a given place, at what point would you be happy to use the word replication?

Bolton: You need to be able to define what it is in the agent that is being replicated, then with the proper molecular probes you can determine which cells are actually replicating the agent. Up to that point it's really not accurate to define the sites of replication, although we can easily look at sites of accumulation.

Kimberlin: Well I am happy with that, if the Chairman thinks it is reasonable to apply the same principle to virology as a whole. Is it usual to apply the word replication to a virus only after it has been completely characterized?

F. Brown: I don't think we need to have characterized a virus completely before we apply the word replication to it. It is usual to use the term replication when there is an increase in the amount of virus.

*Dickinson:*What David (Bolton) said is formally correct. It would certainly be a big problem so far as the early accumulation of titre in spleen was concerned, if we knew that there was a lot of accumulation going on somewhere else. However, when the early events are coming to a plateau in the spleen you are not getting lots of infectivity somewhere else from which it could be spreading into the spleen.

F. Brown: I didn't mean that the infectivity should go elsewhere, I meant that it might be inactivated in some way.

Bolton: I think it's most important when you look in the brain, particularly in different regions of the brain, to remember that there may be spread of the agent and accumulation along the flow as you discussed earlier, but the site of synthesis may be a different region of the brain.

Kimberlin: I agree, and I outlined ideas on the neuronal targeting of infectivity within the CNS. But for over 20 years the term replication has been used to describe the accumulation of infectivity in different tissues. It would be nice to be more precise, but you may confuse people by using terms like accumulation rather than multiplication or replication, if that's probably what it is.

F. Brown: It could be that you produce the agent, which can be measured by its infectivity, it is then converted into material that cannot be measured by infectivity titration but which spreads to more cells until eventually enough cells become involved for clinical symptoms to appear.

Dickinson: In terms of a focalization of the lesions, that argument does not hold. You really need to think about the biological implications of the detailed pathology.

Prusiner: You are looking at synthesis, which can be followed by degradation or by transport, and what you measure is the end result of these processes—that is, accumulation or levels.

Carp: We have some data which relate to Richard's (Kimberlin) concept of clinical target areas. We bypassed the invasion of the brain by putting 5 µl of a scrapie inoculum into specific areas within the central nervous system: the cerebral cortex, caudate nucleus, thalamus, substantia nigra and the cerebellum (Kim et al 1987). With the 22L scrapie agent, the cerebellar incubation period is much shorter than that for other areas, particularly the cortex, caudate nucleus and thalamus. So, at least with these five areas, the clinical target area for the 22L strain of scrapie is the cerebellum. We also observed ataxia in the mice injected in the cerebellum with the 22L strain several weeks before the typical clinical symptoms of scrapie. In contrast, with the ME7 strain of scrapie, injection into the thalamus and the cerebellum gives much shorter incubation periods than injection into the cortex, caudate nucleus or substantia nigra. With 139A, injection into the four brain areas other than the cortex gives similar incubation periods and all are much shorter than that in the cerebral cortex. These are the only five areas we studied, there may be other areas where injection would lead to even shorter incubation periods. These experiments were all done with the same strain of mice (C57BL) at the same time. At other times we have done experiments injecting ME7 into the hypothalamus, and have suggestive evidence that ME7 in the hypothalamus may give very short incubation periods, at least as short as the incubation period for mice infected with ME7 in the thalamus or cerebellum.

Kimberlin: The Marseilles group did a pilot experiment which illustrates the converse of this situation (Gorde et al 1982). They stereotactically injected 263K into hamsters, into the nigrostriatal region. This produced local effects which clearly indicated replication of infection, but in some animals clinical disease did not develop during a normal dose-response end-point. I find that fascinating because Richard Carp's data show that you can speed up incubation period by injecting scrapie into the right part of the CNS, whereas the Marseilles study says you can almost avoid clinical scrapie by putting it into the wrong part of the CNS; the infection may not reach the clinical target areas.

F. Brown: A comment from a 'non-scrapieologist': the lengths of incubation period that Richard Carp is describing all seem so similar, is a difference of plus or minus a few days significant?

Carp: Yes, these are standard errors and they are statistically significant.

F. Brown: The inoculum you used was five microlitres, which is difficult to inject accurately into a defined target area. Is this a source of error?

Carp: The volume of inoculum was determined by measuring movement along very fine tubing, which is quite accurate, and the material was injected slowly to prevent overspill into other areas.

Kimberlin: With non-stereotactic injection of 20 µl of inoculum the errors are considerable but they don't seem to matter a great deal; the concentration of the inoculum is much more important than the volume.

Dickinson: The degree of control in these long incubation period models is one of the most fascinating aspects of scrapie. It all depends on the quality of data. Since I have used incubation period and incubation period assays for at least a decade longer than anybody else, I have to justify the quality of those data. Initially, we were so distrustful of this that we devised an elaborate coding system, which we have used ever since, to randomize all possible influential factors. 20 years ago we published that in the lymphoreticular system, using the ME7 strain of scrapie, the effect of the *Sinc* gene makes an even finer difference than the small differences described by Richard Carp. With a large dose, for example 10000 intracerebral infectious units, injected i.c. or i.p., replication starts in the spleen, say after a week in one *Sinc* genotype but after a month in the other, whereas the end-point times of the incubations differ by 140 days, so there is this marked amplification. The maximum rate of replication in the spleen, even though the starting points were different, is very similar, irrespective of *Sinc* genotype. *Sinc* seems to control delays, and in our early experiments this was seen as the delay before the start of similar rates of replication. We now have a scrapie model which is a long one, 22A scrapie in C57BL mice. If the *Sinc* genotype changes (for example from s7s7 to p7p7), the incubation instead of ending at 500 days ends at 200 days. The amount of 22A infectivity in the brain of a C57BL mouse virtually plateaus for 200 days starting about 200 days after injection; that is, for over half the incubation period. The *Sinc*-controlled difference is effected mainly in the brain: what happens right at the end of the incubation is loss of control, accompanied by a 10-fold increase in infectivity. Scrapie as a clinical disease has always fascinated me, because of these strict controls and then the sudden loss of control.

Prusiner: I disagree with the accuracy being claimed for these small differences in the length of the incubation period. Let me describe our recent results with scrapie in the hamster. Our bioassay measures the time from inoculation to the onset of illness and then we let the animals go to death. I think most people would agree that the clinical phase is fairly uniform in the hamster. Recently, some people questioned us about the use of this assay, so we did an experiment to determine whether or not we needed to let animals die: this is the objective point in the bioassay, the clinical assessment of these animals is subjective. We decided to see if we could consistently determine a point prior to but near death, i.e. within 2 days, when the animals were no longer able to right themselves, at which time we would sacrifice them. We performed 50 bioassays with four animals per assay and tried to predict this time point: we said 'this animal can no longer right itself and we would kill it in our new assay', but then we let it die. The interval between when we predicted they would die within the next two days and death ranged from one day to 15 days. Therefore we have to be extremely careful when looking at two week differences in these animals. We see the same thing in mice except, as Alan Dickinson pointed out, different inbred strains of mice have different clinical phases. For example, many of the I/Ln mice develop clinical scrapie very rapidly; whereas the Swiss mice have a very prolonged clinical phase. I think it's very important to try to be objective, and to claim that these data are absolute is wrong.

Kimberlin: Richard Carp showed differences between numbers which represent incubation periods. All Richard is claiming, is that the system is such that he can measure differences between numbers and I think a lot of the time the data are perfectly believable. What is more important and much more difficult, is when you try, for example in the bioassay systems, to convert measured incubation periods into infectivity titres.

Prusiner: I would agree completely.

Carp: Let me just comment on my own data: (1) those numbers are based on 10 to 15 animals, and (2) we have let animals go to death and we see the same differences with regard to the clinical target areas, that is, the animals injected in the cerebellum with 22L die long before the animals injected in the cortex with 22L (Kim et al 1987). Stan, don't your comments dispute your own original data (Prusiner et al 1982) in which you did curves of assay for clinical disease and for death, and found that these curves were parallel?

Prusiner: Not at all; I am saying that the onset of illness is the point that can be measured with a reasonable degree of reliability. As these animals progress, to find a time point in the middle is very difficult. We check this all the time by measuring the two points. There are a lot of data in the scrapie literature where incubation periods of scrapie-infected animals are measured at only one point—this is a point well into the clinical phase of the illness of these animals where they are scored as ill. This is a very difficult point to judge clinically in a reproducible and consistent manner.

Dickinson: That is not true of our data; we give an end-point after a sequence of observations.

Carp: We require three positive scores before we say that the animal is ill; three examinations separated by one week each.

Prusiner: The only time points that we believe to be reliable and internally consistent are the onset of illness and death, not some period in between where you see progression of the disease.

Carp: This is not a time point in between—this is a time point based on the first demonstration of clinical disease. If the animal is sick again the following week and the week after, then we call that the end of the incubation period. The basic assessment was made on that first appearance of clinical disease i.e. the onset of illness, to use your terms. We do not do our assessment for scrapie at some point after the start of clinical disease.

F. Brown: When virus is produced in culture, one gets high titres and then the infectivity titre levels out, but the amount of virus particles continues to increase because some of the virus is being inactivated. Do you know the number of cells that are affected at different stages of the infection?

Kimberlin: I cannot answer your question because there is no way to identify which cells in a tissue support replication at any one time.

Merz: Richard, you talked about clinical target areas with respect to scrapie. In scrapie, you measure infectivity changes in the cerebellum, pons or medulla but vacuolation occurs throughout the entire brain. In human CJD, particularly the iatrogenic growth hormone cases versus the i.c. iatrogenic inoculations, there are dementia and cerebellar ataxia with a long duration of the postulated time after inoculation with the growth hormone: how do you use clinical target areas to explain these human cases?

Kimberlin: I think that exactly the same principles apply. 'Clinical target areas' simply refers to those parts of the CNS which are necessarily damaged by the infectious agent to produce the clinical signs by which scrapie or CJD is recognized. However, the greater complexity of the human brain compared to rodents gives scope for a greater range of diagnostic clinical signs. The signs actually exhibited by individual human cases will in part depend on the site of injection or invasion of the CNS because this will enable infectivity to spread to some potential clinical target areas more easily than to others. I think there are situations in which some of the microscopic lesions could indicate where these clinical target areas are, but there are also situations in which lesions are so widespread as to confuse everything, because many sites of tissue damage will be outside clinical target areas. I would suggest that in cases caused by 'wild-type' infections, for example, Paul Brown's story about iatrogenic growth hormone cases and Hugh Fraser's comments about distinguishing between 'wild-type' and mutant strains, the pathology might reveal more about the location of clinical target areas than in cases with mutant strains, where pathological changes occur throughout the brain.

Merz: The term you use is clinical target area. Clinical means onset of signs: in human cases there can be dementia or no dementia yet the brain shows a lot of vacuolation.

Kimberlin: I am saying that some areas of vacuolation may correlate with the clinical target areas but others will be irrelevant to the clinical disease.

Merz: I would like to see you expand clinical target areas such that you can use the phrase with respect to disease in animals and humans, because I think it's very valuable.

Kimberlin: The idea of clinical target areas applies equally well to animals and humans. The problem is correlating pathological lesions like vacuolation with a particular type of clinical disease because lesions will often occur in non-clinical target areas. It is also possible that some clinical target areas may have no vacuolar lesions even though there is disease.

Wisniewski: In neurology, the function of the brain is related to a given topography. The brain is a multi-organ organ, it has many areas that could be termed clinically silent and many clinically active areas. Replication of agent in a given area will depend upon the agent reaching that area and upon the selective vulnerability of the cells in that area. The induction of clinical disease depends then on the replication of agent, the ability of agent to damage the function of important cells and how important the cells in that area are for normal function of the organism. In an important area the titre may not have to be very high in order to produce a lot of clinical symptoms and the animal dies before the agent has multiplied extensively. So the concept of clinical target areas relates to the functional activity of neurons in a particular area. Clinical target areas refer to correlations between agent-induced pathological effects in specific areas, and clinical manifestations of disease. In a way, the whole neurological examination is based on clinical target areas. You measure time of incubation, which is the direct measurement of clinical manifestation. However, pathoclisis is also very important: it refers to areas of the brain where there is selective vulnerability of important neurons which leads to the expression of pathology. Clinical target areas and pathoclisis are not necessarily correlated because certain areas may have extensive pathology but they are silent in terms of clinical expression. You must remember that the brain is a multi-organ organ. Your clinical target areas represent clinical disease–agent replication correlates, which are easy to make in complex brains, much harder to make in simple brains.

Kimberlin: I agree with most of that, Henryk. Initially the idea of using the phrase clinical target area was to emphasize your first point, that the brain is functionally and anatomically a complicated system. We need to start thinking in more precise terms and recognize that the presence of infectivity and of pathological lesions in many brain areas is not directly related to the clinical disease. However, even in the clinical target areas, the presence of infectivity may not necessarily lead to microscopic lesions; the concepts of clinical target areas and of pathoclisis are different.

Wisniewski: Pathoclisis is pertinent to the distribution of pathology. Hugh Fraser talks about pathoclisis in terms of which strains show what pathology and that's fine. I think we agree that clinical target areas involve the replication of agent and induction of changes in one or more specific areas that then lead to clinical changes. One aspect of the concept of pathoclisis that is important in this context is the selective vulnerability of specific neurons for chemical and/or infectious (as in this case) agents. The selective vulnerability of neurons may lead to the differences seen in clinical target areas of different scrapie strains. Thus, cells in one clinical target area may be selectively vulnerable (because of replication of agent and/or the induction of damaged function) to one scrapie strain and not others, whereas cells in another area are vulnerable to a different scrapie strain. In each instance these 'vulnerable' cells would play an important role in maintaining the function of one organism.

*Kimberlin:*I deliberately refrained from talking about pathoclisis to avoid confusion with clinical target areas. I wanted to develop ideas about replication and spread of infectivity in relation to the incubation time and the clinical disease. I said nothing about clinical target areas and Hugh Fraser's results on the distribution of lesions. There is another layer of dynamics relating to the appearance of vacuolation and other lesions in areas to which infectivity has spread.

References

Bruce ME 1985 Agent replication dynamics in a long incubation period model of mouse scrapie. J Gen Virol 66:2517–2522

Carp RI Callahan SM 1981 In vitro interaction of scrapie agent and mouse peritoneal macrophages. Intervirology 16:8–13

Carp RI, Callahan SM 1982 Effect of mouse peritoneal macrophages on scrapie infectivity during extended in vitro incubation. Intervirology 17:201–207

Carp RI, Callahan SM 1985 Effect of prior treatment with thioglycolate on the incubation period of intraperitoneally injected scrapie. Intervirology 24:170–173

Gorde JM, Tamalet J, Toga M, Bert J 1982 Changes in the nigrostriatal system following microinjection of an unconventional agent. Brain Res 240:87–93

Kim YS, Carp RI, Callahan SM, Wisniewski HM 1987 Incubation periods and survival times for mice injected stereotaxically with three scrapie strains in different brain regions. J Gen Virol 68:695–702

Moreau-Dubois MC, Brown P, Rohwer RG, Masters CL, Franko M, Gajdusek DC 1982 Experimental scrapie in golden Syrian hamsters: temporal comparison of in vitro cell-fusing activity with brain infectivity and histopathological changes. Infect Immun 37:195–199

Prusiner B, Cochran SP, Groth DF, Downey DE, Bowman KA, Martinez HM 1982 Measurement of the scrapie agent using an incubation time interval assay. Ann Neurol 11:353–358

Genetic aspects of unconventional virus infections: the basis of the virino hypothesis

A.G. Dickinson and G.W. Outram

AFRC & MRC Neuropathogenesis Unit, West Mains Road, Edinburgh EH9 3JF, UK

Abstract. The properties of genes involved directly or indirectly in the pathogenesis of scrapie and other unconventional (UCV) virus infections are reviewed. Reasons are presented for assigning paramount importance to the *Sinc* gene in mice and the *Sip* gene in sheep (the likely homologue of *Sinc*). The rationale is given for concluding that the agents of UCV infections have their own genomic molecules coding for strain differences. The virino hypothesis, which proposes that the infective form of the agent is an informational hybrid between the agent's genome and protective host proteins, is presented in detail, with an explanation of the postulated role of *Sinc*.

1988 Novel infectious agents and the central nervous system. Wiley, Chichester (Ciba Foundation Symposium 135) p 63–83

The genetic aspects of any virus infection involve the genotypes of both the host and the microorganism. In a conventional acute virus disease the host's contribution falls into categories such as the types of cell receptors, the efficiency and persistence of the immune and interferon responses, and the inherited ability to minimize and repair tissue damage. The genetic contribution of the virus includes virion specificities required for cell penetration and various properties leading to replication and host cell disruption.

None of these categories were thought to apply to the disease scrapie when work started in earnest 40 years ago, and we now know that few, if any, of them are relevant to the group of unconventional slow infections for which scrapie is the prototype. Initially it was even doubted whether scrapie was caused by an independent transmissible agent. The disease in commercial flocks often appeared to run in families, but an 'outbreak' could start without any evidence that the sheep had been exposed to a source of infection (within the time scale which then seemed reasonable). There was scepticism about there being a 'transmissible agent' because it had been established that it could not be inactivated by the then accepted decontamination procedures, so there were reasonable grounds for discounting a '1950's-type virus' as the cause. The demonstration of scrapie agent's ability to withstand extreme irradiation led some to conclude that it must be too small to carry the genes required even to code for a coat, and without a coat or general protection it would be difficult to explain the agent's resistance.

Although echoes of this argument persist, there is now a simple hypothesis that accommodates the salient facts — namely, that the infectious agent is produced by the host providing coat proteins to protect the agent's independent genome, which can be very small because it need not code for a protein product. Whatever the nature of the agent's informational molecule, it presumably acts by 'disregulating' or blocking some important step in cell metabolism. This concept of the infectious agent as an informational hybrid between host-coded molecules and the genome of the agent *per se* has been designated 'the virino hypothesis' (Dickinson & Outram 1983, Kimberlin 1982).

This concept is based on two assumptions whose validity needs to be established: (1) that the disease is caused by a naturally infectious agent, not by the host's genotype, and (2) that the agent is essentially independent of its host, as are conventional viruses, and can vary in its properties, these variants being coded independently of the host's genotype.

Genetic approaches have been crucial in the testing of these foundations of the virino concept, but it is still not known whether the agent's genome is nucleic acid or not.

Genes affecting scrapie incubation in mice

Some of the genetic controls exerted by the host (e.g. *Sinc* in mice) operate throughout the incubation of scrapie in tissues of both the lymphoreticular and central nervous systems (CNS) and appear to be closely concerned with aspects of the replication of scrapie agent. Some other genes, even if active throughout incubation, influence only extraneural events and are bypassed by intracerebral (i.c.) injection e.g., *Dh* in mice. *Sinc* (and its putative analogues in other species, such as *Sip* in sheep) is the only gene known to have a large effect on incubation (Dickinson & Meikle 1971, Dickinson 1975) and can prolong it even beyond the natural lifespan of the host (Dickinson et al 1975a). All other genes known to affect incubation have only a relatively small effect, which may be indirect, for the following reasons.

As incubation period is inversely proportional to the effective dose of agent, we need to know whether a gene with a small effect is acting only by facilitating or impairing the initial stage of infection. For example, reduced uptake of infectivity would lengthen the incubation period, but the gene would be controlling susceptibility to infection rather than agent replication during pathogenesis. Alternatively, the host gene could affect the initial routing of infectivity after passive uptake, towards either replication or poss-

TABLE 1 Differences in end-point titres[b] according to the *Sinc* genotype of the recipients for various strains of scrapie

Scrapie strain	Unspun/ spun	i.c. ID_{50} titre			i.p. ID_{50} titre		
		s7s7	s7p7	p7p7	s7s7	s7p7	p7p7
22A	S	4.5		5.7			
22A	U	4.5		5.0			
22A	S	4.8		5.5			
22A	S	4.6	5.0	5.4			
22A	S	5.0		6.4			
22A	S	5.5		5.5			
ME7 s7 $	S	7.0		5.5 (7.0)			
ME7 s7	S	5.9	5.1	4.5	3.6	3.6	2.5
ME7 s7	S	6.6	6.6	5.8			
ME7 s7	S^a	6.3		6.5 (5.5)	4.9		3.5 (2.5)
ME7 p7	S^a	6.5		6.5		3.5	3.8
ME7 p7	S	6.5		6.0			
22C	S	5.4		5.0			
22F	S	5.7		5.5			
22F	S	5.8		5.7			
87V	S	$<1.0^a$	$<1.0^a$	5.8 (5.5)			

$ *Sinc* genotype of donor mouse strain; S, 2000 *g* supernatant; S^a, 500 *g* supernatant used as inoculum. Mice in parentheses are IM strain, all other *Sinc* p7p7 mice are VM strain. All *Sinc* s7s7 mice are C57BL and heterozygotes are C57BL×VM
[a] Titre may be underestimated, because of incubations extending beyond lifespan
All donors and recipients are *H-2*[b]
[b] Negative log titres (Karber) per 0.02 ml dose

ible degradation. Therefore, where a gene's apparent effect on incubation is small relative to the effect of dose of infectivity, one must rule out the possibility that it acts only by changing the effective titre before drawing conclusions about an effect on incubation *per se*. This has not yet been assessed in mice for sex determinants (Outram 1976, Kingsbury et al 1983), the *Dh* gene (Dickinson & Fraser 1972) or a gene linked to the H-2 complex, non-standardly named 'PID-1' (Kingsbury et al 1983). If, as seems probable, *Dh* affects the incubation of scrapie because it produces asplenia, it is likely to determine stages during incubation: splenectomy increases the incubation period without affecting the operational titre of a peripheral injection. In contrast, 'PID-1' may control only initial susceptibility, and even then not to the agent *per se* but to the H-2 type of the donor tissue in which infective agent is likely to be sequestered (the inocula were crude tissue homogenates: see Dickinson & Outram 1983).

The small effect of 'PID-1' on the incubation period is equivalent to a titre difference of two orders of magnitude. This degree of change in the operational titre of a scrapie inoculum according to the genotype of recipient, has

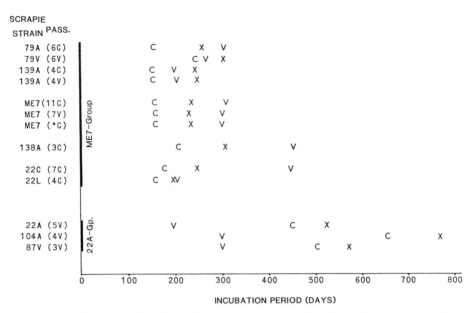

FIG. 1. Incubation periods for various scrapie strains in the three *Sinc* genotypes (C, C57BL *Sinc*^s7; V, VM *Sinc*^p7; X, C×VF₁ cross). 'Pass,' indicates number of consecutive i.c. passages in C or V mice. Data refer to mice injected i.c. with 1% brain homogenates (500 *g* supernatant) from mice with terminal scrapie.

been found after intraperitoneal (i.p.) injection (Carp & Callahan 1987). The 'PID-1' effect was found by i.c. injection of C57BL/10J congenic mice, differing in their H-2 haplotypes, with BALB/c mouse brain homogenate (*H-2*^d) infected with K.Fu Creutzfeldt-Jakob disease (CJD) agent. Lack of two controls prevents clear interpretation of these results: (1) there was no end-point titration to determine whether the effect was entirely due to initial differences in uptake, and (2) no attempt was made to use K.Fu agent donors of different H-2 types to decide whether the effect was simply due to particular donor/recipient differences in H-2. One cannot therefore conclude that 'PID-1' plays 'a central role in controlling the length of the CJD incubation period'. Similar considerations apply to another genetic effect relating to the incubation period of two scrapie strains in NZW and NZB mice (Kingsbury et al 1983).

The Sinc gene in mice

The p7 allele of *Sinc* has been found only twice, initially in randomly bred mice (Dickinson & Meikle 1971) from which three inbred *Sinc*^p7 stocks were made (VM, IM and MB). Mice (I strain) were subsequently found to have a long incubation period when injected with a scrapie subline derived from the 'Chandler' isolate (Kingsbury et al 1983) and this was shown to be due to the p7 allele of *Sinc* (R.I. Carp, unpublished paper, Am Soc Virol 21 July 1985, Carp et al 1987).

The variety of action and degree of control of incubation period which *Sinc* exerts on all strains of scrapie suggested that it directly controls some aspect of agent replication (Dickinson & Meikle 1971). There is, however, no clear evidence that it affects either the maximum rate of replication or the level of the titre plateau in the spleen; it probably alters the time delay before replication (Dickinson & Fraser 1969) or the extent of any titre plateau attained in the brain (see Kimberlin & Walker, this volume). The indirect effect of *Sinc*, arising from the correlation of incubation period with operational dose, is usually only trivial — up to about 30 days (Table 1). The exception is with the 87V strain, where titre may play a relatively important role.

The direct effect of *Sinc* can be enormous: substitution of only one allele can more than double the incubation period (e.g. 1000 i.c. ID_{50} units of 22A injected i.c. in $Sinc^{p7p7}$ mice takes 200 days to end-point but in $Sinc^{s7p7}$ mice takes 550 days: Fig. 1). The scale of the effect of *Sinc* depends on the scrapie strain used. *Sinc* clearly controls both the extraneural and neural stages of the infection, and its effect is greater with peripheral injection routes.

Whether incubation is shorter in s7 or p7 homozygotes depends entirely on the scrapie strain: two sets of strains ('ME7 group' and '22A group') are distinguished by this criterion, and it is of fundamental importance. Because *Sinc* achieves a degree of selective exclusion of strains which are slower in that host's genotype, it provides one technique for separating strains from natural or artificial mixtures. A similar effect is seen between tissues: for example, when a mixed infection of 22A and 22C is given extraneurally, at death both strains are present in the spleen but only the one which kills the mouse is present in the brain — which strain depends on the *Sinc* genotype (D.M. Taylor, personal communication).

Another peculiarity of *Sinc* is its variety of allelic interaction: whether there is any dominance, or even overdominance, depends on the strain of scrapie, but the heterozygote has never been found to have incubations as short as, or shorter than, the faster homozygote. The overdominance (e.g., longer 22A, 22F, 139A or 87V incubation in the heterozygote than in either homozygote) is unusual; it prompted the hypothesis that *Sinc* codes for part or all of a multimeric replication site for scrapie and related agents (Dickinson & Outram 1979). Competition for these sites between scrapie strains injected at widely different times was predicted (Dickinson & Meikle 1971) and a competitive effect has been found which may have this basis (Dickinson et al 1975b).

Recent developments in the molecular biology of scrapie support these interpretations of how *Sinc* operates. The gene, provisionally designated *PrP-p*, coding for the major protein PrP 33–35 of scrapie-associated fibrils is closely linked to *Sinc* in both segregating (Carlson et al 1986) and *Sinc*-congenic mice (Hunter et al 1987). It may turn out that only one gene is involved and that PrP 33–35 is the *Sinc* gene product.

No sequence differences have yet been found in PrP 33–35 from different *Sinc* genotypes. If this continues to be the case, PrP cannot mediate the variety of incubation controls which characterize *Sinc*. This would argue against PrP being its product but not exclude it entirely. It will only be straightforward to prove whether PrP is the *Sinc* gene product if a consistent structural difference is found that correlates with the functionally different alleles.

This situation could be resolved using transgenic mice. However, merely to show that incubation period is altered non-specifically by a cDNA or genomic clone of PrP (say, from another *Sinc* genotype or another species) is insufficient; a controlled change must be shown which reflects the complexities of the differences between the two *Sinc* alleles in conventional mice. In attempts to transfer *Sinc* genomic information between congenic strains, success will depend on a combination of gene dosage and heterozygosity, and the likely incubation phenotype is unknown. It will be essential to show that part of the characteristic pattern of *Sinc* action can be transferred.

There would be clear advantages in using genomic rather than cDNA clones in transgenic work because the control of incubation, presumably mediated through an overall control of agent replication, may entail aspects of *Sinc* not represented at the level of its messenger RNA sequence. It is also possible that the gene is expressed differently in different neuronal (and other) sets, according to the *Sinc* genotype; this could account for some of the observed effects on incubation and lesion profiles (Fig. 1; see Kimberlin & Walker, this volume).

Natural scrapie in sheep

It has become clear over the past 15 years that the genetic control of scrapie in sheep is focused on a gene which shares many features with *Sinc*. Not surprisingly, this has been easier to deduce from experimental than from natural sheep scrapie.

Attempts in the 1950's to analyse the incidence of natural scrapie in terms of its genetic components were complicated by several factors (Dickinson 1976). An initial case was often followed by sporadically distributed cases during the subsequent two or three years, after which the pattern tended to become one of affected maternal lineages. The occurrence of both vertical and lateral transmission of infection was deduced from breeding data for natural scrapie (Dickinson et al 1965) together with a re-analysis of the data of Parry (1962), whose original contention that scrapie was not infectious but due entirely to a mutant sheep gene was based on flawed methods of analysis. At that time there was no decisive evidence that scrapie was infectious vertically, from ewe to lamb, or laterally, to flock mates: proof came later (Gordon 1966, Dickinson et al 1974, Hourrigan et al 1979), as did evidence for different strains of scrapie agent.

When assessing an apparently normal sheep, one must take into account not only its genetic potential but also whether it has been exposed to scrapie infection, the type and time of exposure and, ideally, the strains involved. Genetic analysis yields clear-cut information about major genes only after a high degree of exposure to infection. We therefore bred a flock of Suffolk sheep with maximum opportunities for maternal transmission, in order to produce a large number of cases over many years. One group of foundation stock had at least one parent affected and came from many farms where exposure levels had generally been low. The other group was from flocks reliably free from scrapie. The two groups were mated in all four combinations, including reciprocal crosses. The initial generations, when exposure levels were still relatively low, showed large reciprocal differences in the incidence of scrapie — the maternal scrapie status accounted for almost all the variation, irrespective of the sire-type used. Over the years this pattern became less pronounced, presumably as the level of lateral exposure increased. The other striking trend, perhaps also due to increasing exposure, was that the mean age at death from scrapie decreased gradually from 41 to 18.5 months over 14 years (J.D. Foster, personal communication; see Kimberlin 1979). This finally achieved self-limitation of the disease, with females dying before leaving progeny, but in the intermediate high-exposure years it was clear that segregation of a single gene accounted for the distribution of almost all the cases. For example, 274/277 progeny developed natural scrapie in matings where both parents became affected, whereas 37/66 were affected when only the sire became affected and the dam remained unaffected but had an affected sire. In our flock, where scrapie strains 87A, 87V and ME7 (or their precursors) are the ones most commonly isolated, the gene acts with full dominance and the homozygous recessive Suffolks are the ones liable to develop the natural disease. Careful analysis in another breed has shown the same (Millot et al 1987).

Further breeding experiments have shown that this gene is *Sip*, which was first identified in Cheviot sheep infected with the SSBP/1 complex of scrapie strains (Dickinson et al 1968). Similar findings following SSBP/1 injection have been made in Herdwicks and Swaledales (Davies & Kimberlin 1985, Nussbaum et al 1975). *Sip* does not act uniformly in all circumstances, in terms of which allele is recessive or which confers the greater susceptibility or shorter incubation: these peculiarities are strikingly like those of *Sinc*, which suggests that the two genes are homologues.

TABLE 2 Incubation period (days ± SE) for Cheviot sheep and Anglo-Nubian goats injected i.c. with 0.5 ml 10% Cheviot brain suspension infected with scrapie strain CH1641

Passage	Sheep with high frequency of Sip^{sA} allele[a]			Sip pA/pA sheep			Goats		
	No.	Scrapie cases	Incubation period	No.	Scrapie cases	Incubation period	No.	Scrapie cases	Incubation period
Primary	2	50%	395[b]	11	45%	751 ± 252		—	
2	15	60%	856 ± 84	16	37%	360 ± 147	10	100%	987 ± 72
3	3	67%	595 ± 122	59	31%	360 ± 15	6	100%	525 ± 90

[a] Population selected for high frequency of Sip^{sA} allele ([b] possibly a pA/pA segregant individual)

The Sip gene in sheep

The two alleles of the *Sip* gene are designated *Sip*[sA] and *Sip*[pA]. In sheep injected i.c. with scrapie-infected tissue homogenate, the gene determines incubation period: *Sip* sA/sA and sA/pA genotypes have short incubations with scrapie brain pool SSBP/1, the pA/pA sheep have extremely long incubations that extend beyond the normal lifespan of the host. When SSBP/1 is given subcutaneously (s.c.) to young adult Cheviots, only those carrying the sA allele develop scrapie; the pA homozygotes survive for a full lifespan (Dickinson et al 1968). The *Sip* gene therefore acts with full dominance for the A-group of scrapie strains (i.e. the majority of those known). However, with the C-group scrapie strain, CH1641, the position is reversed.

The CH1641 strain was isolated from a natural-scrapie Cheviot carrying *Sip*[sA]. With this strain the disease in Cheviots is virtually restricted to those injected i.c., a massive s.c. dose being required to achieve infection. Two types of Cheviot were available for testing i.c. with CH1641: (1) sheep known to be *Sip* pA/pA, and (2) sheep from a segregating population with a large excess of the sA allele but including a small proportion of pA homozygotes (Table 2). Results from primary passage to sheep are difficult to compare with the later passages because of the shortage of sheep known to be carrying *Sip*[sA]; also there is a hint that the pA homozygotes have longer incubation at primary than later passages. For the second and third passages incubation is much shorter in the pA/pA group than in the other sheep (three of these sheep are presumably the expected pA homozygotes because their incubations overlap with those of sheep known to be of this genotype).

Another striking aspect of these results is the survival of about half of the sheep, from all groups. If, as seems likely, another major gene is responsible for this survivorship, the consistently lower proportion of scrapie cases at all three passages among the *Sip* pA/pA group is not significant, because the two groups of sheep have been separate for more than 15 generations (it suggests that the second gene, conferring C-group resistance, is not closely linked to *Sip*). Evidence for this second gene stems from the significantly higher proportion of CH1641 cases of scrapie among the progeny of CH1641-positive *Sip* pA/pA rams than among those of CH1641-negative rams mated to equivalent groups of ewes. More progeny tests are required to confirm this. There is no evidence of a second gene conferring this type of survivorship in our Anglo-Nubian goat flock; all of them develop scrapie with the doses of SSBP/1 or CH1641 used in the Cheviots. Nor is there any evidence for segregation of the goat homologue of *Sip*.

In order to show that *Sip* controls the major events not only in experimental scrapie but also in the natural disease, one should be able to predict the segregation ratios in a group of sheep with experimental scrapie from knowledge of the parental genotypes in terms of the natural disease.

TABLE 3   Incidence and incubation of natural or experimental scrapie in sheep of different *Sip* genotypes

Sip genotype	*sAsA*	*sApA*	*pApA*	*Dominant allele*
		→————————————→		
Natural scrapie*	+	−	−	pA
Infection by maternal transmission	+	(+)	−	(sA)
SSBP/1 injected s.c.	+	+	−	sA
SSBP/1 injected i.c.	+[a]	+[a]	+[b]	sA
CH1641 injected i.c.	+[b]	+[b]	+[c]	sA
	←—————————————			

+, affected; −, unaffected; *, Suffolk and Ile-de-France data; ( ), postulated; [a], short incubation; [b], long incubation, partial incidence; [c], short incubation, partial incidence.
Arrows indicate direction of increase in incubation period/resistance

An uninfected pApA Cheviot ram was mated with sApA Suffolk ewes (these were the progeny of uninfected mothers so there was no infection by maternal transmission). The lambs were therefore an equal mixture of pA homozygotes and heterozygotes. Half were injected s.c. with SSBP/1 scrapie and half s.c. with SUF81. The SUF81 brain pool came from naturally infected Suffolks in our flock and would be expected to be more representative of the strains involved in natural scrapie than SSBP/1. 5/12 and 4/9 sheep, respectively, developed scrapie, which is close to the 50% expected if *Sip* controls both experimental and natural scrapie.

Thus the *Sip* heterozygotes developed scrapie when injected with a pool of natural strains but would not have become infected naturally (other than possibly by the maternal route). However, given the variable gene action of *Sip* and the reciprocal differences in incidence in the early years of our Suffolk flock and in Suffolk × Blackface sheep (Dickinson et al 1974), the overall results suggest that heterozygotes can develop natural scrapie if infected early by the maternal route (Table 3). Further matings are needed to prove this.

Agent variants are coded independently of the host's genome

Having examined the evidence for a conserved gene which controls overall agent replication (and might contribute directly to the host component of a virino), we now turn to the question of the *sine qua non* of the agent, namely its genomic replicating informational molecule. We will summarize the evidence that this genome can vary independently and, although replicated by normal host mechanisms, is not coded by the host (Bruce & Dickinson 1979, 1987, Dickinson & Outram 1979, 1983, Dickinson et al 1984, 1987, Kimberlin & Walker 1978, Kimberlin et al 1986, 1987).

Although the mismatching of donor and recipient phenotypes in such properties as antigenic specificities may influence the degree of infectivity, and the *Sinc* genotype of each host may influence the agent selectively (Bruce & Dickinson 1979), no host-coded properties have been found that determine agent strain differences, despite extensive searches.

The nub of the issue is whether different scrapie strains exist, like conventional virus strains. That they do, is proved by the fact that an infected animal replicates, in a predictable manner, the strain, or mixture of strains, introduced in the inoculum. As would be expected for an agent with an independent genome, variants can arise during incubation. Given the constraints that *Sinc* can exercise on the injected strain, if a strain with shorter incubation arises, it is at a selective advantage and either is preserved in a mixture with its parent strain or, if very much quicker in that *Sinc* genotype, rapidly supersedes its parent. Several examples of this type are known (Bruce & Dickinson 1979, Dickinson et al 1984). In a deliberately mixed infection arising from a mixed inoculum, or by infection with different strains on separate occasions, the outcome can be predicted in terms of either differential replication centering on the details of *Sinc* action in those particular strains (Dickinson 1975), or competition between the two strains (Dickinson et al 1975b, Dickinson & Outram 1979, Kimberlin & Walker 1985).

Proof that strains of scrapie exist also requires that an individual strain, separated from others by suitable microbiological cloning techniques, can retain its characteristics (in terms of Class II changes, see Bruce & Dickinson 1979). Some strains are fully stable when passaged in one *Sinc* homozygote but not the other (Table 4). Several strains have not yet been tested in both genotypes and none has been tested by serial passage in the *Sinc* heterozygote.

Mutation from strain 87A to strain ME7 is a repeatable event and occurred in all the independent reisolations of 87A from different sheep breeds. It

TABLE 4 The stability[a] of different strains of scrapie when passaged in inbred mice carrying different alleles of *Sinc*

Properties stable in *Sinc*^s7 stocks	Properties stable in both homozygotes	Properties stable in *Sinc*^p7 stocks
22F	ME7	22A
22L $	22C	79V $
79A $	139A[b]	87V $
87A $[b]		22H
124A		111A
		124V

[a] Class II stability (Bruce & Dickinson, 1979)
[b] Class III mutations occur
$ stability untested in alternative *Sinc* genotype

recurred even after purification of 87A by extremely rigorous end-point cloning (Bruce & Dickinson 1987 and unpublished). Furthermore, this mutation is dose dependent, as expected for an event with a finite probability. The most clinching evidence favouring a mutational interpretation is that this also provides a simple explanation for the asymmetrical foci of brain vacuolation which are a unique feature of 87A. These foci would be near the location of each mutational event during incubation in the brain and most foci would therefore lie asymmetrically. All these events take place without any change in the host genotype.

In cases of mixed infections, where two contrasting strains have been injected on different occasions (sometimes over a year apart), there can be competition between the strains, the first tending to 'block' the second. This is further proof that different scrapie strains exist and preserve their identities even in the same host. In some competition experiments the genotypes of the donors and the recipients have been the same (Dickinson & Outram 1979).

Single strains can preserve their identities after more than one passage between species e.g., ME7 from mice to Cheviot sheep and back to mice. Natural or experimental mixtures of certain strains can be separated by passaging in particular *Sinc* or *Sip* genotypes; other mixtures are difficult to separate and can persist through more than one interspecific passage e.g., 22A and 22H when passaged, several times in each species, either from sheep to mice or from sheep to goats to mice (Dickinson et al 1987).

Finally, it is important to have established that the same strain (by present criteria) of natural scrapie can be reisolated from different natural cases, even from widely different breeds, and that it is possible to isolate different strains from cases within the same flock. Some of these genetic arguments for scrapie strain differences are complex but we consider the evidence for their existence to be convincing, and any hypothesis concerning the nature of the scrapie agent must be able to account for these.

The virino hypothesis: the infectious agent as an informational hybrid

In the absence of any alternative candidate, it seems likely that the agent's informational molecule is a nucleic acid, though this is not a necessary condition for our virino concept. In our model, the life cycle of scrapie agent includes a stage when its genome is bound to host protein, or more probably a host protein multimeric complex, and it seems increasingly possible that this includes a *Sinc*-coded enzyme involved in its replication. We predicted that a fuller understanding of the way in which *Sinc* acts would explain the nature of the infective agent (Dickinson & Meikle 1971) and much subsequent genetic and molecular evidence supports this hypothesis.

Binding of the agent genome to host protein would provide the resistance to inactivation for which scrapie is renowned and render it immunologically invisible to the host. Any stage of the agent's life cycle in which the genome exists as an unprotected nucleic acid could be labile, and therefore relatively uninfectious and difficult to detect. The main (or only) transmissible unit would be a virino, with its genomic molecule (presumably too small to code for protein), acting simply by disrupting the normal function of *Sinc* and other cellular processes.

The way in which *Sinc* normally functions in the physiology of the animal presumably involves the replication of a host informational molecule which is probably nucleic acid but could be of a novel type. This molecule may have much in common with the agent's genomic molecule, because of the functions of *Sinc* they are able to share: the similarity could stem from their phylogenetic relationship. If these speculations are correct they would account for the difficulty of isolating the genome of scrapie and related agents.

References

Bruce M, Dickinson AG 1979 Biological stability of different classes of scrapie agent. In: Prusiner SB, Hadlow WJ (eds) Slow transmissible diseases of the nervous system. Academic Press, New York, vol 2: p 71–86

Bruce M, Dickinson AG 1987 Biological evidence that scrapie agent has an independent genome. J Gen Virol 68:79–89

Carlson GA, Kingsbury DT, Goodmann PA et al 1986 Prion protein and scrapie incubation time genes are linked. Cell 46:503–511

Carp RI, Callahan SM 1987 Scrapie incubation periods and end-point titers in mouse strains differing at the *H-2D* locus. Int Virol 26:85–92

Carp RI, Moretz RC, Natelli N, Dickinson AG 1987 Genetic control of scrapie: incubation period and plaque formation in I mice. J Gen Virol 68:401–407

Davies DC, Kimberlin RH 1985 Selections of Swaledale sheep of reduced susceptibility to experimental scrapie. Vet Rec 116:211–214

Dickinson AG 1975 Host-pathogen interactions in scrapie. Genetics 79:387–395

Dickinson AG 1976 Scrapie in sheep and goats. In: Kimberlin RH (ed) Slow virus diseases of animals and man. Elsevier/North-Holland, Amsterdam, p 209–241

Dickinson AG, Fraser H 1969 Genetical control of the concentration of ME7 scrapie agent in mouse spleen. J Comp Pathol 79:363–366

Dickinson AG, Fraser H 1972 Scrapie: effect of *Dh* gene on incubation period of extraneurally injected agent. Heredity 29:91–93

Dickinson AG, Meikle VMH 1971 Host-genotype and agent effects in scrapie incubation: change in allelic interaction with different strains of agent. Mol & Gen Genet 112:73–79

Dickinson AG, Outram GW 1979 The scrapie replication-site hypothesis and its implications for pathogenesis. In: Prusiner SB, Hadlow WJ (eds) Slow transmissible diseases of the nervous system. Academic Press, New York, vol 2:13–31

Dickinson AG, Outram GW 1983 Operational limitations in the characterisation of the infective units of scrapie. In: Court LA, Cathala F (eds) Virus non-conventionnels et affections du système nerveux central. Masson, Paris, p 3–16

Dickinson AG, Young GB, Stamp JT, Renwick CC 1965 An analysis of natural scrapie in Suffolk sheep. Heredity 20:485–503

Dickinson AG, Stamp JT, Renwick CC, Rennie JC 1968 Some factors controlling the incidence of scrapie in Cheviot sheep injected with a Cheviot-passaged scrapie agent. J Comp Pathol 78:313–321

Dickinson AG, Stamp JT, Renwick CC 1974 Maternal and lateral transmission of scrapie in sheep. J Comp Pathol 84:19–25

Dickinson AG, Fraser H, Outram GW 1975a Scrapie incubation time can exceed natural lifespan. Nature (Lond) 256:732–733

Dickinson AG, Fraser H, McConnell I, Outram GW, Sales DI, Taylor DM 1975b Extraneural competition between different scrapie agents leading to loss of infectivity. Nature (Lond) 253:556

Dickinson AG, Bruce ME, Outram GW, Kimberlin RH 1984 Scrapie strain differences: the implications of stability and mutation. In: Tateishi J (ed) Proc Workshop on slow transmissible diseases, Tokyo. Jpn Min Health & Welfare Publ, p 105–118

Dickinson AG, Outram GW, Taylor DM, Foster JD 1988 Further evidence that scrapie agent has an independent genome. In: Court LA et al (eds) Unconventional viruses and central nervous system diseases. Atelier d'Arts Graphiques, Abbaye de Melleray, in press

Gordon WS 1966 Review of work on scrapie at Compton, England 1952–1964. In: Report of Scrapie Seminar ARS 91–53, USDA, Washington p 19–40

Hunter N, Hope J, McConnell I, Dickinson AG 1987 Linkage of the SAF protein (PrP) gene and *Sinc* using congenic mice and restriction fragment length polymorphism analysis. J Gen Virol 68:2711–2716

Hourrigan J, Klingsporn A, Clark WW, de Camp M 1979 Epidemiology of scrapie in the United States. In: Prusiner SB, Hadlow WJ (eds) Slow transmissible disease of the nervous system. Academic Press, New York, vol 2:331–356

Kimberlin RH 1979 An assessment of genetic methods in the control of scrapie. Livest Prod Sci 6:233–242

Kimberlin RH 1982 Scrapie agent: Prions or virinos? Nature (Lond) 297:107–108

Kimberlin RH, Walker CA 1978 Evidence that the transmission of one source of scrapie agent to hamsters involves separation of agent strains from a mixture. J Gen Virol 39:487–496

Kimberlin RH, Walker CA 1985 Competition between strains of scrapie depends on the blocking agent being infectious. Int Virol 23:74–81

Kimberlin RH, Walker CA 1988 Pathogenesis of experimental scrapie. In: Novel infectious agents and the central nervous system. Wiley, Chichester (Ciba Found Symp 135) p 37–62

Kimberlin RH, Cole S, Walker CA 1986 Transmissible mink encephalopathy (TME) in Chinese Hamsters: identification of two strains of TME and comparisons with scrapie. Neuropathol Appl Neurobiol 12:197–206

Kimberlin RH, Cole S, Walker CA 1987 Temporary and permanent modifications of a single strain of mouse scrapie on transmission to rats and hamsters. J Gen Virol 68:1875–1881

Kingsbury DT, Kasper KC, Stites DP, Watson JD, Hogan RN, Prusiner SB 1983 Genetic control of scrapie and Creutzfeldt-Jakob Disease in mice. J Immunol 131:391–396

Millot P, Chatelain J, Dautheville C, Salmon D, Cathala F 1988 Etude genetique de la tremblente (scrapie) dans des descendances de moutons Ile-de-France. Liason d'un locus Scr de susceptibilite/resistance avec le complexe majeur OLA d'histocompatibilite. In: Court LA et al (eds) Unconventional viruses and central nervous system diseases. Atelier d'Arts Graphiques, Abbaye de Melleray, in press

Nussbaum RE, Henderson WM, Pattison IH, Elcock NV, Davies DC 1975 The establishment of sheep flocks of predictable susceptibility to experimental scrapie. Res Vet Sci 18:49–58

Outram GW 1976 The pathogenesis of scrapie in mice. In: Kimberlin RH (ed) Slow
    virus diseases of animals and man. Elsevier/North-Holland, Amsterdam, p 325–357
Parry HB 1962 Scrapie: a transmissible and hereditary disease of sheep. Heredity
    17:75–105

DISCUSSION

Carlson: When showing phenomena such as overdominance, or attempting
to show homology between *Sinc* in mice and *Sip* in sheep, I would like to point
out the importance of linked markers. It doesn't matter whether it is a coat
colour gene or a cell surface antigen, it is useful to be able to follow the
probable genotype of the animal before assigning the alleles. All your data are
based on inference, for example that *Sinc* overdominance occurs in an F1. Are
the same results seen in the congenics of these strains?

Dickinson: Yes, but they have not been published yet. I agree that we need
better linkage markers, but in the case of the sheep I am trying to present the
current state of play on very difficult, costly data.

Carlson: You describe a longer incubation period in an F1 than in the two
parents and conclude that it is due to overdominance of *Sinc*. In F1 mice it could
be simply hybrid vigour; an F1 animal is healthier than an inbred animal. If it
has a slightly longer incubation period, that does not mean that there is an
overdominant effect of *Sinc*.

Dickinson: If that happened in all combinations, then I might agree. But for
a single gene, where overdominance is not constant, there is no mammalian
example and only one avian example. In yeast there are enzymes which fold
differently and change their enzymic efficiencies as single gene effects, according to the pH or temperature. This is the sort of tertiary conformation system
that I think we are dealing with.

Carlson: I am not saying that overdominance does not occur but that it
cannot be shown from the data you have presented without a linked marker for
that gene or its isolation in the congenic stain.

Chesebro: Alan, I disagree. The *trans* complementation between the I-A and
I-E regions of the major histocompatibility locus are an example where F1 mice
are immunological responders, whereas both parental strains are non-
responders. In any situation where two genes from different parents could have
trans complementary effects you can get this kind of situation.

Dickinson: That point is met by the observation that the congenics do exactly
the same.

Chesebro: It isn't, because the congenics cannot be precisely defined–the H2
congenics do this too. Until Jack Stimpfling and others found recombinants
within the H2 complex, they didn't recognize that recombination was taking
place.

Carlson: We don't know how many genes there are within this prion gene
complex.

Chesebro: There may be a large amount of genetic material being transferred in the congenic mice.

Dickinson: Are you saying that there could be multiple copies of the marker you have?

*Carlson:*No, not of the prion protein, but I have never said that the prion protein controls the incubation period, just that this is one possibility. It is clear that there are differences between the different scrapie isolates but it is not true to say that different scrapie isolates have been cloned. It has not been shown by the initial criteria established by Luria and Delbruck (1943) that mutants pre-exist the selection. I appreciate the difficulties of doing this with scrapie but I think it's inappropriate to use the words 'cloning' and 'mutation' because these terms pre-judge the nature of the agent.

Dickinson: Aggregation is the main complicating factor. One can examine the question of aggregation by making artificial mixtures of two separate scrapie strains. We haven't presented those data at this meeting but you can separate two strains more easily than worries about aggregation would have led you to expect. We recently published a broadly comparable example involving the separation of 87A from its mutant progeny, 7D (Bruce & Dickinson 1987). The mutant and its parent obviously co-exist in the same brain and direct evidence for this is the characteristic asymmetrical foci of vacuolation present in this model, which Moira Bruce has suggested represent the location in the brain where a mutation occurred. Inclusion of a large mutant focus would hinder our attempt to separate the 87A parent strain by microbiological cloning. Therefore, we almost always use very small brain tissue samples for passage, with all our scrapie strains, rather than homogenized whole brains.

Carp: Our work on genetics confirms much of what Alan (Dickinson) says concerning the different scrapie strains passaged in the same host, that is, the material that is injected has all been derived after multiple passages in C57BL mice. We were struck by the fact that when we looked at a variety of biological parameters of several scrapie strains (including some new parameters which had not been examined previously) we found differences based on the strain of scrapie.

For example, we compared two strains, 139A and ME7. We found that the differences between 139A and ME7 in the distribution of vacuolation essentially confirm Alan's results. The incubation periods following i.c. or i.p. injection of the same dose are shorter for 139A than for ME7. White matter vacuolation occurs with 139A, not with ME7. Amyloid plaques are formed in $Sinc^{p7p7}$ after infection with ME7, not in the case of 139A. Pre-clinical weight gain in SJL and CBA mice is not seen after injection of 139A into any area of the brain. If ME7 is injected into the cortex of a C57BL mouse, there is no weight increase; however, if it is injected into the hypothalamus, there is. The clinical target areas are another difference between 139A and ME7. In the case of ME7, the shortest incubation periods are after injection into the thalamus or cerebellum.

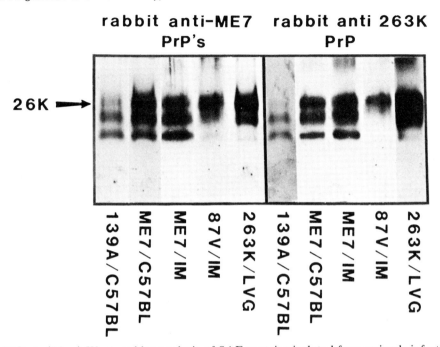

rabbit anti-ME7 PrP's   **rabbit anti 263K PrP**

26K ➡

Lanes: 139A/C57BL · ME7/C57BL · ME7/IM · 87V/IM · 263K/LVG · 139A/C57BL · ME7/C57BL · ME7/IM · 87V/IM · 263K/LVG

FIG. 1. (*Merz*) Western blot analysis of SAF proteins isolated from animals infected with four different scrapie strains. SAF from mouse or hamster brains infected with strain ME7, 139A, 87V or 263K were isolated. SAF proteins (approximately 200 ng) were solubilized and electrophoresed on 12% Laemmli gels. Proteins were electrophoretically transferred to nitrocellulose with a Bio-Rad trans-blot apparatus. Blots were reacted with antisera raised against ME7 and 263K SAF proteins. Lane designations indicate scrapie strain/host strain. The profile of SAF proteins from 139A/C57BL and ME7/C57BL are immunologically distinct, as are the SAF proteins of ME7/IM from those of 87V/IM. (Reprinted from Kacscak et al 1986.)

With the same scrapie strain in C57BL mice (*Sinc*^{s7s7}), and in IM mice (Sinc ^{p7p7}) kindly provided by Alan Dickinson, differences in the SAF and antigen differences in the PrPs are consistent with the strain inoculated into the animal. There are differences in the biological properties of the strains: the SAF that are isolated differ both morphologically and in their protease sensitivity (Kascsak et al 1985). There are also Western blot profile differences in the proteins, which are characteristic for individual scrapie strains (Kascsak et al 1986). In material from GSS-affected individuals the antigens related to PrP are different from those observed in CJD-affected individuals (Fig. 2).

With 139A, all four regions other than the cortex give much shorter incubation periods, by at least 15 or 20 days.

In another set of comparisons, we used ME7 and 22L in *Sinc*^{s7s7} mice. The incubation period of ME7 is slightly longer than that of the 22L agent in *Sinc*^{s7s7} mice. The incubation periods in *Sinc*^{p7p7} mice are 300 days for ME7, 200 days for 22L. The vacuolation pattern after i.c. injection is highest in the anterior section of the brain with ME7, highest in the posterior section of the brain in the

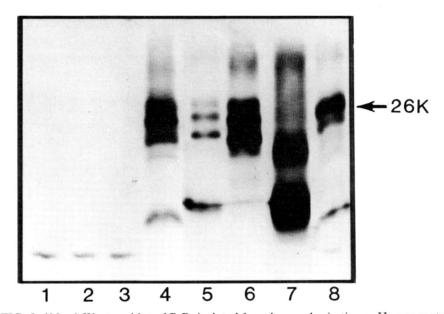

FIG. 2. (*Merz*) Western blot of PrPs isolated from human brain tissue. Homogenates were prepared in 10% sarcosyl and SAF isolated by differential centrifugation using a Beckman airfuge. Samples were treated with proteinase K and electrophoresed on 12% Laemmli gels. Proteins were electrophoretically transferred to nitrocellulose and Western blotted using monoclonal antibody 263K-3F4. Lanes: 1,2,3, preparations from patients with Alzheimer's disease; 4,5,6, preparations from individual CJD patients; 7, preparation from a GSS patient; 8, positive control of a preparation from hamsters infected with scrapie strain 263K. Note the variety in the Western blot profiles in the spongiform encephalopathy cases (lanes 4–8), potentially reflecting different strains of spongiform encephalopathy agents infecting each case. Note the absence of the PrPs in the cases with Alzheimer's disease (lanes 1–3). 26K indicates the position of the 26–30kDa PrP protein. (Reprinted from: Merz & Wisniewski, in press.)

case of 22L. The brain vacuolation pattern after intracerebellar injection is really quite striking. If ME7 or 139A is injected into any of the five brain regions that I mentioned (cortex, caudate nucleus, substantia nigra, thalamus and cerebellum), the pattern essentially looks the same. With 22L, the pattern looks the same, except when the agent is injected directly into the cerebellum, in which case vacuolation is limited to the posterior portion of the brain, particularly the cerebellum. With ME7 injected into the cerebellum, vacuolation occurs throughout the brain. Again, we should emphasize that these differences were seen after extensive passages of these three strains in the same strain of mouse, C57BL.

Merz: We have run Western blots of SAF isolated from CJD-infected and scrapie-infected brains, which illustrate that the antigens present in the material are different, depending on which scrapie strain is used (Fig. 1).

Carlson: By antigen differences you mean migration differences on gels, not differences in the antigenicity.

Oesch: There is only one PrP gene, so these differences in the protein probably represent degradation products. The differences in the protease sensitivity of SAF isolated from different human individuals may be due to polymorphism of the PrP coding sequence. I don't think these Western blots prove anything with regard to scrapie or CJD strains.

Merz: We looked at three cases of Alzheimer's disease (cortex received from Colin Masters); these are samples from Paul Brown of primary CJD in humans (Fig. 2). The material was not treated with proteinase K before being studied for the presence of SAF. For the Western blots the samples were all treated with proteinase K.

In two of the cases of primary human CJD there were similarities and in one of the cases there were differences in the Western blotting antigenicity. The SAF yield in these cases was similar, measured by SAF counts per square by electron microscopy. All of these samples react with monoclonal antibody 3F4, which is specific for scrapie PrP in the hamster and the human (Kacscak et al 1987). The antibody reacted with a band of 26 kDa and lower molecular weight bands. This pattern is similar to that seen with SAF from the scrapie strain 139A in C57BL mice. Proteins from the other primary CJD cases react more strongly with these monoclonal antibodies, suggesting that more sites are present on these proteins than on those from the previous case. SAF for the GSS case of Paul Brown (there are also amyloid fibrils in this case) contain only two bands that react with monoclonal antibody 3F4, proteins in the range of 20 kDa and 14 kDa.

Gabizon: The host is different.

Merz: I have the same data with scrapie in *Sinc* ^{s7s7} mice (Fig. 1).

Gabizon: You cannot apply the mouse data to humans because humans are not inbred and different individuals may have slightly different proteins.

F. Brown: How are the protein extracts processed before examination by electron microscopy?

Merz: The isolation procedure employed for the human cases involved treatment with the detergent sarcosyl and differential centrifugation in a Beckman airfuge. Dilutions of these samples were examined by electron microscopy for the presence of abnormal fibrils: SAF, paired helical filaments or amyloid fibrils. The number of fibrils were counted per 10 squares of the grid. An aliquot of undiluted sample was treated with proteinase K to remove any contaminating proteins. This procedure does not isolate the normal protein of 33–35 kDa and a protease inhibitor cocktail was used to block endogenous protease activity (Merz & Wisniewski, in press).

Oesch: Are these purified SAF?

Merz: These are crude purified SAF, some of which were obtained by biopsy. The scrapie SAF are purified SAF.

Oesch: You don't know what portion is truly PrP. When you say that the second CJD case reacts more strongly with the antibody, you may have loaded more protein than in the first example.

Merz: That may be true for some of the human biopsy cases but it does not seem to be true for experimental scrapie, since those samples were adjusted for their protein content.

Dickinson: Stan (Prusiner), some years ago we gave you three of our strains of scrapie. Have you studied them?

Prusiner: Yes, we have inoculated C57BL mice with the three strains and we cannot see any differences in incubation periods.

Dickinson: If your methods are not sensitive enough, you will fail to detect differences.

Fraser: Did you look for the differences in neuropathology of the strains.

Prusiner: We have not looked at the pathology.

Chesebro: If Alan sees differences and the Prusiner group do not, it may be that the mice are different. It is very hard to maintain a constant mouse genotype. Unless each group is buying mice regularly from a single supplier and doing experiments at the same time it is difficult to make comparisons.

Diringer: There is no doubt that *Sinc* is important for incubation period but is there any hard evidence that *Sinc* regulates replication?

Dickinson: Sinc must regulate overall replication dynamics, because of the effects we see on incubation period. In terms of things like maximum rates of replication, where you might expect *Sinc* to operate, it doesn't seem to have any effect. It seems to operate more by extending the duration of the plateau period or the delay before replication starts.

Kimberlin: This issue of replication and replication rates differing in different scrapie models has not been satisfatorily explored experimentally and much more work is required in the future. I predict that replication rate in the CNS will turn out to be important in distinguishing some of the longer incubation models from the very short ones.

Wisniewski: I would like to draw attention to the way in which the technique used to study the morphology can affect our interpretation of the data. Colin (Masters) started with historical slides stained by Nissl technique, which did not show vacuolation. By recutting those sections and staining with haematoxylin and eosine he could demonstrate vacuolar pathology. Alan Dickinson mentioned that in some animals he doesn't see vacuolation at all. It all may depend on the thickness of the sections. In the Nissl technique one usually cuts 15 to 30 µm thick sections in which the initial stages of vacuolation are not detectable. Colin cut 7 µm sections and saw the vacuolation. I think that if Alan cuts 1 µm thick sections in those animals which show no vacuolation, changes will be found.

DeArmond: I agree. We have looked at a GSS case in which there was no apparent vacuolar degeneration in the cortex by light microscopy but electron microscopy of those same regions showed the classic spongiform degeneration of post-synaptic processes.

Dickinson: The terminology which has been used was often 'I do not see spongiform change therefore I don't need to entertain these possibilities'. The task of trying to look for infective processes in the absence of vacuolation by light microscopy has not been tackled.

Wisniewski: Always look at the methodology used and the thickness of the section, then it is much easier to interpret the data.

Roberts: Dr Fraser, you described the lesion patterns that you find in different strains—have you checked other brain areas by electron microscopy to see if you can find more subtle changes? What thickness sections were you looking at?

Fraser: 7 μm sections. Another point is that Richard Kimberlin's work on pathogenesis shows the importance of the spinal cord following non-cerebral infections (Kimberlin & Walker 1980). I suggest that in some of these situations where little pathology is found in the brainstem we have not cut though the spinal cord. The central nervous system involves both the brain and the spinal cord!

Dickinson: They show that there is variety arising independently of host differences.

References

Bruce M, Dickinson AG 1987 Biological evidence that scrapie agent has an independent genome. J Gen Virol 68:79–89

Kascsak RJ, Rubenstein R, Merz PA, Carp RI, Wisniewski HM, Diringer H 1985 Biochemical differences among scrapie associated fibrils support the biological diversity of scrapie agents. J Gen Virol 66:1715–1722

Kascsak RJ, Rubenstein R, Merz PA, Carp RI, Robakis N, Wisniewski HM, Diringer H 1986 Immunological analysis of scrapie associated fibrils isolated from four different scrapie agents. J Virol 59:676–683

Kascsak RJ, Rubenstein R, Merz PA, Carp RI, Wisniewski HM 1987 Production and characterization of mouse polyclonal and monoclonal antibodies to scrapie associated fibrils. J Virol 61:3688–3693

Kimberlin RH, Walker CA 1980 Pathogenesis of mouse scrapie: evidence for neural spread of infection to the CNS. J Gen Virol 51:183–187

Luria SE, Delbruck M 1943 Mutations in bacteria from virus sensitivity to resistance. Genetics 28:491–511

Merz PA, Wisniewski HM 1987 Spongiform encephalopathies. In: Lennette EH et al (eds) Laboratory diagnosis of infectious diseases, principles and practices. Vol 11 Viral rickettsial and chlamydial diseases. Springer-Verlag, New York, chap 46, in press

Genetic control of prion incubation period in mice

George A. Carlson[1], David Westaway[2], Patricia A. Goodman[2], Marilyn Peterson[2], Susan T. Marshall[1] and Stanley B. Prusiner[2]

[1]The Jackson Laboratory, Bar Harbor, Maine 04609 and [2]Departments of Neurology and of Biochemistry and Biophysics, University of California, San Francisco, California 94143 USA

Abstract. The prion gene complex (*Prn*) is located on mouse chromosome 2 between the beta-2-microglobulin (*B2m*) and agouti (*A*) genes. Within this complex are the prion protein gene (*Prn-p*), which encodes the only identified macromolecule (PrP) that purifies with infectious scrapie agent, and a scrapie incubation time gene (*Prn-i*). Using a variety of restriction endonucleases, six allelic forms of the *Prn-p* gene have been distinguished by their patterns of restriction fragment length polymorphisms. We had previously shown that the exceptionally long scrapie incubation period of I/LnJ mice inoculated with the Chandler isolate (over 200 days) was due to the effects of a scrapie incubation time gene tightly linked to *Prn-p*. So far, this long scrapie incubation time allele has been found only in those inbred mouse strains (I/LnJ, P/J and IM) that have the *b* allele of *Prn-p*. It is not known whether the incubation time gene and prion protein gene are two distinct loci or are one and the same. Putative recombinants between the incubation time phenotype and *Prn-p* genotype have been observed, but this could be due to effects of other genes segregating in the population. Regardless of whether or not the incubation time and PrP genes are identical, if any differences were found in the amino acid sequences of PrP encoded by the different *Prn-p* alleles there would be important implications for interpretation of results on 'strains' of scrapie agent. It would not be necessary to invoke nucleic acid as the informational macromolecule of the scrapie agent because differences in prion 'strains' recovered from mice with different *Prn-p* genotypes need not be the result of host selection but could be due to differences in host-encoded PrP.

1988 Novel infectious agents and the central nervous system. Wiley, Chichester (Ciba Foundation Symposium 135) p 84–99

The only macromolecule that has been identified in preparations of infectious scrapie agent is prion protein (PrP) (McKinley et al 1983). PrP is encoded by a single-copy host gene rather than by any nucleic acid that may be present in the infectious agent (Oesch et al 1985). Two isoforms of PrP have been identified (Meyer et al 1986, Barry et al 1986): PrP^C is approximately 33–35 kDa, is the normal cellular form and is highly sensitive to digestion with proteinase K. PrP^{Sc} is also 33–35 kDa but is found only in scrapie-infected animals; limited proteinase K digestion yields PrP molecules of 27–30 kDa apparent molecular weight. Both isoforms are encoded by the prion protein gene (*Prn-p*); no alternative splice sites within hamster *Prn-p* have been identified and the entire open reading frame is encoded in a single exon, making it likely that the formation of PrP^{Sc} is due to post-translational modification (Basler et al 1986).

The proteinaceous nature of the scrapie agent and its resistance to treatments that inactivate nucleic acids led to the term prion as an appropriate descriptive name for this novel type of infectious particle (Prusiner 1982). Extensive biochemical analyses have indicated that PrP^{Sc} is a functional, and possibly the only, component of scrapie prions (reviewed in Prusiner & DeArmond 1987). However, work on the isolation and characterization of 'strains' of scrapie agent indicates that there are informational macromolecules in prions (Dickinson & Meikle 1971, Dickinson & Fraser 1977, Bruce & Dickinson 1979). The possibility that scrapie prions contain cryptic nucleic acids has not been excluded, but the conclusion that the agent contains an independent genome needs to be re-evaluated in view of our finding (Carlson et al 1986) that a gene (*Prn-i*) with a profound effect on scrapie incubation period is tightly linked and possibly identical to the prion protein gene (*Prn-p*).

Restriction fragment polymorphisms for the prion protein gene

Using hamster (Oesch et al 1985) and mouse (Chesebro et al 1985) PrP cDNA clones, and synthetic oligonucleotides for the 5' untranslated sequence, we identified six allelic patterns of restriction fragment length polymorphisms (RFLP) for the prion protein gene (*Prn-p*) among inbred strains of mice. Fragment sizes obtained with several restriction endonucleases for each allelic pattern are shown in Table 1. As shown in Table 2, most inbred strains that have been typed have the *a* RFLP pattern; I/LnJ, P/J, IM and BDP/J mice have the *b* pattern. RIIIS/J and MA/MyJ are the sole representatives of the *c* and *d* patterns; both had been previously classified as *Prn-p*^{b} based solely on the polymorphism detected with *Xba*I (Carlson et al 1986). The *e* and *f* alleles are found in CAST/Ei and MOLF/Ei, inbred strains derived from wild *castaneus* and *molossinus* mice. I/LnJ mice have exceptionally long incubation periods following inoculation with scrapie prions due to the effects of a single gene (*Prn-i*^{i}) that is tightly linked or possibly identical to *Prn-p* (Carlson et al 1986); these results will be discussed in more detail.

It is not known whether any of the differences in nucleic acid sequence that have been detected in our analyses have any biological significance; however, these polymorphisms do provide convenient markers for linkage analysis.

TABLE 1   Restriction fragments (in kilobase pairs) that distinguish alleles of the prion protein gene (Prn-p)

Allele	XbaI	TaqI	SacI	EcoRI	BamHI
	ORF and 3' untranslated (UT) probes				5' UT oligo probe
a	3.8	11.0	10.9	4.2	10.9
b	5.5	9.1	12.9	9.4	12.2
c	5.5	11.0	12.9	4.2	12.2
d	5.5	13.5	10.9	4.2	10.9
e	5.5	9.1	12.9	10.0	10.9
f	5.5	9.1	12.9	4.2	12.2

Chromosomal location of *Prn-p*

Previous work using somatic cell hybrids had localized the human prion protein gene (PRNP) to chromosome 20p and the mouse *Prn-p* gene to chromosome 2 (Sparkes et al 1986). The position of *Prn-p* on chromosome 2 in relation to the agouti (*a*) and beta-2-microglobulin (*B2m*) genes was determined using (B6 × MA/MyJ) F1 × C57BL/6J (B6) backcross mice. B6 is *a*, *Prn-p*^{a}, *B2m*^{b} and MA/MyJ is +, *Prn-p*^{d}, *B2m*^{a}. The two alleles of *B2m* were distinguished by the presence of a *Bgl*I site within the open reading frame of the *b* allele using a *B2m* probe (Parnes & Seidman 1982), while the *Xba*I polymorphism between the *a* and *d* alleles (Table 1) was used to type for *Prn-p*. The agouti locus controls the relative amount and distribution of yellow pigment and black pigment in the hairs of the coat. The recessive nonagouti (*a*) allele causes a lack of yellow banding in the hairs. The genotype

TABLE 2   Alleles for Prn-p based on restriction fragment polymorphisms

Allele	Strain
Prn-p^a	A/J, AKR/J, AU/SsJ, **BALB/cJ**, BUB/BnJ, **CBA/J**, CE/J, **C3H/HeSn**, **C57BL/6J**, C57BL/10Sn, C57L/J, C58/J, DBA/2J, HRS/J, LG/J, LP/J, LT/SvEi, **NZB/BINJ**, **NZW/LacJ**, PL/J, **RIII/Dm**, SEA/GnJ, SEC/1ReJ, **SJL/J**, SM/J, ST/bJ, **SWR/J**, V/Le, WB/ReJ, WC/ReJ, YBR/Ei, 129/J
Prn-p^b	**I/LnJ**, BDP/J, **P/J**, **IM/Dk**
Prn-p^c	**RIIIS/J**
Prn-p^d	**MA/MyJ**
Prn-p^e	**CAST/Ei**
Prn-p^f	MOLF/Ei

Scrapie incubation time has been determined for the strains in bold type

TABLE 3 Mapping of Prn-p using (B6 × MA/MyJ)F1 × B6 backcross mice

Region type	Gametes produced by F1 parent			Number of mice
	B2m	Prn-p	a	
B6 parental	b	a	a	31
MA parental	a	d	+	31
B2m–Prn-p	a	a	a	3
recombinants	b	d	+	2
Prn-p—a	b	a	+	6
recombinants	a	d	a	7

	Recombination frequencies	
B2m	Prn-p	a
	0.0625 ± 0.027	0.1625 ± 0.041

for agouti was determined by coat colour: a/a mice are black and $+/a$ mice are agouti (wild-type). The results are shown in Table 3. The provisional location of the prion protein gene on chromosome 2 is shown in Fig. 1. Inosine triphosphatase (Itp) maps between $B2m$ and a (Taylor et al 1987); the homologous human gene (ITP) is located on chromosome 20p, as is the prion protein gene (PRNP). This suggests that the mouse and human chromosomes may be homologous in this region (Sparkes et al 1986). In mice, a prion incubation time gene ($Prn-i$) is tightly linked to $Prn-p$, and a homologous gene probably exists in humans.

TABLE 4 Scrapie incubation times in inbred and F1 hybrid mice carrying different Prn-p alleles

Mice	Prn-p	n	Onset of illness	Death (days ± SE)
NZW/LacJ	a	20	113.2 ± 2	119.9 ± 2.3
I/LnJ	b	11	314.4 ± 13.9	322.4 ± 15.2
P/J	b	13	>240 no signs of illness	
RIIIS/J	c	4	136.2 ± 2.9	141.2 ± 1.7
MA/MyJ	d	6	170 (all)	189.7 ± 5.2
CAST/Ei	e	5	172.2 ± 5.9	216 (n = 1)
(NZW × I/Ln)F1	a/b	24	222.6 ± 2.8	233.8 ± 2.2
(B6 × RIIIS)F1	a/c	5	157.6 ± 1.2	161.6 ± 0.9
(B6 × MA/MyJ)F1	a/d	4	204.0 ± 5.4	215.5 ± 3.3
(NZW × CAST)F1	a/e	13	182.0 ± 4.1	203 ± 6.6

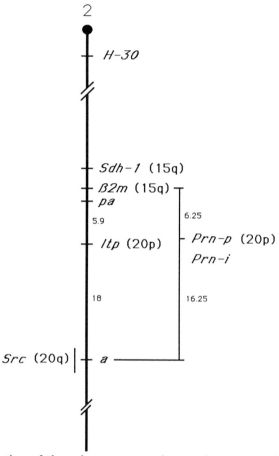

FIG. 1. Location of the prion gene complex on chromosome 2 between the β-2-microglobulin (*B2m*) and agouti genes (*a*). The map distances (in centimorgans) between pallid (*pa*), *Itp*, and *a* are from Taylor and coworkers (1987), and the *B2m—Prn-p—a* distances are from the data shown in Table 3. The position of *Prn-p* relative to *Itp* has not been determined. The human chromosomal locations of homologous genes are given in parentheses.

Linkage of prion incubation time with the prion protein gene — the prion gene complex (*Prn*)

As shown in Table 4, the only inbred mice with scrapie incubation times in excess of 200 days following inoculation with the Chandler scrapie isolate are those with the *b* allele of the prion protein gene. I/LnJ mice have scrapie incubation times ranging from 200 to 385 days; 13 P/J mice (also *Prn-p*[b]) inoculated with the Chandler scrapie prion isolate showed no signs of scrapie up to 240 days after inoculation.

In a previous study (Carlson et al 1986), we demonstrated that the long scrapie incubation period of I/LnJ mice was due to the effects of a single prion incubation time gene (*Prn-i*^{i}) that co-segregated with the *Prn-p*^{b} allele. (NZW × I/LnJ) F1 × NZW/LacJ backcross progeny were inoculated with scrapie prions and the resultant incubation periods segregated into two groups, indicating single gene control. One possible recombinant between *Prn-p* and *Prn-i* was seen among the 66 mice that were typed for *Prn-p* in this study. The results also suggested that longer incubation times were dominant.

To further assess the influence of *Prn-i* on scrapie incubation period and to determine whether there is recombination between *Prn-i* and *Prn-p*, (NZW × I/LnJ) F2 mice were inoculated with the Chandler isolate of scrapie prions. Scrapie incubation times in *Prn-p*^{a}, *Prn-p*^{a}/*Prn-p*^{b}, and *Prn-p*^{b} F2 mice are illustrated in Fig. 2. The results clearly indicated that incubation time in *Prn-p* heterozygotes was intermediate between that of *a* and *b* homozygotes. Three possible *Prn-i–Prn-p* recombinants were seen among 62 inoculated mice; one *Prn-p*^{a}/*Prn-p*^{b} mouse had an incubation time of 126 days, two *Prn-p*^{a} mice had incubation times of 232 and 275 days. If these mice were true recombinants, this would indicate that *Prn-i* and *Prn-p* are roughly 2.7 ± 1.7 centimorgans apart. However, this conclusion ignores the possibility that cumulative effects of other genes segregating in the population caused the divergence of incubation time from *Prn-p* genotype.

The long incubation time *Prn-i*^{i} allele has been found only in *Prn-p*^{b} mice

The incubation times of some inbred strains of mice with the *a*, *b*, *c*, *d* and *e* alleles at *Prn-p* and of *Prn-p* heterozygous F1 hybrid mice are given in Table 4. MA/MyJ (*Prn-p*^{d}) and CAST/Ei (*Prn-p*^{e}) mice had longer incubation times than *Prn-p*^{a} strains (170 and 172 days); F1 hybrids with B6 or NZW had even longer incubation times. In order to determine whether prolongation of scrapie incubation time in MA/MyJ and CAST/Ei mice was due to the effects of a gene linked to *Prn-p*^{d} and *Prn-p*^{e}, backcross mice were typed for *Prn-p* and inoculated with scrapie prions. The incubation times for (B6 × MA/MyJ) F1 × B6 mice are shown in Fig. 3. Incubation times in the 18 mice that were inoculated ranged from 159 to 195 days, regardless of *Prn-p* genotype; clearly other genes in addition to *Prn-p* can influence scrapie incubation times. Similar results were seen in (NZW × CAST) F1 × NZW backcross mice (data not shown). Our data indicate that only *Prn-p*^{b} mice have the long incubation time *Prn-i*^{i} allele; it is not known whether the prion incubation time allele in mice with the *c*, *d*, and *e* alleles of the PrP gene is the same (*Prn-i*^{n}) or different from that in *Prn-p*^{a} strains.

Carp and his colleagues (1987) and Hope & Kimberlin (1987) have suggested that *Prn-i* is identical to the scrapie incubation time gene, *Sinc*, identified over 20 years ago by Dickinson and coworkers (Dickinson &

MacKay 1964). When I/LnJ mice were crossed to the $Sinc^{p7}$ strain, IM, after inoculation with the ME7 scrapie isolate the F1 hybrid had the long incubation time that is characteristic of $Sinc^{p7}$ homozygotes (Dickinson et al 1968). This result did not rule out the possibility of two distinct dominant genes, but this interpretation was made less likely by the characteristic $Sinc$-controlled incubation times of I/LnJ and its F1 hybrids following inoculation with a variety of scrapie 'strains'. $Sinc^{p7}$ VM and IM mice are thought to have the same 5.5 kb Prn-p^b restriction fragment as I/LnJ, and VM $Sinc^{s7}$ congenic mice to have the smaller Prn-p^a fragment (Hope & Kimberlin 1987).

Although it is possible that Prn-i and $Sinc$ are identical, the use of the prion gene complex (Prn-i and Prn-p) nomenclature offers some advantages even though the discovery of $Sinc$ predates that of Prn-i. First, Prn-i (or $Sinc$) controls not only scrapie incubation phenotype but also the incubation time following inoculation with mouse-adapted Creutzfeldt-Jakob disease prions (Kingsbury et al 1987). Second, it is not yet known whether Prn-i and Prn-p are two distinct genes or whether Prn-p itself controls prion incubation period. A cDNA encoding mouse PrP has been cloned and sequenced (Chesebro et al 1986). The nomenclature for a gene should be an indication of its product, hence, Prn-p is an appropriate symbol though this could change once the physiological and biochemical functions of PrP have been elucidated. The symbols Prn-i and Prn-p do not prejudge whether the incubation time phenotype is a reflection of Prn-p genotype.

'Strains' of scrapie agent — influence of host Prn-p genotype

Differential behaviour of scrapie agent 'strains' has been used as an argument that prions contain nucleic acid that is capable of stable replication but is also susceptible to mutation (Bruce & Dickinson 1979). Much of the data on 'strains' of mouse scrapie agent came from experiments using $Sinc^{p7}$ (VM and IM) and $Sinc^{s7}$ mice. The ME7 scrapie agent, which is related to the Chandler isolate, is stable, regardless of previous passage history. That is, scrapie agent isolated from VM mice produces the long incubation period in VM and the short incubation period in other mouse strains, as does the original inoculum. The behaviour of other 'strains' of scrapie agent is more complex. Although VM mice have a long incubation period when inoculated with the ME7 isolate, they have a shorter incubation time (about 200 days) than $Sinc^{s7}$ mice after inoculation of the 22A 'strain' of scrapie agent (Dickinson & Meikle 1971). Given that all $Sinc^{s7}$ homozygous mouse strains have long incubation periods (over 400 days) after inoculation with the 22A strain it is likely that $Sinc$ controls the incubation period for both ME7 and 22A. 'Strains' of another class of scrapie agent, including 22A, are stable in mice of the $Sinc$ genotype in which they were isolated but change on serial passage in mice of the other $Sinc$ genotype. For example, 87A that had been passaged three times in C57BL ($s7$) mice had a shorter incubation period in C57BL mice than in VM ($p7$) mice, but 87V (passaged five times in VM mice) had a shorter incubation period in VM than in C57BL (Dickinson & Fraser 1977). These results have been interpreted as indicating preferential outgrowth of genetic variants capable of most rapid proliferation in mice of a given *Sinc* genotype. Although it has been suggested that this mouse strain-dependent change in scrapie agent behaviour is gradual, almost all the change occurred in the first passage (Bruce & Dickinson 1979).

The finding of different alleles encoding PrP, which are linked to a gene controlling scrapie incubation period, could provide an alternative explanation. The scrapie PrP isoform is the major component of the scrapie prion, and clearly is host encoded (Oesch et al 1985). If the DNA polymorphisms for *Prn-p* are reflected in the proteins, then prions isolated from *Prn-p*[a] mice will differ from those isolated from *Prn-p*[b] mice, raising the possibility that much of the 'genetics' of the scrapie agent is due to allelic variants of a host-encoded gene. Nonetheless, it is clear that the prion contains an informational macromolecule that influences its behaviour; whether this is due to genetically distinct prion 'strains' or to epigenetic variation between 'strains' caused by host-encoded genes has not been determined.

What is the informational macromolecule of prions?

It is extremely unlikely that the prion is a conventional virus with a nucleic acid encoding virus-specific proteins. Gabizon and her colleagues (1987) showed that highly purified PrP 27–30 and scrapie infectivity co-partition into liposomes; no rod-shaped or filamentous particles were found among the liposomes, even though small amounts of added tobacco mosaic virus could be readily detected. Although nuclease and Zn^{2+} treatment of the PrP-liposomes had no effect on scrapie infectivity, the possibility that a scrapie-specific nucleic acid is bound and protected by PrP has not been excluded.

In addition to the genetic evidence summarized here, extensive biochemical analysis indicates that PrP[Sc] is required for scrapie infectivity. There are two major possibilities for the informational molecule of the prion that is responsible for differential behaviour of scrapie 'strains'. It could be either a nucleic acid that may be hidden and protected by PrP[Sc] (although unlikely, a conventional virus has not been totally eliminated as a possibility), or PrP itself. At present, there are insufficient data for definitive discrimination between the two alternatives, but testing of predictions about the behaviour of the scrapie agent and the nature of the disease should determine whether a protein or nucleic acid is responsible. Some of the predictions favoured by the protein-only or nucleic acid hypotheses are summarized in Table 5.

The mutational basis for the generation of strains of microorganisms is well established. However, the long incubation period of scrapie makes genetic

TABLE 5   What is the informational macromolecule in the prion?

Nucleic acid	Protein
Mutagens can induce variant agents	Mutagenesis of agent would have no effect
Biological cloning of agent possible	Host gene sole determinant of agent behaviour
Host genes exert selective pressure on agent	Host gene encodes the agent
Labile scrapie strains due to selection	Labile 'strains' reflect host $Prn-p$ genotype
Stable scrapie strains exist regardless of host passage	Different PrP^{Sc} isoforms
Disease requires inoculation of agent	Transmissible disease can occur without inoculation of agent
Impossible to transmit disease with protein product of cloned host gene	Disease transmissible with PrP^{Sc} alone

analysis of the agent extremely difficult; for example, there is no evidence which fulfils the criteria established by Luria and Delbruck (1943) for biological cloning of the scrapie agent or for mutations in the agent.

Existing biochemical information on the nature of the post-translational modifications responsible for converting PrP^C to PrP^{Sc} is not sufficient to construct a detailed hypothesis to account for 'strains' of protein-only prions. However, in many respects a protein-only model for the infectious agent is less complicated than one involving an agent-specific nucleic acid that interacts with a host-encoded protein. PrP mRNA levels do not increase during the course of infection (Oesch et al 1985, Chesebro et al 1985) but the amount of PrP^{Sc} in the brains of infected animals increases in parallel with infectivity (McKinley et al 1983). PrP^{Sc} accumulates extracellularly, often as amyloid deposits (Prusiner et al 1983). This suggests that scrapie may be a disease of protein catabolism due to positive feedback induced by the inoculated PrP^{Sc}, rather than an induction of PrP by a replicating agent with an independent genome. The existence of scrapie 'strains' could be explained by different post-translational modifications of PrP; differences in mobility of PrP^{Sc} fragments after limited proteinase K digestion between different scrapie 'strains' isolated from the same strain of mouse (Kascsak et al 1986) support this contention. If the different $Prn-p$ alleles encode different proteins, this could explain the lability of certain 'strains' following passage in mice of different $Prn-p$ genotype, with homologous PrP favouring shorter incubation times (Kingsbury et al 1987).

Recent results emphasize the similarities between accumulation of PrP^{Sc} in prion-induced diseases and accumulation of the A4 or amyloid β-protein in

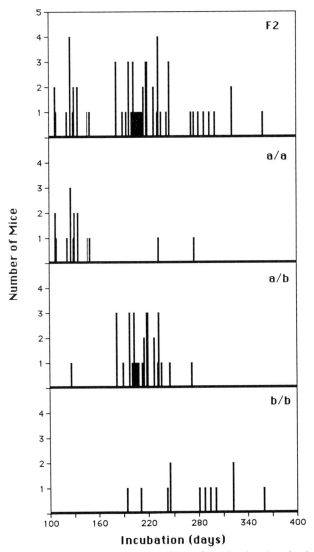

FIG. 2. Linkage of the prion protein gene (*Prn-p*) and prion incubation time gene (*Prn-i*) in (NZW/LacJ × I/LnJ) F2 mice inoculated with the Chandler scrapie isolate. The incubation times for the total F2 population and for mice of each *Prn-p* genotype are shown. See text for details.

Alzheimer's disease (Kang et al 1987, Goldgaber et al 1987). In familial Alzheimer's disease, a RLFP near the A4 precursor gene has been found in affected individuals (Tanzi et al 1987); if protein sequence differences between affected and non-affected family members are found in the A4 precursor protein, this would suggest that the altered protein itself might trigger its

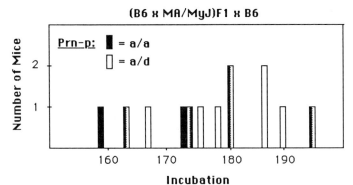

FIG. 3. Prion incubation time and prion protein gene are not linked in (B6 × MA/MyJ) F1 × B6 backcross mice inoculated with the Chandler scrapie isolate. The incubation times of $Prn\text{-}p^a$ homozygous mice are indicated by closed bars and the times for $Prn\text{-}p^a/Prn\text{-}p^d$ heterozygotes are represented by open bars. See text for details.

own pathological accumulation as amyloid. The concept of scrapie as a degenerative disease that happens to be infectious warrants consideration.

References

Barry RA, Kent SBH, McKinley MP et al 1986 Scrapie and cellular PrP isoforms share polypeptide isoforms. J Infect Dis 153:848–854

Basler K, Oesch B, Scott B et al 1986 Scrapie and cellular PrP isoforms are encoded by the same chromosomal gene. Cell 46:417–428

Bruce ME, Dickinson AG 1978 Biological stability of different classes of scrapie agent. In: Prusiner SB, Hadlow WJ (eds) Slow transmissible disease of the nervous system. Academic Press, New York, vol 2:71–86

Carlson GA, Kingsbury DT, Goodman PA et al 1986 Linkage of prion protein and scrapie incubation time genes. Cell 46:503–511

Carp RI, Moretz RC, Natelli M, Dickinson AG 1987 Genetic control of scrapie: Incubation period and plaque formation in I mice. J Gen Virol 68:401–407

Chesebro B, Race R, Wehrly K et al 1985 Identification of scrapie prion protein-specific mRNA in scrapie-infected and uninfected brain. Nature (Lond) 315:331–333

Dickinson AG, Fraser H 1977 The pathogenesis of scrapie in inbred mice: an assessment of host control and response involving many strains of agent. In: terMulen V, Katz M (eds) Slow virus infections of the central nervous system. Springer-Verlag, New York, p 3–14

Dickinson AG, MacKay JMK 1964 Genetical control of the incubation period in mice of the neurological disease, scrapie. Heredity 19:279–288

Dickinson AG, Meikle VMH 1971 Host genotype and agent effects in scrapie incubation: change in allelic interaction with different strains of agent. Mol & Gen Genet 112:73–79

Dickinson AG, Meikle VMH, Fraser HG 1968 Identification of a gene which controls the incubation period of some strains of scrapie agent in mice. J Comp Pathol 78:293–299

Gabizon R, McKinley MP, Prusiner SB 1987 Purified prion proteins and scrapie infectivity copartition into liposomes. Proc Natl Acad Sci USA 84:4017–4021

Goldgaber D, Lerman MI, McBride OW, Saffiotti U, Gajdusek DC 1987 Characterization and chromosomal localization of a cDNA encoding brain amyloid of Alzheimer's disease. Science (Wash DC) 235:877–880

Hope J, Kimberlin RH 1987 The molecular biology of scrapie: the last two years. Trends Neurosci 4:149–151

Kang J, Lemaire H-G, Unterbeck A et al 1987 The precursor of Alzheimer's disease amyloid A4 protein resembles a cell-surface receptor. Nature (Lond) 325:733–736

Kascsak RJ, Rubenstein R, Merz PA et al 1986 Immunological comparison of scrapie-associated fibrils isolated from animals infected with four different scrapie strains. J Virol 59:676–683

Kingsbury DT, Carlson GA, Prusiner SB 1987 Genetic control of prion replication. In: McKinley MP, Prusiner SB (eds) Prions: novel infectious pathogens causing scrapie and Creutzfeldt-Jakob disease. Academic Press, New York, p 315–329

Luria SE, Delbruck M 1943 Mutations in bacteria from virus sensitivity to resistance. Genetics 28:491–511

McKinley MP, Bolton DC, Prusiner SB 1983 A protease-resistant protein is a structural component of the scrapie prion. Cell 35:57–62

Meyer RK, McKinley MP, Bowman KA, Barry RA, Prusiner SB 1986 Separation and properties of cellular and scrapie prion proteins. Proc Natl Acad Sci USA 83:2310–2314

Oesch B, Westaway D, Wälchli M et al 1985 A cellular gene encodes scrapie PrP 27–30 protein. Cell 40:735–746

Parnes JR, Seidman JG 1982 Structure of wild-type and mutant β2-microglobulin genes. Cell 29:661–669

Prusiner SB 1982 Novel proteinaceous infectious particles cause scrapie. Science (Wash DC) 216:136–144

Prusiner SB, DeArmond SJ 1987 Prions causing nervous system degeneration. Lab Invest 56:349–363

Prusiner SB, McKinley MP, Bowman KA et al 1983 Scrapie prions aggregate to form amyloid-like birefringent rods. Cell 35:349–358

Sparkes RF, Simon M, Cohn VH et al 1986 Assignment of the mouse and human prion protein genes to homologous chromosomes. Proc Natl Acad Sci USA 83:7358–7362

Tanzi RE, Gusella JF, Watkins PC et al 1987 Amyloid β protein gene: cDNA, mRNA distribution, and genetic linkage near the Alzheimer locus. Science (Wash DC) 235:880–884

Taylor BA, Walls DM, Wimsatt MJ 1987 Localization of the inosine triphosphatase locus (Itp) on chromosome 2 of the mouse. Biochem Genet 25:267–274

DISCUSSION

Diringer: I understand your correlation between this gene and the prion protein but what is the genetic evidence that this gene correlates with infectivity or with agent replication?

Carlson: There is no direct evidence that the prion protein gene itself has anything to do with infectivity or incubation period, at present it is just a linked marker.

*Dickinson:*There is a variety in the scrapie inoculum due to strain differences in the agent, even when the host is constant. There is no need to invoke complicated arguments about mixtures, competition or changes of selective environment according to the *Sinc* allele being carried. We are talking about a uniform passage history for two different strains and their behaviour when you passage them again, without changing the host. That immediately cancels some of your predictions (Table 5) for a protein as the informational molecule, for example, the proposal that a host gene encodes the agent.

Carlson: At the molecular level there is no explanation for how this agent replicates. A single host gene can encode two apparently different proteins, for example prealbumin and albumin or trypsin and trypsinogen.

Dickinson: Solid data do exist, but you are saying let's speculate rather than come to terms with the data.

Carlson: There are no clear data that, for example, the prion protein of ME7 in C57BL mice is the same in every respect as the prion protein of 22A in C57BL mice.

Manuelidis: I thought that the sequencing data show that the protein is the same in every case examined thus far.

Carlson: That's right. If there's no difference between the prion protein sequences encoded by the *Prn-p*^{a} and *Prn-p*^{b} alleles then the proposition that the lability of certain scrapie isolates following passage across 'mouse strain barriers' is due to allotypic differences in PrP cannot be true. (See p 99.)

Dickinson: But I am saying that when the host is constant, through numerous passages, strain differences of scrapie do exist.

Carlson: There are two ways to explain that result: nucleic acid changes or different conformational or post-translational modifications of the prion protein.

Dickinson: But where does this the specification of difference come from in the 'protein only' model?

Bolton: In the same host inoculated with the same agent there are at least 15 to 20 different isoforms of this protein. Within different regions of the brain inoculated with one agent different amounts of these different isoforms are produced. Similarly, different agents inoculated into the same strain of mouse lead to the production of different isoforms of the protein.

Manuelidis: What do you mean by isoform, a different cleavage product derived from the same amino acid sequence?

Bolton: No, these are not cleaved by any protease *in vitro*. By 'isoform' I mean the different charge and size variants of the scrapie protein detected by gel electrophoresis. Many of these forms, if not most of them, appear to arise from variations in post-translational modifications other than proteolysis.

Manuelidis: But a preparation from a particular brain gives four bands on a

Western blot which all have the same antibody-binding characteristics. To the best of our knowledge these are made from the same protein, so how can you call them isoforms? They are simply different proteolytic cleavage products, possibly produced by endogenous proteases activated in the brain during disease or as a consequence of isolation procedures.

Dickinson: The starting point, presumably, is differences in different regions of the brain and different patterns of damage. Therefore altered patterns on a Western blot are a consequence of different exposure to host proteases.

Bolton: That is the point, there are other host genes that may operate on the agent. The products of these genes may be protein kinases, glycosyl transferases, glycosidases, etcetera, as well as proteases.

Dickinson: No, because those variables stay constant when the host is kept the same. The difference is only explicable in terms of agent strain differences in the inoculum. The problem for your model is therefore to explain how there can be replication of the difference in the inoculum by a constant host.

Carlson: I agree. Can you explain how nucleic acid is using this host protein to replicate? I can't explain how a protein can use a protein to replicate.

Manuelidis: If it is.

Carlson: I am not saying that one or the other of these models is true, but I think that they are going to be distinguishable. The available data do not necessarily say that there has to be a nucleic acid in the scrapie agent.

Hope: We have a silver-stained polyacrylamide gel of PrP in SAF from the brains of VM mice infected with the 22L, 22A, 87V or 177A strains of scrapie (Fig. 1). The incubation periods produced by a standard dose (10^{-2} terminal brain homogenate) of 22L, 22A and 177A in VM mice are very similar, approximately 200 days, in contrast to 87V in VM mice which gives an incubation period of around 300 days. There is no scrapie strain-dependent, qualitative difference in the pattern of PrP obtained from SAF purified without the use of proteinase K. There is variation in the susceptibility of PrP in SAF to proteinase K digestion; this variation depends on the strain of scrapie, since these samples were prepared using the same mouse strain (VM). It's most noticeable in 87V-induced SAF protein, where proteinase K hydrolysis gives essentially one molecular weight variant of PrP, similar to the PrP 27-30 variant found in 263K-induced SAF; in contrast, three variants are produced by proteolysis of 22L-, 22A- or 177A-induced SAF (Fig 1).

Gabizon: So what are the differences in the proteins from the different strains?

Hope: We have not yet found differences by 1D and 2D polyacrylamide gel analysis between PrP in SAF prepared without the use of proteinase K. The only difference about which I'm confident so far is that PrP in SAF shows a scrapie strain-specific susceptibility to hydrolysis by proteinase K.

Gabizon: What is the difference between these strains?

Hope: They produce different pathologies in the brains of terminally

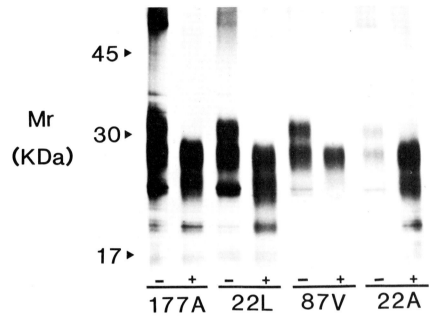

FIG. 1. (*Hope*) SAF protein from VM (*Sinc*[p7]) mice: effect of scrapie strain and proteinase K. SAF fractions were purified with (+) or without (−) the use of proteinase K (Hope et al 1986) from brains of VM mice at the clinical stage of infection with four different strains of scrapie: 177A, 22L, 87V and 22A. Proteins were analysed as previously described (Hope et al 1986); each track contains 0.1 mouse brain equivalents.

affected mice. There are two criteria for strain typing : 1) incubation period, and 2) the induction of different vacuolar lesion profiles in the brain (Fraser et al 1973).

Masters: What is your conclusion?

Hope: We've confirmed the observation of Kascsak and colleagues (Kascsak et al 1986) that there are differences in proteinase K sensitivity of SAF protein prepared from different scrapie models–even though you keep the host genotype constant. Kascsak also showed strain-specific differences in SAF morphology and sedimentation properties.

Masters: This doesn't say anything about the agent itself.

Hope: I agree that it may not tell you about the biochemical structure of scrapie strains; but, in parallel with the biological evidence for many different strains of scrapie, it adds further to the idea that there are replicable differences in scrapie inoculum, which are independent of the host genome (Bruce & Dickinson 1987).

Manuelidis: George (Carlson), does it not bother you that this is a housekeeping gene that is highly conserved in evolution, and that it suddenly becomes infectious when inoculated into an animal?

Carlson: I am not sure that it is a house-keeping protein.

Oesch: This idea of the house-keeping gene is derived from the observation that the promoter does not have a TATA box or a CAAT box, but it does have these GC boxes, which are often found in the promoter regions of house-keeping genes (Basler et al 1986). The *in situ* hybridizations done by Hans Kretzschmar, Stephen DeArmond and others (Kretzschmar et al 1986) showed that the expression of this gene is not uniform throughout the body as you would expect for a house-keeping gene. It is localized, the highest level of expression is in neurons in the brain. It is not correct to say it is a house-keeping gene, because a house-keeping gene is expressed in all cells.

F. Brown: Can't house-keeping genes have localized effects as well? For example, brain house-keeping genes?

Oesch: That is not a true house-keeping gene, that is tissue-specific expression.

Carlson: Selection is important. How would a host gene evolve to become infectious? I think the answer is that its basic physiological function has nothing to do with scrapie. Scrapie, Alzheimer's and CJD are diseases that occur after reproductive age so there would be no selective pressure exerted on deleterious effects of these genes in old age.

Note added in proof by Dr Carlson. Since this symposium, we have sequenced the *Prn-p*[a] and *Prn-p*[b] alleles from NZW/LacJ and I/LnJ mice, and found that the predicted proteins differ from one another at the amino acids coded by codons 108 and 189 (Westaway et al 1987).

References

Basler K, Oesch B, Scott M et al 1986 Scrapie and cellular PrP isoforms are encoded by the same chromosomal gene. Cell 46:417–428

Bruce M, Dickinson AG 1987 Biological evidence that scrapie agent has an independent genome. J Gen Virol 68:79–89

Fraser H, Dickinson AG 1973 Scrapie in mice: agent strain differences in the distribution and intensity of grey matter vacuolation. J Comp Pathol 83:29–40

Kascsak RJ, Rubenstein R, Merz PA et al 1986 Immunological comparison of scrapie-associated fibrils isolated from animals infected with four different scrapie strains. J Virol 59:676–683

Kretzschmar HA, Prusiner SB, Stowring LE, DeArmond SJ 1986 Scrapie prion proteins are synthesized in neurons. Am J Pathol 122:1–5

Westaway D, Goodman PA, Mirenda CA et al 1987 Distinct prion proteins in short and long incubation period mice. Cell 51:651–662

Developmental regulation of prion protein mRNA in brain

Michael P. McKinley*+, Vishwanath R. Lingappa† and Stanley B. Prusiner*‡

Departments of *Neurology, +Anatomy, †Physiology and Medicine, and ‡Biochemistry and Biophysics, University of California, San Francisco, California 94143, USA

Abstract. During development of the hamster brain, synthesis of the cellular isoform of the scrapie prion protein (PrP^C) was found to be regulated. Low levels of PrP poly(A)$^+$ mRNA were detectable one day after birth. PrP poly(A)$^+$ mRNA reached maximal levels between 10 and 20 days post-partum; thereafter, no change in its level could be detected at ages up to 13 months. In contrast, myelin basic protein poly(A)$^+$ mRNA was shown to reach maximal levels by 30 days of age and thereafter steadily declined in adult brain. Using monospecific PrP antisera, immunoprecipitable cell-free translation products were detected at low levels two days after birth and progressively increased up to 10 days of age. How the PrP mRNA participates in brain development and its function in scrapie prion infection are being investigated.

1988 Novel infectious agents and the central nervous system. Wiley, Chichester (Ciba Foundation Symposium 135) p 101–116

The unique molecular properties of the scrapie agent prompted introduction of the term 'prion' to describe this class of infectious pathogens (Prusiner 1982). Purification of scrapie prions led to the identification of a protease-resistant sialoglycoprotein, PrP 27–30, which was subsequently found to be a component of the prion (Bolton et al 1982, Prusiner et al 1982, McKinley et al 1983, Bolton et al 1985). After molecular cloning of a cDNA encoding PrP 27–30 it was shown that a 2.1 kilobase (kb) PrP mRNA is present in both scrapie-infected and uninfected hamster brains (Oesch et al 1985). Antibodies raised against either PrP 27–30 or a synthetic peptide corresponding to the amino terminus of PrP 27–30 (Bendheim et al 1984, Barry et al 1986), identified a cellular isoform of the scrapie prion protein. Its apparent molecular weight (M_r) of 33–35 kilodaltons (kDa) was determined by immunoblotting (Oesch et al 1985, Barry et al 1986). Subsequent studies showed that the molecular weights of both the cellular (PrP^C) and scrapie (PrP^{Sc}) prion protein isoforms are similar (Meyer et al 1986). Proteinase K digestion destroys PrP^C, whereas PrP^{Sc} is only partially hydrolysed to form PrP 27–30.

Identification of the cellular isoform, PrP^C, suggested that studies on this protein might provide insight into the structure and function of the scrapie PrP isoform. Since PrP mRNA was found at constant levels in both scrapie-infected and uninfected adult hamster brains (Oesch et al 1985, Kretzschmar et al 1986), we chose to investigate the regulation of PrP mRNA accumulation in developing hamster brain. PrP mRNA is undetectable until one day after birth and it remains at low levels until about 10 days of age. Between 10 and 20 days after birth, PrP mRNA attains maximal concentrations which appear to be maintained throughout life.

Methods

Total RNA was isolated from the brains of uninfected hamsters using the guanidinium/caesium chloride method of Glisin et al (1974). Poly(A)$^+$ mRNA for Northern analysis was recovered by one cycle of oligo(dT)-chromatography (Aviv & Leder 1972). RNA samples (5 μg) were ethanol precipitated, washed once with absolute ethanol, and dissolved in 50% formamide, 2.2 M formaldehyde. After the addition of one-fifth volume 10% Ficoll, 1% bromophenol blue, the samples were electrophoresed on a 1% agarose gel. The running buffer was 20 mM MOPS (pH 7.0), 1 mM EDTA, 2.2 M formaldehyde. After electrophoresis, the gel was soaked in 20× saline sodium citrate (SSC), and the RNA transferred to nitrocellulose (Thomas 1980). The filters were pre-hybridized and hybridized essentially as described by Shank et al (1978). The *Sau*I to *Taq*I fragment of the pHaPrPcDNA-1 insert (Oesch et al 1985) was labelled to a specific activity of 10^8 d.p.m./μg using random priming with oligonucleotides purchased from BIORAD Laboratories (Taylor et al 1976), as modified by Payne et al (1981). Hybridizations were performed at 42°C in 3× SSC, 50% formamide, 0.05 M HEPES (pH 7.4), 0.2 mg/ml salmon sperm DNA, 0.15 mg/ml yeast RNA, 0.02% bovine serum albumin, 0.02% polyvinyl pyrrolidone. Filters were washed in 0.1× SSC, 0.1% sodium dodecyl sulphate (SDS) at 60°C and autoradiographed for 1–5 days at −70°C using Dupont Cronex intensifying screens and Kodak XAR-5 film.

Cell-free translations were performed on RNA extracted as described above from freshly dissected brains of hamsters of various ages. One A_{260} unit of RNA was diluted into a translation reaction pre-mix with a final volume of 100 μl and final concentration of 20 mM HEPES (pH 7.5), 140 mM K acetate, 3 mM dithiothreitol (DTT), 2.2 mM Mg acetate plus Mg chloride, 10 mM Tris-HCl (pH 7.5), 0.4 mM spermidine, 1 mM ATP and GTP, 10 mM creatine phosphate, 40 mM of each of 19 L-amino acids except methionine, 1 mCi/ml [^{35}S]methionine (1200 Ci/mmole), 0.1 mg/ml calf liver tRNA, 20 μg/ml creatine phosphokinase, 1 U/ml ribonuclease inhibitor and 20% by volume wheat-germ extract prepared according to the method of Erikson & Blobel (1983) at a concentration of 2.5 A_{280} units/ml. Translations were incubated for 1 h at 24°C. Samples (2 µl) to be analysed for total products were dissolved directly in 15 µl of SDS sample buffer (10% SDS, 0.1 M Tris-acetate pH 8.9, 0.5 M DTT), and boiled for two minutes before SDS polyacrylamide gel electrophoresis and fluorography by a modification of the method of Bonner & Laskey (1974). Samples to be immunoprecipitated (98 µl) were precipitated with trichloroacetic acid, washed with ethanol:ether (1:1), and solubilized in 100 µl of 1% SDS, 0.1 M Tris-acetate pH 8, 0.1 M NaC1, 10 mM EDTA, 1 mM phenylmethylsulphonylchloride before addition of PrP 27–30 antisera (Bendheim et al 1984). Antigen-antibody complexes were pelleted with Protein A Sepharose, washed and resuspended in SDS sample buffer.

The presence of myelin basic protein (MBP) mRNA in hamster brain samples was detected using a cDNA encoding rat MBP (Roach et al 1983). MBP cDNA was labelled by random priming as above. Hybridizations were performed as described except formamide was at 40% concentration. Filters were washed in 1× SSC, 0.1% SDS at 55°C before autoradiography.

Results

We investigated the possibility that the expression of PrP mRNA is developmentally regulated, since a prion protein cellular isoform and its mRNA were found in adult animals (Oesch et al 1985). Poly(A)+ mRNA was prepared from the brains of uninfected hamsters at one day before birth, as well as at post-natal days 1, 2, 4, 6, 8, 10 and 20. Ethidium bromide profiles showed that RNA was not degraded. Northern blotting with a labelled cDNA fragment derived principally from the open reading frame identified a 2.1 kb transcript in samples prepared from animals at 10 and 20 days of age (Fig. 1). In other studies described below, the level of the PrP transcript remained unchanged throughout the lifetime of the animal. No difference between the levels of PrP mRNA at 20 days of age and 13 months was found.

Cell-free translation studies were undertaken using total RNA isolated from hamster brains at various times before and after birth. No PrP-related translation products were seen with the prenatal RNA isolated one day before birth. The translation products were precipitated using monospecific antiserum raised against a synthetic peptide corresponding to the N-terminal 13 amino acids of PrP 27–30 (Barry et al 1986). At two and four days after birth a faint PrP-related translation product of approximately 23 kDa was found (Fig. 2). By six days of age this product was readily discerned and continued to increase at eight and ten days of age. The lanes with preimmune serum showed no immunoprecipitable products from the translation mixture. When the total RNA used in these cell-free translation studies was blotted for Northern analysis without prior purification on an oligo(dT) cellulose column, an RNA of 2.1 kb was identified at eight days after birth which hybrid-

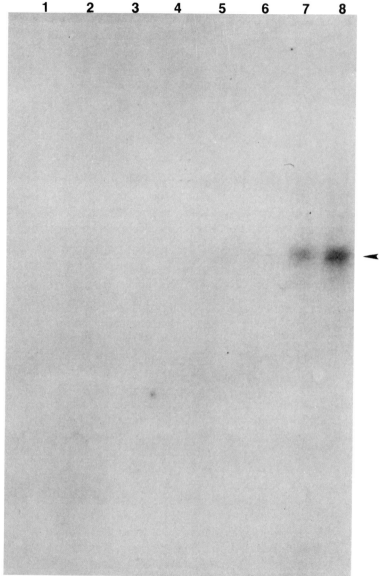

FIG. 1. Northern analysis of PrP mRNA during early development of the hamster brain. Lane 1 contains poly(A)⁺ mRNA from uninfected hamster brains at one day before birth. Lanes 2–8 contain poly(A)⁺ mRNA from hamster brains at 1, 2, 4, 6, 8, 10 and 20 days after birth, respectively. The arrow indicates 2.1 kb.

ized with a PrP cDNA. Again, the level of PrP mRNA did not change throughout the next 13 months.

When 5 μg of poly(A)⁺ mRNA was analysed by Northern blots from

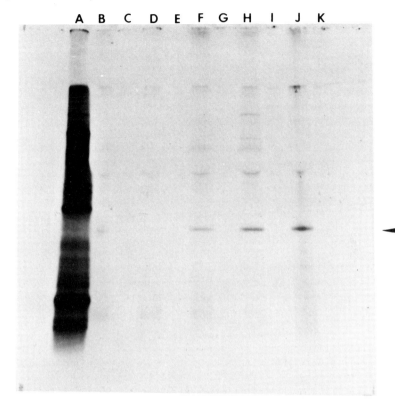

FIG. 2. Developmental profile of RNA encoding PrP immunoreactive products. Autoradiography revealed a very small amount of PrP immunoreactive product from 2- and 4-day-old brain extracts (B and D), and much higher levels in the immune lanes for days 6, 8 and 10 (F, H, J). A, total translation products; B, 2-day immune; C, 2-day preimmune; D, 4-day immune; E, 4-day preimmune; F, 6-day immune; G, 6-day preimmune; H, 8-day immune; I, 8-day preimmune; J, 10-day immune; K, 10-day preimmune. Arrow is 23 kDa product.

animals one day of age, no PrP-related transcript could be detected (Figs. 1 and 3). Increasing the poly(A)$^+$ mRNA concentration fivefold from 5 μg to 25 μg per lane resulted in a faint but detectable signal (Fig. 3A, lane 2). These results are consistent with those observed with the cell-free translation described in Fig. 2. As shown in Fig. 3A (lanes 3–6), there was no change in the level of the PrP mRNA between one and four months of age. As noted above, the level of PrP mRNA was the same at both one and 13 months.

In contrast to PrP mRNA, which is detected at one day after birth when five times as much poly(A)$^+$ mRNA is loaded onto the gel, no detectable signal is found with a hybridization probe which encodes rat MBP. As shown in Fig. 3B, there is an intense MBP mRNA signal for 30-day-old animals,

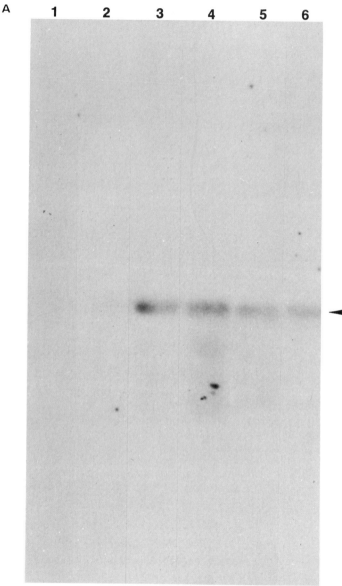

FIG. 3.   Northern analysis of PrP and MBP poly(A)$^+$ mRNA during development of
the hamster brain. (A) PrP poly(A)$^+$ mRNA. Lane 1 is 5 μg of poly(A)$^+$ mRNA from
1-day old hamster brain. Lane 2 is 25 μg of poly(A)$^+$ mRNA from 1-day-old hamster
brain. Lanes 3–6 contain 5 μg of poly(A)$^+$ mRNA from 30-day, 60-day, 90-day and

which decreases progressively as the animals age. This agrees with the developmental regulation of MBP and its mRNA levels in the rodent brain
(Zeller et al 1984).

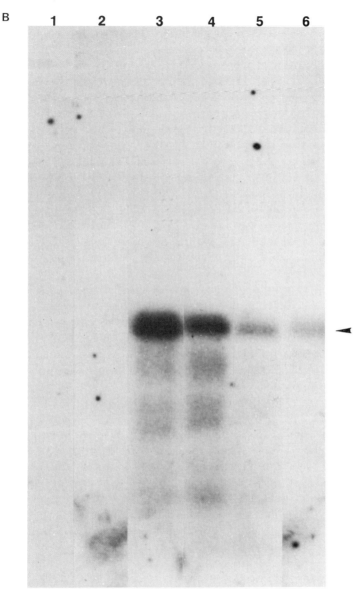

120-day-old hamster brains, respectively. Arrow indicates 2.1 kb. (B) MBP poly(A)$^+$ mRNA. Lanes 1–6 contained samples identical to those described in (A). Arrow indicates 2.0 kb.

Discussion

The role of PrP^C in cellular metabolism is unknown. The highest concentrations of PrP mRNA are found in brain, with other organs showing significant but lower levels of the transcript (Oesch et al 1985). It is not known whether the PrP mRNA detected in organs other than brain reflects the presence of the transcript in the stroma of these organs or in the peripheral nerves which innervate the organs. In the brain, PrP^C is synthesized primarily in neurons (Kretzschmar et al 1986). PrP^C is a membrane-associated protein, while PrP^{Sc} is amphipathic (Meyer et al 1986). Late during scrapie infection a small portion of PrP^{Sc} is detected within extracellular spaces in the form of amyloid filaments (DeArmond et al 1985). Although PrP^C and PrP^{Sc} have profoundly different properties, the molecular basis for their differences remains to be established. PrP^{Sc} is protease resistant and is found only in infected animals; PrP^C is protease sensitive and is found in both uninfected controls and infected animals. Interestingly, the only PrP transcript identified in scrapie-infected hamster brain is a 2.1 kb mRNA which is apparently identical to that present in uninfected control brain. While PrP poly(A)$^+$ mRNA increases during the early development of the brain, it does not change following scrapie infection even though the level of PrP^{Sc} increases in parallel with the titre of prions.

The marked morphological and physiological changes which occur during mammalian brain development are accompanied by or result from changes in gene expression. The temporal correlation between the synthesis of specific proteins and neuronal differentiation strongly suggests that brain-specific functions are accompanied by precisely regulated steady-state levels of specific brain mRNAs (Morrison et al 1981). As neurons differentiate in rodents, after post-natal day six, the rates of synaptogenesis and myelination of neurons increase (Morrison et al 1981).

The adult mouse brain contains both poly(A)$^+$ and poly(A)$^-$ mRNAs which exhibit similar degrees of complexity. It has been suggested that virtually all adult brain poly(A)$^+$ mRNAs are present at birth, whereas most poly(A)$^-$ mRNAs are absent (Chaudhari & Hahn 1983). Interestingly, poly(A)$^-$ mRNAs appear soon after birth, suggesting that they specify proteins required for brain functions that emerge during the course of post-natal development (Chaudhari & Hahn 1983). Although the levels are low, PrP poly(A)$^+$ mRNA is clearly present at one day of age. There is no evidence for a poly(A)$^-$ mRNA encoding PrP. Approximately 35% of the poly(A)$^+$ mRNA found in brain is also found in other tissues, suggesting 'housekeeping' functions for the encoded proteins. Recent studies have shown that the hamster PrP gene lacks a TATA box promoter but does contain GC rich repeats which are typical of 'housekeeping' gene promoters (Basler et al 1986).

The low level of PrP mRNA at birth is an interesting observation with respect to the development of scrapie infection. When newborn mice were inoculated peripherally with scrapie prions during the first six hours after birth, the incubation period was increased nearly threefold (Hotchin &

Buckley 1977). Whether or not this delay in scrapie infection is related to the expression or regulation of PrP mRNA remains to be established. Intracerebral inoculation of newborn mice abolished the delay in scrapie infection, suggesting that systemic transport or processing of injected prions may be responsible for this delay and not the level of intraneuronal PrP mRNA.

Whether or not the regulation of PrP mRNA expression is coordinated with that of other neuronal proteins remains to be determined. The mechanism by which the levels of PrP transcripts are modulated is unknown. Although PrP^C does not assemble into filaments, PrP^{Sc} does, and transcriptional regulation of the gene for intermediate filament proteins during development is well documented (Capoetanski et al 1984).

The developmental regulation of the mammalian brain is certainly the most complex and highly programmed phase of differentiation in all living organisms. The large number of cell types and their extensive connections in the central nervous system present a fascinating problem in deciphering the controlling elements in brain development. Our finding that PrP^C in brain is under developmental control poses many interesting questions with respect to neuronal maturation, the control of synaptogenesis and susceptibility to scrapie prion infection. We are currently investigating (1) the regulation of PrP mRNA levels in developing hamster brain, (2) expression of PrP mRNA in various brain regions during maturation of the neonatal hamsters, and (3) the effect on scrapie incubation time of inoculation of scrapie into newborn hamsters. These studies are being pursued to try to acquire some understanding of the appearance and regulation of brain levels of PrP^C, the relationship of PrP^C and PrP^{Sc} in newly infected animals, and the role that other, as yet undetermined, factors may have in scrapie pathogenesis in rodents.

Acknowledgements

The authors thank L. Gallagher for manuscript production assistance. This work was supported by research grants from the National Institutes of Health (AG02132 and NS14069) and a Senator Jacob Javits Center of Excellence in Neuroscience (NS22786) as well as by gifts from Sherman Fairchild Foundation and RJR-Nabisco, Inc.

References

Aviv H, Leder P 1972 Purification of biologically active globin messenger RNA by chromatography on oligothymidylic acid-cellulose. Proc Natl Acad Sci USA 69:1408–1412

Barry RA, Kent SBH, McKinley MP et al 1986 Scrapie and cellular prion proteins share polypeptide epitopes. J Infect Dis 153:848–854

Basler KB, Oesch B, Scott M et al 1986 Scrapie and cellular PrP isoforms are encoded by the same chromosomal gene. Cell 46:417–428

Bendheim PE, Barry RA, DeArmond SJ, Stites DP, Prusiner SB 1984 Antibodies to a scrapie prion protein. Nature (Lond) 310:418–421

Bolton DC, McKinley MP, Prusiner SB 1982 Identification of a protein that purifies with the scrapie prion. Science (Wash DC) 218:1309–1311

Bolton DC, Meyer RK, Prusiner SB 1985 Scrapie PrP 27–30 is a sialoglycoprotein. J Virol 53:596–606

Bonner W, Laskey R 1974 A film detection method for tritium-labeled proteins and nucleic acids in polyacrylamide gels. Eur J Biochem 46:83–88

Capoetanski YG, Ngai J, Lazarides E 1984 Regulation of the expression of genes coding for the intermediate filament subunits vimentin, desmin, and glial fibrillary acidic protein. In: Brisy G et al (eds) Molecular biology of the cytoskeleton. Cold Spring Harbor Laboratory, Cold Spring Harbor, New York, p 415–434

Chaudhari N, Hahn W 1983 Genetic expression in the developing brain. Science (Wash DC) 220:924–928

DeArmond SJ, McKinley MP, Barry RA, Braunfeld MB, McCulloch JR, Prusiner SB 1985 Identification of prion amyloid filaments in scrapie-infected brain. Cell 41:221–235

Erikson A, Blobel G 1983 Cell-free translation of messenger RNA in a wheat germ system. Methods Enzymol 96:38–49

Glisin V, Crkvenjakov R, Byus C 1974 Ribonucleic acid isolated by cesium chloride centrifugation. Biochemistry 13:2633–2641

Hotchin J, Buckley R 1977 Latent form of scrapie virus: a new factor in slow virus disease. Science (Wash DC) 196:668–671

Kretzschmar HA, Prusiner SB, Stowring LE, DeArmond SJ 1986 Scrapie prion proteins are synthesized in neurons. Am J Pathol 122:1–5

McKinley MP, Bolton DC, Prusiner SB 1983 A protease resistant protein is a structural component of the scrapie prion. Cell 35:57–62

Meyer RK, McKinley MP, Bowman KA, Barry RA, Prusiner SB 1986 Separation and properties of cellular and scrapie prion proteins. Proc Natl Acad Sci USA 83:2310–2314

Morrison M, Pardue S, Griffin WST 1981 Developmental alterations in the levels of translationally active messenger RNAs in the postnatal rat cerebellum. J Biol Chem 256:3550–3556

Oesch B, Westaway D, Wälchli M et al 1985 A cellular gene encodes scrapie PrP 27–30 protein. Cell 40:735–746

Payne GS, Courtneidge SA, Crittenden LB, Fadly AM, Bishop JM, Varmus HE 1981 Analysis of avian leukosis virus DNA and RNA in bousal tumors: viral gene expression is not required for maintenance of the tumor state. Cell 23:311–322

Prusiner SB 1982 Novel proteinaceous infectious particles cause scrapie. Science (Wash DC) 216:136–144

Prusiner SB, Bolton DC, Groth DF, Bowman KA, Cochran SP, McKinley MP 1982 Further purification and characterization of scrapie prions. Biochemistry 21:6942–6950

Roach A, Boylan K, Horvath S, Prusiner SB, Hood LE 1983 Characterization of cloned cDNA representing rat myelin basic protein: absence of expression in brain of shiverer mutant mice. Cell 34:799–806

Shank PR, Hughes SH, Kung HJ et al 1978 Mapping integrates avian sarcoma virus DNA: termini of linear DNA bear 300 nucleotides present once or twice in two species of circular DNA. Cell 15:1383–1395

Taylor JM, Illmensee R, Summers J 1976 Efficient transcription of RNA into DNA by avian sarcoma virus polymerase. Biochim Biophys Acta 442:324–330

Thomas PS 1980 Hybridization of denatured RNA and small DNA fragments to nitrocellulose. Proc Natl Acad Sci USA 77:5201–5205

Zeller NK, Hunkeller MJ, Campagnoni AT, Sprague J, Lazzarini RA 1984 Characterization of mouse myelin basic protein messenger RNAs with a myelin basic protein
cDNA clone. Proc Natl Acad Sci USA 81:18–22

DISCUSSION

F. Brown: Did you measure infectivity titres in spleen versus brain when you
had those differences in the mRNA?

McKinley: Those are currently being repeated in animals. We have done it
more than once.

Roberts: It seems that the less prion you have being made in the brain, the
faster the animals die of scrapie. This is rather paradoxical.

McKinley: Our developmental studies showed that there is very little or no
detectable PrP messenger RNA in the brain during the first few days of life in
hamsters. Hotchin had found that if you inoculated newborn mice i.p., there
was a latency—it took three times longer for the animals to become sick with
scrapie; however, their i.c. data were no different when comparing time and
route of inoculation (Hotchin & Buckley 1977). We obtained the opposite
results: incubation times in neonatal hamsters were reduced in both i.c. and i.p.
inoculated animals when PrP mRNA was very low. It is a bit confusing. We
don't understand the relationship between PrP^{Sc} and PrP^C at this point. It
would be nice to postulate that PrP^{Sc} merely converts PrP^C to more PrP^{Sc}, so
PrP^C might interact with the PrP^{Sc} in the inoculum. We don't know what the
mechanism is for replication of the scrapie agent, but if you challenge hamsters
with an inoculation, either i.c. or i.p., before they are 10–14 days old, before
there is much PrP^C present, they become sick more rapidly than do older
animals in which PrP^C has reached a constant level.

Dickinson: In 1978 I criticized the Hotchin and Buckley work that you are
quoting as deficient in many respects, including intercurrent deaths. Outram et
al (1973) found that as age decreased before weaning so the population of
incubation periods became progressively bimodal, and as titre of infectivity
increased there was a trend towards short incubation models predominating
over long incubation models. As Outram et al showed, this is not a small effect:
within the 0–1 day, 1–2 day intervals in the mouse changes of greater than three
standard deviations are occurring. One problem is that you can't give an
intraperitoneal injection without being in danger of giving a subcutaneous
injection. If you review your own data in the light of that, you might interpret
them rather differently.

Carp: Surely the shortening of the incubation period in a system where there
is little or no detectable PrP mRNA is suggestive evidence that the PrP has
nothing to do with incubation period or with scrapie agent!

McKinley: There is some PrP messenger RNA there. One day before birth we can detect it in the brainstem. In neocortex (we looked for PrP mRNA in 11 different regions of the brain) there are low levels of PrP mRNA. One hypothesis is that, if you inoculate animals after PrP^C has reached its maximal amount, PrP^C competes with PrP^{Sc} for a finite number of receptors. It could be that the interval from the time of inoculation until onset of clinical symptoms would be comparable to that found in neonates, if one could decrease this pool of PrP^C present in the brain of weanling hamsters. When PrP^C is present, the prions in the inoculum take longer to bring on the disease.

Prusiner: I would interpret this slightly differently. I think it reflects what Richard Kimberlin was saying, that there are several phases of scrapie infection. One is this initiation phase and what we have probably accomplished is to separate this from subsequent phases. We find low PrP mRNA and low PrP^C expression during the early phase of infection and the initiation is accelerated by these conditions—it seems to be paradoxical. You have to remember that during most of the incubation period in these animals there are maximal PrP mRNA levels. There is an initiation phase followed by a replication phase; indeed, it may be even more complicated.

Kimberlin: I think it is relevant to remind people of the wonderful paradox about the intrasciatic route of infection. It is a very inefficient route but when it works it gives very short incubations! Indeed, successful infection of the sciatic nerve gave shorter incubation periods than by intracerebral inoculation. You cannot interpret incubation period differences by themselves because you don't know whether you are altering the initial infection process, local replication and spread to neighbouring cells, or affecting later events such as spread to clinical target areas.

Masters: Is the highest concentration of PrP mRNA and protein in the brain and the least in the liver?

McKinley: The problem with our studies on liver is that the animals were not starved prior to tissue isolation and glycogen in the liver contaminated the RNA preparations, so the amount of PrP mRNA there was probably underestimated.

Masters: What's the next organ in the scale downwards?

McKinley: I think heart and lung are next in terms of PrP mRNA.

Masters: Did you find PrP^{Sc} in the heart?

McKinley: I haven't looked for it.

Bolton: We have looked for Cp 33–37 and Sp 33–37 in the heart and don't find either. We do find a protein that we call p54, which reacts specifically with the antibody raised against scrapie protein (A Potempska, D C Bolton, P E Bendheim, unpublished). We can't tell if it is structurally related to the PrP protein or whether it is just an antigenic relationship.

Diringer: Mike, you said that PrP^C is not related to infectivity, but PrP^{Sc} is.

McKinley: I said that PrP 27–30 was associated with infectivity.

Diringer: You also showed that PrP mRNA is present in the spleen, but you should have shown that PrP^{Sc} is present there, if you want to relate this to infectivity. We could not find any PrP^{Sc} in the spleen.

McKinley: Shinagawa and his colleagues (1986) published a Western blot showing that PrP is present in the spleen of mice. We showed that the messenger RNA is there in mice and hamsters, and they have demonstrated that the protein is present.

Diringer: We tried to relate SAF protein (or PrP^{Sc} as you call it) to infectivity titres in a quantitative manner. We could not find this pathological protein at all in spleen, even if we immunoblotted a purified preparation derived from two grams of spleen tissue (Czub et al 1986).

McKinley: It could be your purification protocol.

Merz: SAF have been reported in the spleen (Merz et al 1983,1984,1985) and PrPs have been detected in the spleens of scrapie-infected animals (Rubenstein et al 1986,1987, Shinagawa et al 1986).

*Chesebro:*I think we should go back and repeat these experiments of the same preparations, quantitatively. The Japanese group has found PrP^{Sc} but they don't have your samples and are not necessarily measuring titres of infectivity. We need the quantitative comparison; this is difficult because the quantitative range for accurate assay of the protein is not the same range as the assay for infectivity. We can measure titres of infectivity plus or minus tenfold over 6 or 7 logs but we can only measure protein titres over one order of magnitude.

F. Brown: Can't you titrate the protein serologically?

Chesebro: The concentration is so low that we are already near the limit of detection.

Bolton: Using quantitative Western blotting we can measure about a fifty thousandfold difference in the amount of the protein purified from brain. However, in the spleen the amount is reduced by a factor of 100 or 1000.

F. Brown: What would you expect the infectivity to be in the spleen under these conditions?

Gabizon: It is about a 100-fold lower.

Prusiner: In summary, there are at least two groups that agree independently that PrP mRNA is present in the spleen, that's in San Francisco (Oesch et al 1985) and in Hamilton, Montana (Caughey et al, this volume). There are three groups that agree that the protein is there in the spleen: Staten Island, NY (Rubenstein et al 1986), Hokaido, Japan, (Shinagawa et al 1986) and Bethesda, MD (Gibbs et al, American Society of Virology meeting 1986). We all agree that the titre in spleen is at least 10-fold lower than in brain, sometimes as much as 100-fold lower.

Kimberlin: The biggest differential is with 263K scrapie in hamsters - there is a 3 to 4 log difference between maximum brain titres and plateau spleen titres. 139A or ME7 scrapie in *Sinc*^{s7} mice would be about 10 to 100-fold lower in spleen than in brain.

Carp: In our experience with 263K in the hamster we get about 5 or 6 logs difference between brain titre and spleen titre.

Chesebro: You can't approach the comparison of PrP concentration and infectivity titre in the hamster spleen because of the very low infectivity titre, it is only possible in the mouse where the titre in spleen is relatively high.

Dormont: We also detected PrP mRNA in spleen in mice, at the same level in normal, scrapie-infected and CJD-infected animals. We have different results in newborn mice inoculated i.c. or i.p. We observed an increase in incubation period when we inoculated i.p. before mice were 12 hours old. With i.c. injection it is less evident. The pathology is very different in newborn mice inoculated i.c. or i.p.: spongiosis and vacuolation are dramatically increased in comparison with mice which were adult at the time of the inoculation.

*Dickinson:*There is a technical point: because titre goes up so quickly in spleen and reaches a plateau long before anything happens in the brain, the question should be asked at the early stage. That excludes Pat Merz's data, which show SAF in the spleen later. The question is, whether you can find PrP message and protein in the spleen before events have started in the brain after inoculation by a peripheral route. That avoids the problem of something coming out of damaged brain and localizing in the spleen.

Kimberlin: What you find in early spleen is likely to be a true reflection of events in the LRS, uncomplicated by any contribution from damaged CNS or peripheral nerves because infectivity won't have progressed that far.

Prusiner: No, I disagree with you completely. If you inoculate indian ink or labelled bacteriophage i.c., 95 or 99% of the inoculum will pass into the circulation within an hour.

Kimberlin: That's not the point; we are talking about i.p. inoculations.

Chesebro: I agree with Alan that if we want a good association we need to do a peripheral inoculation and then show the association of infectivity and PrP^{Sc} in the spleen early, before late pathological effects develop.

Merz: We did such an experiment. We inoculated an animal i.c. with a 1% brain homogenate, removed the spleen at 70 days when you have achieved maximum replication of the agent and minimal contamination with brain material, and inoculated it i.p. into C57BL mice. Extremely low levels of SAF were detected in the spleen three to four weeks after that inoculation; we could not detect PrP. We have only recently begun to determine the levels of SAF needed by our criteria to obtain a positive Western blot for PrP.

Diringer: Mike, you showed Western blots of PrP^{C} and PrP^{Sc} in brain homogenates. In brain from scrapie-infected hamsters without treatment with proteinase K you find no PrP 27-30 (Lane 3).

McKinley: For this experiment we didn't see a band that we could identify as PrP 27-30 when the sample was not pre-treated with proteinase K. The brain was homogenized in the presence of protease inhibitors.

Diringer: So it is not necessary to degrade this protein to make it infectious?

McKinley: We don't know what happens to a sample when the inoculum is put into the brain of the animal.

Hope: We have immunoblots of 87V in IM mice which look exactly like that (see Fig. 1a, lane 3: Hope & Hunter, this volume); you can't see any degraded products in total brain homogenate. However, if you take the preparation through a purification procedure you begin to see those degraded products. The degradation is not occurring during purification, but there is so much protein in the crude homogenate that it is blocking the binding of components which are present in much lower amounts (see also Discussion after Hope & Hunter).

Prusiner: What do you think its significance is?

Hope: I don't know; it may be related to the aggregation of the SAF.

Bolton: But by N-terminal sequencing at least 90% of the sequences have the predicted amino acid sequence, Lys-Lys-Arg-Pro-Lys. We do not see the predicted PrP 27-30 sequence appearing. So even though there are these lower molecular weight forms, they may not be the result of peptide degradation, they may be incomplete post-translational modifications.

Hope: The majority of the protein starts with the Lys-Lys-Arg sequence but we do find minor amounts of variant forms (Hope & Hunter, this volume).

*Wisniewski:*Mike McKinley said that antibody against PrP can neutralize infectivity. This is remarkable, because the infectivity is resistant to almost every other means of inactivation.

Prusiner: The PrP antibody neutralization studies of scrapie infectivity are still at a preliminary stage but the results look encouraging.

Kimberlin: I was intrigued, Michael, by the fact that NGF given on the same day as scrapie shortened the incubation by two weeks, whereas NGF given two days before scrapie didn't give that shortening. What is NGF doing which wears off after two days?

McKinley: If we gave NGF either by a three day regimen of injections or by a single injection, two days after the last injection there was a massive increase in the amount of PrP messenger RNA in the septum. That suggests that this process occurs in the basal forebrain. If we inject newborn animals with NGF and then inoculate scrapie two days later, that acceleration of incubation period is markedly reduced.

Kimberlin: So whatever NGF is doing, it has stopped two days later?

McKinley: No, we know that NGF increases the amount of PrP messenger RNA in specific areas of the brain, i.e. septum. This effect continues to work for several days.

Masters: Mike, are you saying that the PrP^C has something to do with the cholinergic system because of this response to NGF? Is there a selective localization of PrP^C in the cholinergic system? What about the cerebral cortex or other areas of the brain?

McKinley: Certainly PrP^C occurs outside the cholinergic system.

*DeArmond:*We (DeArmond et al 1987) see a lot of PrP^C in the septal cholinergic neurons and in the cholinergic neurons which extend into the septo-hypothalamic area in normal hamsters. In the cerebellar cortex, scattered Purkinje cells that are not cholinergic contain PrP^C, as do neurons throughout the hippocampal formation which are also not cholinergic. Therefore, the prion protein is also expressed in many non-cholinergic neurons. However, it appears that NGF stimulates PrP messenger RNA production in cholinergic neurons; if we knew the stimulating factors for the other neuronal systems, we might get a similar increase in PrP mRNA in them.

McKinley: Another experiment that we are doing now is inoculating with NGF then regionally dissecting the brain and looking for PrP^C by Western blotting.

References

Caughey B, Race, Vogel M, Buchmeier M, Chesebro B 1988 In vitro expression of cloned PrP cDNA derived from scrapie-infected mouse brain: lack of transmission of scrapie infectivity. In: Novel infectious agents and the central nervous system. Wiley, Chichester (Ciba Found Symp 135) p 197–208

Czub M, Braig HR, Blode H, Diringer H 1986 The major protein of SAF is absent from spleen and thus not an essential part of the scrapie agent. Arch Virol 91:383–386

DeArmond SJ, Mobley WC, DeMott DL, Barry RA, Beckstead JH, Prusiner SB 1987 Changes in the localization of brain prion proteins during scrapie infection. Neurology 37:1271–1280

Hope J, Hunter N 1988 Scrapie-associated fibrils, PrP protein and the sinc gene. In: Novel infectious agents and the central nervous system. Wiley, Chichester (Ciba Found Symp 135) p 146–163

Hotchin J, Buckley R 1977 Latent form of scrapie virus: a new factor in slow virus disease. Science (Wash DC) 196:668–671

Merz PA, Somerville RA, Wisniewski HM, Manuelidis L, Manuelidis EE 1983 Scrapie associated fibrils in Creutzfeldt-Jakob disease. Nature (Lond) 306:474–476

Merz PA, Rohwer RR, Somerville RA, Wisniewski HM, Gibbs Jr CJ, Gadjusek DC 1984 Infection-specific particle from the unconventional slow virus diseases. Science 225:437–440

Merz PA, Kascsak R, Rubenstein R, Carp RI, Wisniewski HM 1985 Variations in SAF from different scrapie agents. In: Tateishi J (ed) Proc Workshop on slow transmissible diseases. Japanese Ministry of Health and Welfare, Tokyo, p 137–145

Oesch B, Westaway D, Wälchli M et al 1985 A cellular gene encodes scrapie PrP 27–30 protein. Cell 40:735–746

Outram GW, Dickinson AG, Fraser H 1973 Developmental maturation of susceptibility to scrapie in mice. Nature (Lond) 241:536–537

Rubenstein R, Kascsak RJ, Merz PA et al 1986 Detection of scrapie associated fibril (SAF) proteins using anti-SAF antibody in non-purified tissue preparations. J Gen Virol 67:671–681

Rubenstein R, Merz PA, Kascsak R et al 1987 Detection of scrapie associated fibrils (SAF) and SAF proteins from scrapie affected sheep. J Infect Dis 156:36–42

Shinagawa M, Munekata E, Doi S, Takahashi K, Gato H, Sato G 1986 Immunoreactivity of a synthetic pentadecapeptide corresponding to the N-terminal region of the scrapie prion protein. J Gen Virol 67:1745-1750

Potential involvement of retroviral elements in human dementias

Laura Manuelidis, Geoffrey Murdoch and Elias E. Manuelidis

Yale University School of Medicine, 310 Cedar Street, New Haven, Connecticut 06510, USA

Abstract. Creutzfeldt-Jakob disease (CJD) is a dementia of humans caused by a class of infectious agents with several biological properties similar to those of conventional viruses. The molecular nature of this group of agents is enigmatic, for neither an agent-specific nucleic acid nor a non-host protein has yet been identified. Recent transmissions of familial CJD dementias to rodents suggest that this class of agent can be integrated into the germline. Furthermore, tissue culture studies indicate that CJD causes transformation of cells in a manner reminiscent of slowly oncogenic retroviruses. Currently characterized retroviral-like elements include many forms that do not have 'typical' retroviral ultra-structural morphology; several forms are also known to be resistant to various types of standard physicochemical inactivation. We suggest that CJD agents are either constituted by retroviral-like nucleic acids or interact with endogenous retroviral sequences to elicit a slowly progressive disease of the central nervous system. Several overlapping properties between infectious CJD and 'non-infectious' dementias, such as Alzheimer's disease, implicate potential common pathogenic mechanisms.

1988 Novel infectious agents and the central nervous system. Wiley, Chichester (Ciba Foundation Symposium 135) p 117–134

Disparate hypotheses concerning the nature of the 'unconventional' agents are possible depending on which data are chosen for citation. On the one hand, biological and virological data are most compatible with a conventional viral assembly, i.e. a protein-nucleic acid complex (Manuelidis & Manuelidis 1986). On the other hand, physicochemical studies support the concept of an infectious moiety that lacks significant nucleic acid (Prusiner 1987). In this paper we consider recent compelling biological data in Creutzfeldt-Jakob disease (CJD) that emphasize the requirement for an agent-specific nucleic acid, and we propose a model that 1) encompasses the array of virological and biochemical evidence accumulated to date, 2) is experimentally testable, and 3) has potential implications for the aetiology and mechanisms involved in the more common human dementias such as Alzheimer's disease (AD).

A few well known but salient biological properties of the unconventional viral diseases are worth reiterating, as they clearly imply an entity that contains significant nucleic acid. Scrapie, shown as early as 1936 to be an infectious disease by inoculation studies by Cuillé and Chelle, replicates with a typical exponential progression (Kimberlin & Walker 1986, Czub et al 1986). These findings are difficult to reconcile with known properties of proteins. Although there are model systems in which a protein derepresses its own synthesis, these mechanisms result in accumulation of protein with only an arithmetic progression, not a geometric (log) one. A second scenario involves the production of a modified version of a normal host protein that allows it to behave as an infectious entity; this is the current version of the 'prion' (infectious protein) hypothesis (Prusiner 1987). In this case the modified protein would have to elicit a cascade of identical self-alterations in a unique tissue-specific pattern. Because the CJD agent is present in blood (E.E. Manuelidis et al 1978b), all organs are exposed to the infectious agent. It is therefore difficult to explain the lack of correlation between infectivity and the levels of 'prion' protein in different tissues. For example, the lung is rich in this protein but is very low in infectivity, while spleen tissue is reasonably infectious and contains, at most, only traces of this protein (Locht et al 1986, Robakis et al 1986). Furthermore, purified forms of this protein, including those made from an expression vector (Caughey et al, this volume) are not infectious. Another biological feature which indicates that nucleic acid is a constituent of these agents is that different agent isolates show distinct clinical and pathological characteristics. In scrapie for example, incubation time, development of plaques in inbred strains of mice (Bruce et al 1976) and pathological targeting of different neuronal regions (Fraser & Dickinson 1973) appear to depend at least in part on the derivation of the infectious isolate. Furthermore, cross-species transmissions of CJD and the behaviour of these human agents in serial rodent passages (Manuelidis & Manuelidis 1986) also suggest that there are distinct agent isolates, most consistent with a mutable or adaptable nucleic acid component. Some of our more recent transmission studies in CJD extend these observations.

Transmission studies

Individual CJD isolates have distinguishing properties. We have transmitted 21/23 human subacute and chronic CJD dementia cases to rodents. These accumulated transmissions represent a success rate of 90%, and no transmissions were observed with a variety of control human and rodent samples. Our western hemisphere CJD isolates are clearly different from several Japanese CJD isolates with respect to incubation time characteristics in mice; the Japanese CJD material can cause a relatively rapid (~120 day) incubation in mice, whereas none of our CJD isolates tested to date cause clinically apparent disease in less than 250 days in any of six mouse strains, including some of those used for the Japanese CJD transmissions (Tateishi et al 1981). Although all of our CJD isolates are slow in mice, several of the isolates tested do have distinguishing strain-specific patterns in incubation time (Fig. 1A). Additionally, some of our CJD isolates also cause pathological sequelae in distinct anatomical regions of hamster brain (E.E. Manuelidis et al 1978a). None of our CJD isolates behave identically to scrapie isolates.

In scrapie, incubation time appears to be strongly influenced by a major mouse genetic locus (*Sinc*), and characteristic restriction fragment length polymorphisms within this locus have been linked to scrapie incubation time (Bruce et al 1976, Carlson et al 1986). Although this genetic locus may not be as critical for western hemisphere CJD isolates (Fig. 1A), specific host genetic parameters can strongly influence the course of CJD in rodents regardless of the source of the inoculum. For example, CJD-induced demyelination is prominent only in certain strains of mice. In these mouse strains demyelination occurs irrespective of the CJD isolate inoculated (E.E. Manuelidis et al 1987a). The influence of host factors is also illustrated by the strong species effect on incubation time. Fig. 1B shows that CJD serially passaged in mice is slow. However, the agent again displays the characteristic short hamster incubation time even in the first transfer to hamsters. These observations raise the intriguing question of whether an agent-specific nucleic acid can interact with host genetic sequences. The retroviral restrictions in different inbred mouse strains and in hamsters deserve further investigation in this context (vide infra).

Gerstmann-Sträussler-Sheinker disease (GSS), a 'familial' human dementia with a chronic course, provides an opportunity to examine potential agent/ genome interactions. This rare disease has been documented in several families, and in at least five well studied families an autosomal dominant inheritance pattern is observed (Seitelberger 1981). The inheritance pattern of GSS (and also of familial CJD) is similar to that of familial Alzheimer's disease.

We have transmitted two cases of human GSS to rodents. One of these cases was from an English family where 18 family members were affected by the disease within four generations. The second GSS case we transmitted was from a 25-year-old woman who had clinical dementia for three years. Remarkably, 13 of 31 family members were afflicted by a similar neurological disease, with an average age at death of 35 years. Fig. 2 shows that one of these familial cases had a shorter primary incubation time than typical sporadic CJD cases, a feature we would not have predicted. (These transmissions will be reported in detail elsewhere.) In GSS there is no evidence for horizontal transmission, and all human and rodent studies to date indicate no maternal (placental) transmission of these human agents (Manuelidis & Manuelidis 1979, Amyx et al 1981). Thus, we have transmitted an apparently genetic disease and have shown that it is the result of an infectious unconventional agent. Other independent transmissions of GSS agree with these findings

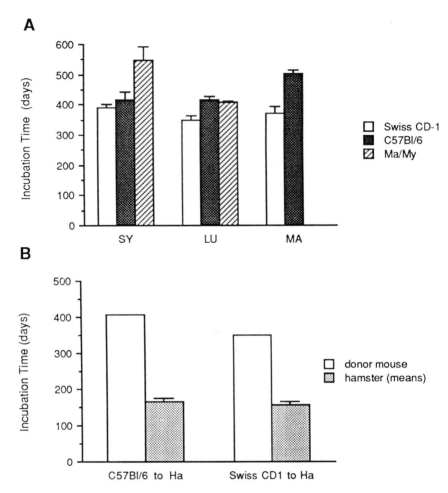

FIG. 1. Influence of host genetic factors on CJD incubation time. (A) Distinct CJD isolates show reproducible characteristic patterns of incubation time when inoculated into different inbred mouse strains. Some isolates (but not all) have prolonged incubation times in Ma/My mice (presumed $Sinc^P$ by PrP Xba-RFLP). Interestingly, no CJD isolates showed a prolonged incubation time in RIIIS/J mice, which also has the $Sinc^P$ allele of PrP. Incubation times are reproducibly longer in C57BL mice but the extent of prolongation varies greatly with the CJD isolate. The figure shows a representative study of three separate CJD isolates (SY, LU, MA) inoculated i.c. with maximal doses. (B) There are strong species effects on CJD incubation time. Incubation times of CJD passaged in mice are significantly longer than in hamsters. However, even after serial passage in mice, the agent has a characteristic short incubation period when introduced into hamster. The figure shows a representative study of CJD (LU isolate) serially passaged in C57BL or Swiss mice. Maximum doses of infectious brain homogenate from a single mouse with characteristic incubation time (white bar) were inoculated i.c. into 10 hamsters (mean incubation time +/− SD).

(Baker et al 1985). These results indicate that the CJD agent, at least in rare instances, can integrate into the host germline and from this locus can produce a complete infectious entity. These results also beg the question of whether Alzheimer's disease involves a similar integrated element which loses its ability to produce a complete infectious entity.

In human GSS there are numerous amyloid plaques in the brain. Similarly, the major pathological hallmark of AD is the accumulation of senile plaques. Although rodents infected with human GSS isolates showed characteristic spongiform changes of CJD, the florid plaques of the human GSS specimen were not reproduced in the hamster model. This absence of plaques in the experimental rodent model may relate to species-specific genetic restrictions; it is notable that aged rodents do not display obvious amyloid plaques in the central nervous system (CNS). In unconventional viral diseases, plaques can be formed at least in part from a glycoprotein that is distinct from the major glycoprotein deposited in senile plaques in AD. However, in both AD and unconventional viral infections, plaque formation appears to involve proteolytic cleavage of specific membrane glycoproteins (L. Manuelidis et al 1987a, 1988, Masters & Beyreuther, 1988). Thus, common mechanisms may underlie these pathological (processing) events in GSS and AD. One potential common pathway for plaque deposition in both diseases would involve the activation of a specific class of proteases of either cellular or viral origin (vide infra).

Alper's disease is a progressive infantile neurological disorder of unknown aetiology that probably encompasses a heterogeneous group of diseases (Friede 1975). Wefring & Lamvik (1967) reported laminar spongy degeneration of the cerebral cortex in two siblings with Alper's disease, and Crompton speculated that Alper's disease of infants may represent a variant of CJD (1968). We received from Dr Lucy Rorke a case of Alper's disease showing spongiform changes in a 2½-year-old infant. We have successfully transmitted this case of Alper's disease, and thus can unambiguously link some cases of infantile spongy degeneration to an infectious CJD-like agent. With the exception of iatrogenically induced CJD cases, the incubation time in human CJD is generally thought to exceed 2.5 years. Because CJD-like agents do not cross the placenta in humans, the most likely source of infection in this case of Alper's disease is via activation of an agent integrated into the host germline. A genetic inbred strain of mice with inherited early-onset CNS disease is especially relevant for these transmissible human infantile diseases, since an infectious agent can be recovered from the brains of these mice (Kinney & Sidman 1986).

The above transmissions raise the intriguing question of whether a significant proportion of the human population has integrated copies of a CJD-like agent. Such an integrated element need not be produced as an infectious entity until some other factor or group of factors (e.g. toxins, ageing changes,

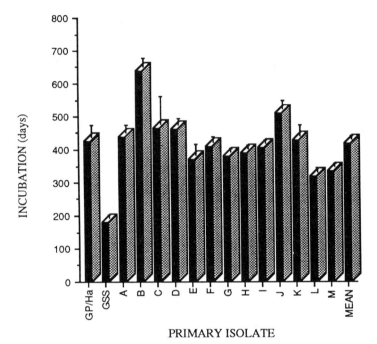

PRIMARY ISOLATE

FIG. 2.   Incubation periods of human CJD isolates inoculated into hamsters. Brain inocula from different subacute and chronic human CJD cases (A-M) characteristically show a long incubation period [mean = 425 days ± 12 (SEM), n ≥ 6] on primary passage. A GSS inoculum shows a significantly shorter incubation time. GP/Ha is derived from a guinea pig passage of human CJD. Subsequent serial passages of many of these isolates in hamsters typically showed a characteristic short incubation time (< 160 days).

other infections, hormones) incites its expression. The latter idea is useful for conceptualizing the late onset expression of pathological sequelae in both GSS and Alzheimer's disease.

Tissue culture studies

An independent group of *in vitro* experiments in our laboratory also implicates the potential integration or interaction of a CJD-specific nucleic acid with host genetic elements. Tissue cultures established from CJD-infected brains of either mice or hamsters readily become permanent cell lines and express transformed characteristics after passage *in vitro*. Notably, rodent-passaged familial GSS behaved in these studies similarly to rodent-passaged CJD isolates (E. Manuelidis et al 1987); cell lines derived from control brains did not. Furthermore, two transformed tissue culture cell lines inoculated into hamsters for bioassay of the CJD agent both showed low, but detectable,

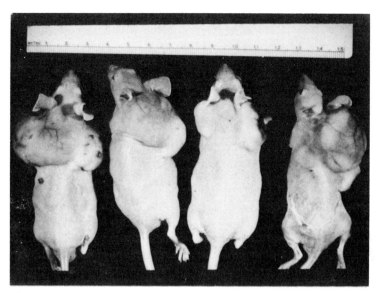

FIG. 3. Cell lines derived from CJD-infected brains induce tumours in nude mice. Above is a typical example. Cell lines derived from CJD-infected brains or by exposure to infectious CJD fractions *in vitro* have a transformed phenotype.

levels of agent which could not have been derived from the original brain material as it was diluted more than 10^{20}-fold during serial propagation. Fig. 3 shows that CJD-infected brain cells were capable of forming huge tumours in nude mice.

In another set of *in vitro* experiments, we briefly exposed contact-inhibited BALB/3T3 as well as other normal (non-permanent) cell lines to identically prepared infectious and control brain fractions. In these assays the CJD-treated cultures, but not the mock-infected cultures, became permanently transformed after passage, as assessed by a variety of criteria (Oleszak et al 1986). Thus transformation was not the direct result of a protein or growth factor in the applied CJD fractions; such factors would be removed with washing and would cause only reversible changes and not permanent trans-formation. The time course to express transformation in these experiments was consistent with the biology of a slowly oncogenic virus, one that is capable of activating cellular proto-oncogenes but would not itself directly encode an oncogene.

All CJD stably transformed cultures, whether derived from CJD-infected brain or from cells exposed to CJD infectious material *in vitro*, produced a TGF-α (transforming growth factor)-like factor that stimulated astroglial cells (E. Oleszak, G. Murdoch, L. Manuelidis, E.E. Manuelidis, in preparation). In animals, increases in the concentration of glial fibrillary acidic protein (GFAP) mRNA and protein in the brain can precede vacuolar changes.

These accumulations correlate with relatively high concentrations of infectious agent (in the absence of pathological changes) and may involve a diffusible humoral factor (L. Manuelidis et al 1987b). Astroglial stimulation in the brain could result from direct agent-induced transcriptional activation of specific cellular mRNAs or indirectly through stimulation of cellular regulatory pathways such as the 'oncogene' activation seen in tissue cultures. It remains to be determined if specific growth factors produced in brain are related to those produced by established CJD cultures. The concentration of GFAP mRNA is also highly elevated in brains from patients with Alzheimer's disease, and could involve similar activation mechanisms that do not simply reflect secondary responses to neuronal damage.

If the CJD agent is capable of genomic integration, why are tumours not found with higher frequency in animals? First, not all retroid (retroviral-like) elements are integrated with equal efficiency, and second, cellular replication, thought to be necessary for integration, is limited in the CNS. Thus, integration leading to the full expression of transformed properties may be a relatively rare event in 'subacute' infections of the brain that cannot be fully realized due to the relatively early demise of the animal. Other examples of known oncogenic integrating viruses, such as the JC papovavirus also lead to demyelinating pathology rather than tumour formation in the CNS, and some oncogenic retroviruses, such as human HTLV-1 or mouse mammary tumour virus, can take many years to induce tumours *in vivo*. In this context it is certainly worth examining in more detail the potential peripheral tumours that may occur in familial human CJD, in rodent CJD models, and in human dementias of 'non-infectious' aetiology.

A retroviral model

The above findings indicate that the CJD infectious agent is capable of integrating into the host genome and evoking the production of tumours. The total biological picture strongly implicates the involvement of a virus, which we define most simply as a protein-nucleic acid complex. It is known that these agents require protein for infectivity (cf Manuelidis & Manuelidis 1986). In CJD such a 'viral' complex is likely to involve a genome of appreciable size, from about one hundred up to 3000 bases in length (Fig. 4 and vide infra). Virusoids (e.g. hepatitis delta virus) and retroid viruses (e.g. retroviruses and hepatitis B-like viruses) fall within this category. When one considers the biological features above, retroid viruses present the more appealing focus of inquiry, since they are commonly capable of genomic integration (Seeger et al 1986, Mason et al 1987). Retroviruses are uniquely capable of integrating into the germline, unlike other integrating transforming viruses, e.g. papovaviruses. Indeed, CJD and other 'unconventional' agents may contain one or several retroviral nucleic acid elements (Fig. 4) and

RETROVIRUS

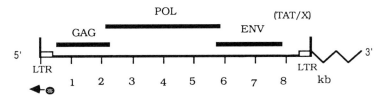

HEPADNAVIRUS

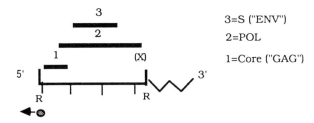

3=S ("ENV")

2=POL

1=Core ("GAG")

POTENTIAL CJD AGENT

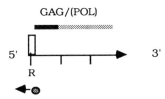

FIG. 4. A simplified map of two retroid viruses with the suggestion that CJD involves at least a portion of equivalent retroid sequence elements. A minimal CJD agent would have a terminal repeat (bar at R) for integration, and may contain a *gag*-like capsid sequence; the *gag* or the *gag-pol* 3' end may be truncated or defective. Only *gag* is required for viral assembly in retroviruses. In hepadnaviruses the complete infectious viral sequence is considerably smaller than that of retroviruses due to overlapping open reading frames. Notably, hepadnaviruses are highly resistant to inactivation, and visible viral structures are virtually undetectable in tissue. LTRs (long terminal repeats) of some retroviruses can confer tissue tropism, and may also contain trans-activating sequences. *Pol* encodes reverse transcriptase and contains the RNAse H necessary for second-strand DNA synthesis. If *Pol* is completely defective, host endogenous retroviruses and retroposons could supply this enzyme, as they contain this coding sequence element. *TAT* (trans-activating region) and *X* are present on some retroid viruses. Circle with arrow denotes the direction of reverse transcription from the RNA genomes. *S* is surface antigen; envelope (*env*)-defective retroviruses may not show characteristic budding particles.

at least one of these should confer an insertional potential. Alternatively, the CJD nucleic acid may be picked up by an endogeneous retroviral sequence, resulting in the same spectrum of action (vide infra).

There are several striking parallels between the established action of several retroviruses and the biology of CJD. Retroviruses can cause a variety of chronic or delayed-onset neurological diseases. For example, HTLV-III (HIV) infections of humans can result in profound dementias early in disease, when no opportunistic infections are detectable and peripheral T cell changes are minimal. Furthermore, in the nervous system there is evidence that the HTLV-III virus can have specific mutations that are peculiar to its residence at that site (Koyanagi et al 1987), and in several cases of AIDS few recognizable viral particles are detected in the brains of severely demented patients. Thus, some dementias may involve CNS-specific defective retroviral variants. HTLV-I, another human retrovirus, has also been aetiologically linked to the development of late-onset neurological disease in cases of spastic tropical paraplegia. Similarly, numerous rodent models of CNS disease are caused by neurotropic murine retroviruses, and in some of these models, as in CJD, there may be little, if any, host inflammatory response (Zachary et al 1986).

Species-specific 'endogenous' retroviral sequences are known to reside in the genome of most mammals (including humans). Some of these endogenous retroviruses can become infectious when they interact with other viral elements, as in the case of mink colony focus virus of mice (Weiss et al 1982). This more indirect route also utilizes or involves retroviral sequences. If either of these routes (direct or indirect) is operational in CJD, it should be possible to detect specific viral sequences and their products, or known cellular products activated by retroviruses (e.g. oncogenes) in the brains of infected animals using defined probes. It may also be propitious to look for and evaluate these sequences in Alzheimer brain samples.

The pathological sequelae in retroviral infections of the CNS include vacuolar changes in the brain, which resemble the spongiform changes seen in both unconventional viral infections and some cases of Alzheimer's disease that are difficult to classify. Such vacuolar changes implicate interaction with a membrane glycoprotein target. The CJD agent is sequestered at membrane sites. Retroviruses and defective retroviral recombinant constructs also target membrane sites. In CJD, the alteration of a host membrane glycoprotein Gp34 (the precursor of 'prion protein') to form amyloid fibrils appears to be a secondary response to agent sequestration at membrane sites (L. Manuelidis et al 1987a, 1988). The retroviral model offers several potential pathways for the production of these host membrane alterations. Retrovirally encoded proteases necessary for viral maturation could be directly responsible for the cleavage of host membrane glycoprotein and the production of amyloid in both GSS and Alzheimer's disease. Alternatively, accumulation of abnormal protein assemblies in the cytoplasm may activate cellular protease systems, such as the ubiquitin-regulated ATP-dependent protease. Additionally, several retroviral sequences contain trans-activating transcriptional regions which provide alternative mechanisms for the activation of cellular proteases and consequent amyloid deposition. Thus, the slowly oncogenic retroviruses provide a useful paradigm, not only for the neurotropic and insertional features of CJD, but also for pathological membrane changes, agent sequestration at membrane sites, and formation of specific cellular products of disease.

Superficially, the lack of visible conventional viral structures in CJD infections of the CNS, and the resistance of this class of agents to a number of inactivation treatments would preclude retroviruses as relevant models. However, several engineered retroviral recombinants, as well as known retroviral intermediates and retroid viruses, are notably resistant to inactivation by nucleases, heat and ionic detergents. For example, subviral particles of retroviral DNA-protein intermediates are resistant to a number of treatments, such as nuclease inactivation and heat (Brown et al 1987). This form of subviral particle would be undetectable in tissue sections. Retroviral *gag* mutants can also result in structurally defective or unrecognizable viral assemblies, and GAG gene products are essentially all that is needed to make an effective viral assembly. Notably, *gag* mutants have also been associated with increased neurotropism (Weiss et al 1982). Typical complete retroviruses in their isolated state, however, do not have the resistance and physical properties of the unconventional agents.

The hepadnaviruses, whose life cycles include small informational retroviral-like RNA genomes, are strikingly resistant to a number of physicochemical treatments, such as nucleases and ionic detergents. These retroid viruses are more parsimonious in sequence utilization due to overlapping open reading frames (see Fig. 4) and encompass structural forms and intermediates that would be virtually impossible to recognize in tissue preparations. Their size (about 40 nM) is in the putative size range of the unconventional viruses. Genomic integration also occurs (as a relatively rare event) in hepadnaviral infections, and tumours are formed probably by selective outgrowth of cells after a very long time span, i.e. these viruses can mimic the biology of slowly oncogenic retroviruses. Interestingly, persistent hepadnaviral infections can be non-cytopathic in the absence of a host immune response. Although all the known viruses of this group are highly tissue-specific for the liver, potential neurotropic members of this class may exist.

In summary, defective retroviruses and hepadnaviruses provide useful examples for the formation of small, stable, and morphologically inapparent infectious molecular structures that are also capable of inserting into the genome. A simplified map of retroviral and retroid elements is depicted in Fig. 4 with the essential sequences of interest. Note that only small regions of retroviral genome are necessary for many of the actions cited above. Thus, retroviral-like elements provide a highly relevant framework for understanding the aetiology and common mechanisms involved in GSS, Alzheimer's disease and Alper's disease. A search for these types of sequences and for the cellular products which they encode or activate is likely to increase our

understanding of both the aetiology and disease mechanisms that underlie the
human dementias.

Acknowledgements

The authors are indebted to Bill Fritch for his fastidious help with cited experiments.
This work was supported by NIH grants AG 03106 and NS 12674. Geoffrey Murdoch
was supported by a Commonwealth Fund fellowship.

References

Amyx HL, Gibbs CJ Jr, Gajdusek DC, Greer WE 1981 Absence of vertical transmission of subacute spongiform viral encephalopathies in experimental primates. Proc
Soc Exp Biol Med 166:469–471
Baker HF, Ridley RM, Crow TJ 1985 Experimental transmission of an autosomal
dominant spongiform encephalopathy: does the infectious agent originate in the
human genome? Br Med J 291:299–302
Brown PO, Bowerman B, Varmus HE, Bishop JM 1987 Correct integration of
retroviral DNA in vitro. Cell 49:347–356
Bruce ME, Dickinson AG, Fraser H 1976 Cerebral amyloidosis in scrapie in the
mouse: effect of agent strain and mouse genotype. Neuropathol Appl Neurobiol
2:471
Carlson GA, Kingsbury DT, Goodman PA et al 1986 Linkage of prion protein and
scrapie incubation time genes. Cell 46:503–511
Caughey B, Race R, Vogel M, Buchmeier M, Chesebro B 1988 In vitro expression of
cloned PrP cDNA derived from scrapie-infected mouse brain: lack of transmission
of scrapie infectivity. In: Novel infectious agents and the central nervous system.
Wiley, Chichester (Ciba Found Symp 135) p 197–208
Crompton MR 1968 Alper's disease — a variant of Creutzfeldt-Jakob disease and
subacute spongiform encephalopathy? Acta Neuropathol 10:99–104
Cuillé J, Chelle PL 1936 Pathologic animale. La maladie dite la tremblante du mouton
est-elle inoculable? CR Acad Sci (D) Paris 203:1552–1554
Czub M, Braig HR, Diringer H 1986 Pathogenesis of scrapie: study of the temporal
development of clinical symptoms, of infectivity titers and scrapie associated fibrils
in brains of hamsters infected intraperitoneally. J Gen Virol 67:2005–2009
Fraser H, Dickinson AG 1973 Scrapie in mice: agent strain differences in the distribution and intensity of grey matter vacuolation. J Comp Pathol 83:239
Friede RL 1975 Developmental neuropathology. Springer Verlag, New York–Wien, p
93–102
Kimberlin RH, Walker CA 1986 Pathogenesis of scrapie (strain 263K) in hamsters
infected intracerebrally, intraperitoneally or intraocularly. J Gen Virol 67:255–263
Kinney HC, Sidman RL 1986 Pathology of the spongiform encephalopathy in the grey
tremor mutant mouse. J Neuropathol Exp Neurol 45:108–126
Koyanagi Y, Miles S, Mitsuyasu RT, Merrill JE, Vinters HV, Chen JSY 1987 Dual
infection of the central nervous system by AIDS viruses with distinct cellular
tropisms. Science (Wash DC) 236:819–822
Locht C, Chesebro B, Race R, Keith JM 1986 Molecular cloning and complete
sequence of prion protein cDNA from mouse brain infected with the scrapie agent.
Proc Natl Acad Sic USA 83:6372–6376
Manuelidis EE, Manuelidis L 1979 Experiments on maternal transmission of
Creutzfeldt-Jakob disease in guinea pigs. Proc Soc Exp Biol Med 160:233–236

Manuelidis EE, Manuelidis L, Pincus JH, Collins WF 1978a Transmission from man to hamster of Creutzfeldt-Jakob disease with clinical recovery. Lancet 1:40

Manuelidis EE, Gorgacz EJ, Manuelidis L 1978b Viremia in experimental Creutzfeldt-Jakob disease. Science (Wash DC) 200:1069–1071

Manuelidis EE, Kim JH, Manuelidis L 1988 Destructive white matter lesions in experimental Creutzfeldt-Jakob disease. In: Court L et al (eds) Unconventional viruses and central nervous system diseases. Atelier d'Arts Graphiques, Abbaye de Melleray, in press

Manuelidis EE, Fritch WW, Kim JH, Manuelidis L 1987 Immortality of cell cultures derived from brains of mice and hamsters infected with Creutzfeldt-Jakob disease agent. Proc Natl Acad Sic USA 84:871–875

Manuelidis L, Manuelidis EE 1986 Recent developments in scrapie and Creutzfeldt-Jakob disease. Prog Med Virol 33:78–98

Manuelidis L, Sklaviadis T, Manuelidis EE 1988 On the origin and formation of SAF. In: Court L et al (eds) Unconventional viruses and central nervous system diseases. Atelier d'Arts Graphiques, Abbaye de Melleray, in press

Manuelidis L, Sklaviadis T, Manuelidis EE 1987a Evidence suggests that PrP is not the infectious agent in Creutzfeldt-Jakob disease. EMBO (Eur Mol Biol Organ) J 6:341–347

Manuelidis L, Tesin D, Sklaviadis T, Manuelidis EE 1987b Astrocyte gene expression in Creutzfeldt-Jakob disease. Proc Natl Acad Sci USA 84:5937–5941

Mason WS, Taylor JM, Hull R 1987 Retroid virus genome replication. Adv Virus Res 32:35–96

Masters CL, Beyreuther K 1988 Neuropathology of unconventional virus infections: molecular pathology of spongiform change and amyloid plaque deposition. In: Novel infectious agents and the central nervous system. Wiley, Chichester (Ciba Found Symp 135) p 24–36

Oleszak E, Manuelidis L, Manuelidis EE 1986 In vitro transformation elicited by Creutzfeldt-Jakob infected brain material. J Neuropathol Exp Neurol 45:489–502

Prusiner SB 1987 Prions causing degenerative neurological diseases. Annu Rev Med 38:381–398

Robakis NK, Sawh PR, Wolfe GC, Rubenstein R, Carp RI, Innis MA 1986 Isolation of a cDNA clone encoding the leader peptide of prion protein and expression of the homologous gene in various tissues. Proc Natl Acad Sci USA 83:6377–6381

Seeger C, Ganem D, Varmus HE 1986 Biochemical and genetic evidence for the hepatitis B virus replication strategy. Science (Wash DC) 232:477–484

Seitelberger F 1981 Straussler's disease. Acta Neuropathol (Berl) Suppl VII:341–343

Tateishi J, Koga M, Mori R 1981 Experimental transmission of Creutzfeldt-Jakob disease. Acta Pathol Jpn 31:943–951

Wefring KW, Lamvik JO 1967 Familial progressive poliodystrophy with cirrhosis of the liver. Acta Paed Scand 56:295–300

Weiss R, Teich N, Seeger C, Varmus HE 1982 RNA tumor viruses. Cold Spring Harbor Laboratory, Cold Spring Harbor, New York

Zachary JF, Knupp CJ, Wong PKY 1986 Noninflammatory spongiform polioencephalomyelopathy caused by a neurotropic temperature-sensitive mutant of Moloney Murine leukemia virus TB. Am J Pathol 124:457–468

DISCUSSION

Fraser: We have now heard twice about the Richard Sidman claim of transmissibility of genetic *gt* mouse spongiosis. The only evidence is the publication in PNAS (Sidman et al 1985). I wrote to Richard Sidman twice in 1985, pointing out the difficulty of diagnosing pathologically-induced vacuolar degeneration in very old mice. We have shown that old mice suffer from a spongiform change which resembles the pathology seen with scrapie and can be misleading. There are strain differences and there are sex differences in this (Fraser & McBride 1985). The transmission of these things should be rigorously established before the pathology is attributed to an agent comparable to scrapie.

Manuelidis: A second paper on *gt/gt* and *gt* passage 1 infectivity in NFS mice will be published by a separate laboratory and I think that the evidence is reasonably strong (Hoffman et al 1987). Infection with *gt/gt* brain entails a much longer latency than scrapie. They used the Compton strain of scrapie for comparison, which gave clinical signs at about 60 days in NFS mice and the *gt/gt* material produced symptoms at 120 days; vacuolization was found in symptomatic *gt* inoculated mice.

Kimberlin: Have they done repeated serial passage?

Manuelidis: I don't know.

Bolton: My understanding was that the serial passage had not yet been completed (it may be in progress) and that the clinical signs that these mice showed were very slight. I am not convinced by these data that the complete syndrome, including clinical disease, was transmitted.

Fraser: I am unhappy about it as well.

Manuelidis: I thought that the data were fairly convincing.

Almond: Have you looked for typical retroviral signs in your cell lines. For example, after mitomycin C or dexamethasone treatment is there evidence of Hirt DNA, or reverse transcriptase activity.

Manuelidis: We haven't looked for reverse transcriptase because I was told that in a lot of transformed lines reverse transcriptase activity is elevated.

Chesebro: Many transformed lines have been passaged in laboratories for a long time and are contaminated by retroviruses, but you have a very special set of lines that you made yourself. I don't think that retrovirus contamination would apply in your case because you have such good control over the generation of those lines.

Manuelidis: That's interesting: when I ask people in Yale they tell me not to bother because there are sufficient rodent endogenous retroviruses and transcripts that the data would not be readily interpretable. We have not even considered contaminating retroviruses. In about half of the mouse lines that we have there are visible endogeneous retroviruses so those lines would not be worth looking at for reverse transcriptase. In three out of 13 of the hamster lines there is a typical hamster intra-cisternal A-type particle, which I would expect to have a reverse transcriptase.

Almond: In the other 10 hamster lines you see nothing at all by electron microscopy?

Manuelidis: Nothing at all. I went through hundreds of those cells looking for them. However, there may be retroviral gene expression in the absence of complete particle formation. We are looking at retroviral types of sequences other than reverse transcriptase. We are also looking at Hirt DNA.

Almond: You said that there are defective variants of retroviruses which are very resistant to harsh treatments.

Manuelidis: There are retroviral intermediates that are resistant. One paper I am referring to in terms of resistant intermediates is by Brown et al (1987). I am not talking about the mature viral RNA forms. In addition, as I noted, hepatitis B is highly resistant to inactivation and is considered a retroviral-like agent because it utilizes an RNA informational stage and has a molecular structure that is strongly analogous to retroviruses.

F. Brown: To focus your attention on retroviruses is probably a little dangerous because there may be other viruses integrated into the cell genome in the germ line.

Manuelidis: In what size range? Plant viroids and mammalian virusoids (such as hepatitis delta) may be represented in the genome anyway and we have not excluded virusoid-like agents from consideration. The usual DNA transforming viruses, such as the SV40 papova virus group, are not integrated into the germ line.

F. Brown: I was thinking about the general principle of integration and viruses like herpes or measles.

Manuelidis: Herpes is huge; it is latent and can integrate but it would be atypical for herpes viruses to be vertically transmitted. Measles and other myxo/paramyxoviruses are not generally associated with an integrative capacity or insertion into the germ line. Myxoviruses are also quite large and are usually quite sensitive to chemical and physical inactivations. We don't exclude other small conventional viruses from consideration but the overall biological picture favours the involvement of retroviral-like sequence elements in the disease either by a direct or indirect route.

Almond: The point about viral proteases associated with retroviruses and the possibility that these might be involved in either the PrP modification or the Alzheimer's A4 modification is interesting. Have you looked carefully at the recognized amino acid signals for cleavage in known retroviruses and tried to match these to the PrP N-terminus?

Manuelidis: We are going to try that. We have some negative preliminary data which I should also mention in terms of our working hypothesis. Malcolm Martin from the NIH generously gave me an essentially complete set of HIV III (AIDS) clones. We tested these at several stringencies on formaldehyde and glyoxal blots of nucleic acids extracted from brain fractions enriched in infectivity. They did not hybridize to infectious CJD fractions convincingly or specifically. However, when I saw that HTLV III didn't cross-hybridize very well to HTLV IV, I was reassured. Additionally, in collaboration with Michael Phelan at the NIH, we used rabbit polyclonal and other antibodies against different parts of gag, pol and envelope proteins from AIDS viruses. We were never able to detect any protein in CJD infectious fractions that cross-reacted with those particular AIDS antibodies in a reproducible, specific manner, although small samples of each AIDS virus protein were readily detected.

Dormont: Concerning HIV I and HIV II hybridization to DNA extracted from samples of human CJD-infected brains, with partial and total HIV probes we did not get any positive hybridization under conditions of low stringency.

DeArmond: We have some data that demonstrate that PrP^{Sc}, the abnormal form of the prion protein, is the cause of the gliosis in scrapie. Glial fibrillary acidic protein (GFAP) is the protein subunit of glial filaments and is the best indicator of the degree of astrocytic gliosis. In the hamster scrapie model, PrP^{Sc}, the protease K resistant form, can first be detected in whole brain homogenates about 35–40 days after i.c. inoculation, approximately 15–20 days before the animal becomes clinically ill. The amount of PrP^{Sc} rises sharply about a week before clinical signs occur. This sharp rise precedes the sharp rise in reactive astrocytic gliosis determined by histology and the rise in GFAP protein determined by neurochemistry by approximately one week. The GFAP curve also breaks away from the normal animal curve at about 30 days after i.c. inoculation, indicating that there is an undercurrent of gliosis early in the disease, but the main rise occurs about a week after the appearance of PrP^{Sc}. This is consistent with the way we would expect the astrocyte to behave after it's been damaged; it takes approximately a week after injury to detect reactive astrogliosis. Mike McKinley has shown that infectivity has the same temporal relationship to the concentration of PrP^{Sc} in the brain.

Merz: What is the measurement of the PrP 33-35 based on?

DeArmond: Proteinase K digestion of whole brain homogenates.

Masters: You couldn't conclude from your data that PrP is an integral component of the virus.

DeArmond: Of course not, this is a temporal relationship between the two (PrP concentration and the degree of gliosis). Histologically, there is very little change before the rise in scrapie infectivity; all the changes occur after this rise. We have not been able to measure PrP^{Sc} in the early stages of infectivity.

Bolton: We have done time course purifications without proteinase K digestion. We detect the protein in purified fractions as early as 21 days after i.c. inoculation. We have related this to scrapie agent titre and at 21 days the titre is just beginning to increase in the purified fractions.

DeArmond: The degree of gliosis temporally follows the degree of PrP expression. We have other data on the spatial relationship between PrP^{Sc} and astrogliosis. We have determined the conditions for staining PrP in tissue sections. This requires McLeon's fixative, which is a periodate-lysine mixture with a very low concentration (0.5%) of paraformaldehyde. In normal animals PrP^{C} is located in nerve cell bodies and in their proximal dendrites. Immunoreactive neurons are scattered throughout the nervous system; but not all nerve cells stain. The majority of nerve cell bodies stain in the normal thalamus, the dentate gyrus, the hippocampus and the septal nuclei. In the terminal stages of scrapie, the cell body staining disappears; PrP^C and/or PrP^{Sc} are no longer present in the nerve cell body, they now appear in the neuropil where the pathology occurs. For example, spongiform degeneration and reactive astrogliosis are intense in the hippocampal CA4 region and extend into the CA1 region and throughout the thalamus. Immunostaining for PrP^{Sc} was correspondingly very intense in these regions. Other regions of the hippocampus, such as the dentate gyrus, show far less astrogliosis and, correspondingly, have little PrP immunoreactivity. Therefore, there is a regional and even sub-regional co-distribution of PrP^{Sc} and pathology.

Merz: Steve, the staining in the ependymal cells is quite heavy.

DeArmond: There are times when you can see plaque-like material extending from the sub-ependymal region into the ventricle, as if it were going either through the ependymal cells or past the sides of the cells. Otherwise the ependymal cells are negative.

More to the point, the relationship of PrP to astrogliosis is probably best demonstrated by comparing the patterns of staining for GFAP and PrP in the septum and the caudate nucleus. The septal nucleus has a general increase in immunoreactivity for PrP at the terminal stages of scrapie, whereas the caudate nucleus shows no staining except for the accumulation of PrP in amyloid plaques along the ventricular surface, which forms the medial surface of the caudate. The distribution of reactive astrocytes coincides precisely with the distribution of PrP. Reactive astrogliosis occurs throughout the septum but is absent from the body of the caudate. The only gliosis that occurs in relation to the caudate is along its medial ventricular edge where the PrP immunopositive plaques have developed. These results, which were obtained from immunoperoxidase staining of tissue sections, were verified by Western blot analysis of PrP 27-30 (the proteinase K resistant portion of PrP^{Sc}) from dissected brain regions. In order to get enough tissue from each brain region for this analysis, we needed approximately 200 mg of tissue. This required pooling dissected regions from about 10 hamster brains. The immunohistochemical findings were confirmed: for instance, caudate nucleus had very little PrP 27-30 and septum contained 20 times as much. Surprisingly, the thalamus had the highest concentration of protein, approximately 50 times as much as the caudate and the hypothalamus was second.

Therefore, I believe that there is a temporal and spatial relationship between the appearance of PrP^{Sc} and the occurrence of gliosis. Laura (Manuelidis) mentioned that the gliosis precedes the spongiform degeneration. We find spongiform degeneration very difficult to evaluate by light microscopy. One micron-thick plastic-embedded tissues and electron microscopy are often required to demonstrate that this sub-microscopic spongiform degeneration has as much functional significance as the gross spongiform degeneration seen at later stages by light microscopy.

References

Brown PO, Bowerman B, Varmus HE, Bishop JM 1987 Correct integration of retroviral DNA in vitro. Cell 49:347–356

Fraser H, McBride PA 1985 Parallels and contrasts between scrapie and dementia of the Alzheimer type and aging: strategies and problems for experiments involving life-span studies. In: Traber J, Gispen WJ (eds) Advances in applied neurological sciences. Senile dementia of the Alzheimer type and aging. Springer-Verlag, Heidelberg, p 250–268

Hoffman PM, Rohwer RG, MacAuley C, Bilello JA, Hartley JW, Morse HC 1987 Transmission in NFS/N mice of the heritable spongiform encephalopathy associated with the gray tremor mutation. Proc Natl Acad Sci (USA) 84:3866–3870

Sidman RC, Kinney HC, Sweet HO 1985 Transmissible spongiform encephalopathy in the gray tremor mutant mouse. Proc Natl Acad Sci USA 82:253–257

Scrapie: a virus-induced amyloidosis of the brain

Heino Diringer, Henk Ronald Braig and Markus Czub

Robert Koch-Institut des Bundesgesundheitsamtes, Nordufer 20, 1000 Berlin 65, Federal Republic of Germany

Abstract. We have studied the pathogenesis of scrapie in hamsters, in particular the increase of infectivity and the formation of scrapie-associated fibrils in relation to clinical disease. The results of such studies after intraperitoneal or intracerebral infection are consistent with the idea that transmissible spongiform encephalopathies are a type of virus-induced, brain-specific amyloidosis. Therefore, an appropriate name for the class of viruses that cause these diseases might be amyloid-inducing viruses.

1988 Novel infectious agents and the central nervous system. Wiley, Chichester (Ciba Foundation Symposium 135) p 135–145

The pathogenesis of scrapie in its natural and experimental hosts is characterized by an extremely long incubation period followed by chronic progressive disease leading to death. There is no evidence that other transmissible spongiform encephalopathies, such as Creutzfeldt-Jakob disease, Gerstmann-Sträussler disease, kuru, mink encephalopathy, or chronic wasting disease, follow a different course of pathogenesis.

There are different opinions as to whether the disease is caused by a virus (Diringer & Kimberlin 1983, Rohwer 1984, Diringer 1985, Braig & Diringer 1985), a virus-sized, new type of pathogen, termed a virino (Dickinson & Outram 1983), or an infectious protein devoid of a nucleic acid to code for infectivity (Prusiner 1982).

The route of infection, the amount and strain of virus, and the genotype of the host are major determinants affecting the incubation period. There is no doubt that after a peripheral infection, virus replication and pathological changes in the brain are preceded by replication of the virus in peripheral organs without pathological changes or symptoms (see Kimberlin 1979). Furthermore, there is good evidence that a sustained viraemia is not only associated with the peripheral replication of the virus (Diringer 1984) but also persists into the clinical phase of the disease (Manuelidis et al 1978). Thus the infectious agent is very likely to enter the central nervous system through haematogenous spread, although other experiments suggest spread along peripheral nerves (Kimberlin & Walker 1986).

Scrapie-associated fibrils (SAF) and the protein of which they are com-

135

posed are hallmarks of all transmissible encephalopathies and are decisive for the disease. Our recent finding that these disease-specific fibrils do not correlate with infectivity levels in the spleen and brain and, in contrast to the virus, are specifically restricted to brain (Czub et al 1986a) argue against the fibril or the protein in any way representing the infectivity or being an essential part of it.

Kinetic studies in hamsters infected intraperitoneally with the 263K strain of scrapie showed that SAF are virus-induced pathological products (Czub et al 1986b). Such studies have allowed us to distinguish four events that occur in the brain after peritoneal injection of the virus: i) a period of low constant levels of infectivity, ii) rapid replication of the virus, iii) the formation of the amyloid fibril protein, and iv) onset of clinical disease (cell death).

We have described the transmissible spongiform encephalopathies as virus-induced amyloidoses (Diringer 1985, Diringer et al 1986, Braig & Diringer 1985) or according to Glenner (1980) as β-fibrilloses. This possibility was discussed when SAF were discovered (Merz et al 1981) and includes the observation that SAF are derived from a protein encoded within the genome of the host (Chesebro et al 1985, Oesch et al 1985). Here we present further evidence to substantiate this concept.

Results

The kinetic experiment of Czub et al (1986b) posed the question: What is the shortest time in which measurable amounts of SAF protein develop in the brains of hamsters after an intraperitoneal injection? We also asked: What is the shortest time needed for maximum titres of infectivity to develop in brain under these experimental conditions? The results clearly showed an increase of infectivity 55–70 days post infection to almost maximum titres, followed by the onset of formation of SAF at 75 days, which reached high levels around 95 days, when clinical symptoms began to appear. Concerning the increase in infectivity, the results were in contrast to those implicating continuous but slow virus growth throughout the course of the disease after the virus has entered the central nervous system, but agreed with those showing a plateau of infectivity before the onset of clinical symptoms (see Czub et al 1986b). Thus the discrepancy may be in the interpretation of the results.

Fig. 1 shows results from the kinetic experiment just mentioned (Czub et al 1986b), together with new results from experiments with AURA and CLAC hamsters. Individual hamsters of a group of inbred animals infected at the same time with the same amount of the same pool of scrapie material reach different titres of infectivity at given times after infection. Indeed, in the brains of some animals at around 60 days post infection the titre is still as low as in the early days after infection (represented here by six animals at Day 40), although in the brains of other animals in the group a considerable amount of virus replication has already begun.

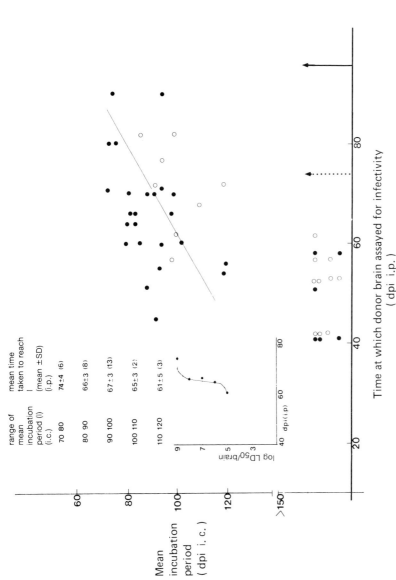

Time at which donor brain assayed for infectivity
(dpi i.p.)

FIG. 1. The development of infectivity in brains of individual hamsters infected i.p. with scrapie. (●) AURA, (○) CLAC hamsters. (↑) start of amyloidosis. (↑) first clinical symptoms. Hamsters were injected i.p. with scrapie and at set times the amount of infectivity that had developed in their brains was assayed by injecting this brain material i.c. into a group of five recipient hamsters and measuring the mean incubation period. These incubation periods are related in an inverse, exponential manner to infectivity titres (Diringer et al 1983). *Inset* Table: mean time (dpi i.p.) taken for a given range of infectivity (as measured by the mean incubation period, dpi i.c.) to develop. No. of donors in each group given in brackets. Graph: infectivity titres (logLD₅₀/brain) derived from the mean incubation periods. dpi, days post infection.

This result could be interpreted as a steady increase in infectivity in the population of hamsters, represented by the line given in Fig. 1. This would suggest that high titres of infectivity do not occur until the later stages of the experiment. However, if one considers the case of a 'standard hamster' the conclusion is different. We asked: At what time does the average infectivity reach a certain level in the population of hamsters? We calculated the infectivity titres for the brain extracts which caused scrapie in i.c. injected hamsters after an incubation period covering a set 10 day range (see Table inset). These infectivity titres were then plotted against the time at which the brain extract was made after injection of the donor animal i.p. (see Graph inset). Thus, animals with brain titres giving incubation periods of 110–120 and 70–80 days in the i.c. assay represent 10^5 and 10^9 infectious units, respectively. From the original data (main graph) it may be seen that the individual hamsters gain these titres at very different times. However, the 'standard' hamster reaches these titres at 61 ± 5 and 74 ± 4 days, respectively. Interpreting our data in this way, we obtain kinetics of virus replication which show that replication occurs during a limited period between 55 and 75 days after i.p. infection. This period precedes the appearance of large amounts of SAF and the onset of clinical symptoms.

It seems unlikely that this type of virus replication in the brain and the time course of SAF formation should depend on the route of infection. We have repeated the kinetic experiment infecting the animals intracerebrally (Czub et al, in preparation). The results are almost identical with those obtained after an intraperitoneal infection, except that the relatively long lag phase before virus replication was not observed. Virus replication begins soon after intracerebral infection with, perhaps, a very short lag phase. Maximum titres are reached at 35–40 days post infection. SAF protein appears at 42 days, increases tenfold about every five days and reaches high levels 56 days post infection. First clinical symptoms are recognized at about 60 days after intracerebral infection. Thus, independent of the route of virus application, i.e. subcutaneously (Eklund et al 1967), intraperitoneally (Czub et al 1986b) or intracerebrally (Baringer et al 1983, Czub et al, in preparation), virus replication is completed long before clinical disease becomes apparent. The kinetics of intracerebral infection is in accordance with scrapie being a virus-induced amyloidosis restricted to the CNS.

Discussion

After a natural infection with an unconventional virus the following sequential steps can be recognized:

1. Replication of virus in peripheral organs (without development of any measurable immune response).
2. Haematogenous spread to the brain.

3. Entrance of virus into the central nervous system.
4. Virus replication in the central nervous system.
5. Induction of a brain-specific amyloidosis.
6. Cell destruction and disease.
7. Death.

This scheme represents a conservative view on the pathogenesis of transmissible spongiform encephalopathies. In all but one item it agrees with what is known about infection of the central nervous system by conventional viruses.

During the replication of virus in the periphery the disease process may be controlled or even stopped (Ehlers & Diringer 1983, Kimberlin 1979). So far, no experimental evidence indicates that steps 2–7 can be influenced. The kinetics presented tells us that blocking of virus replication is ineffective as a cure once the clinical disease has become evident: replication is already complete and the amyloidosis has advanced so far that, even if one were ever able to treat an amyloidosis, patients with a clinical stage unconventional virus infection are unlikely to benefit from it.

A host gene, *Sinc*, influencing the incubation period of the disease (Dickinson & Meikle 1971) seems to be closely related to the process of amyloidosis (Carlson et al 1986), again favouring scrapie as a model to study amyloidoses of the brain (Bruce et al 1976).

Unconventional viruses are the only viruses known to induce an amyloidosis, in this case a brain-specific one. A. Dickinson and G. Outram in 1983 suggested that the long-standing term 'agent' is due for replacement with something more specific. We now have 'prions' or 'virinos' as more speculative names, or 'unconventional viruses' (Gajdusek 1985) as a more conservative term. These viruses have been named 'unconventional' mainly because they do not induce an immune response. We do know that all these viruses induce amyloidoses. Thus, why not, in agreement with the classification and nomenclature of conventional virology, call them 'amyloid-inducing viruses (AIV)', and group them and the amyloid they induce according to their host specificity and — who knows — some time in the future according to their organ specificity.

Acknowledgements

This work was supported by Deutsche Forschungsgemeinschaft and Fonds der Chemischen Industrie.

References

Baringer JR, Bowman KA, Prusiner SB 1983 Replication of scrapie agent in hamster brain precedes neuronal vacuolation. J Neuropathol & Exp Neurol 42:539–547
Braig HR, Diringer H 1985 Scrapie: concept of a virus-induced amyloidosis of the brain. EMBO (Eur Mol Biol Organ) J 4:2309–2312

Bruce ME, Dickinson AG, Fraser H 1976 Cerebral amyloidosis in scrapie in the mouse: effect of agent strain and mouse genotype. Neuropathol Appl Neurobiol 2:471–478

Carlson GA, Kingsbury DT, Goodman PA et al 1986 Linkage of prion protein and scrapie incubation time genes. Cell 46:503–511

Chesebro B, Race R, Wehrly K et al 1985 Identification of scrapie prion protein-specific mRNA in scrapie-infected and uninfected brain. Nature (Lond) 315:331–333

Czub M, Braig HR, Blode H, Diringer H 1986a The major protein of SAF is absent from spleen and thus not an essential part of the scrapie agent. Arch Virol 91:383–386

Czub M, Braig HR, Diringer H 1986b Pathogenesis of scrapie: study of the temporal development of clinical symptoms, of infectivity titres and scrapie-associated fibrils in brains of hamsters infected intraperitoneally. J Gen Virol 67:2005–2009

Dickinson AG, Outram GW 1983 Operational limitations in the characterisation of the infective units of scrapie. In: Court LA, Cathala F (eds) Virus non-conventionnels et affections due système nerveux central. Masson, Paris, p 3–16

Dickinson AG, Meikle VMH 1971 Host-genotype and agent effects in scrapie incubation: change in allelic interaction with different strains of agent. Mol & Gen Genet 112:73–79

Diringer H 1984 Sustained viremia in experimental hamster scrapie. Arch Virol 82:105–109

Diringer H 1985 Ein Modell für Alterungsprozesse und degenerative biochemische Veränderungen des Gehirns — Scrapie. Funkt Biol Med 4:129–140

Diringer H, Kimberlin RH 1983 Infectious scrapie agent is apparently not as small as as recent claims suggest. Bioscience Rep 3:563–568

Diringer H, Hilmert H, Simon D, Werner E, Ehlers B 1983 Towards purification of the scrapie agent. Eur J Biochem 134:556–560

Diringer H, Braig HR, Pocchiari M, Bode L 1986 Scrapie-associated fibrils in the pathogenesis of disease caused by unconventional slow viruses. In: Bignami A et al (eds) Discussion in Neurosciences: Molecular mechanisms of pathogenesis of central nervous system disorders. Fondation pour l'Etude du Système Nerveux Central et Périphérique, Geneva, Switzerland, vol 3[1] p 95–100

Ehlers B, Diringer H 1983 Dextran sulfate 500 delays and prevents mouse scrapie by impairment of agent replication in spleen. J Gen Virol 65:1325–1330

Eklund CM, Kennedy RC, Hadlow WJ 1967 Pathogenesis of scrapie virus infection in the mouse. J Infect Dis 117:15–22

Gajdusek DC 1985 Unconventional virus causing subacute spongiform encephalo-pathies. In: Fields BN et al (eds) Virology. Raven Press, New York, p 1519–1557

Glenner GG 1980 Amyloid. β-Fibrillosis. N Engl J Med 302:1283–1292, 1333–1343

Kimberlin RH 1979 Early events in the pathogenesis of scrapie in mice: biological and biochemical studies. In: Prusiner SB, Hadlow WJ (eds) Slow transmissible disease of the nervous system. Academic Press, New York, vol 2:33–54

Kimberlin RH, Walker CA 1986 Pathogenesis of scrapie (strain 263K) in hamsters infected intracerebrally, intraperitoneally or intraocularly. J Gen Virol 67:255–263

Manuelidis EE, Gorgacz EJ, Manuelidis L 1978 Viremia in experimental Creutzfeldt-Jakob disease. Science (Wash DC) 200:1069–1071

Merz PA, Somerville RA, Wisniewski HM, Iqbal K 1981 Abnormal fibrils from scrapie infected brains. Acta Neuropathol 54:63–74

Oesch B, Westaway D, Wälchli M et al 1985 A cellular gene encodes scrapie PrP 27–30 protein. Cell 40:735–746

Prusiner SB 1982 Novel proteinaceous infectious particles cause scrapie. Science (Wash DC) 216:136–144
Rohwer RG 1984 Scrapie infectious agent is virus-like in size and susceptibility to inactivation. Nature (Lond) 308:658–662

DISCUSSION

Gabizon: How big do you think this virus would be?

Diringer: According to filtration experiments, bigger than 20 nm.

McKinley: Since two groups have published that they found the PrP protein in the spleen and you looked in the spleen at 20-fold greater amount of tissue than needed to find PrP in the brain, and yet you don't find PrP in spleen, do you still believe it's not present in spleen? Does that make you question the validity of some of your other results, such as your reported increase in the virus prior to increase in protein?

Diringer: Of course I believe in our data. Concerning the presence of PrP in spleen, we did the control experiments where we added homogenate from 10 mg of brain to 2 g of spleen tissue and were able to detect SAF protein after purification. SAF protein, PrP^{Sc}, is absent from spleen tissue taken from sick hamsters where the brain contains high infectivity titres and SAF protein. I am convinced that this protein in the aggregated form is absent from the spleen.

McKinley: Do you think that the other two groups had contamination?

Diringer: Probably, or unspecific antibody reactivity, I don't know.

McKinley: Looking at their papers I could not see a possible source of contamination.

F. Brown: Isn't there an issue here about the sensitivity of detection? You can measure the infectivity titre far more easily than the amount of protein.

Diringer: This is true but we have allowed for this. In one example of brain we had 5×10^5 infectious units and easily found SAF protein. In spleen we had 2×10^7 infectious units but found no SAF protein (Czub et al 1986a). Again, infectivity titres and amount of SAF protein do not correspond. They do not correlate if one compares them with materials from two different organs (spleen and brain) nor if they are compared by a kinetic analysis in one organ (brain).

Bolton: Those are not the same fraction–you are comparing a bioassay of an homogenate with a protein measurement in a purified fraction. I suggest that you save the amount that you are inoculating from your homogenate, purify all of that material and bioassay the final fraction. We have repeated those experiments in the i.c. inoculated hamster; in the purified fractions we obtained on the first, seventh and fourteenth days a titre of about 10^4 infectious units. At 21 days it starts to increase and that's the first day we detect the protein HaSp 33-37 on an immunoblot in that purified brain fraction. After that day the amount of the protein increases in parallel with the amount of scrapie infectivity.

Diringer: That doesn't correlate with the data from Steve DeArmond, which correlate exactly with ours.

DeArmond: We used crude whole homogenates, we didn't purify PrP^{Sc} as Dr Bolton did.

Diringer: Even better. Did you use the crude homogenate for SAF determination?

DeArmond: We have only measured the prion protein, PrP 27-30. Western blot analysis of crude whole brain extracts of PrP 27-30 is not very sensitive. Our more recent data show that the PrP 27-30 is regionally distributed. We lose sensitivity of detection by using whole brain homogenates. Tissue isolates from specific areas would yield greater sensitivity.

Bolton: When we have done the experiment we pick up both infectivity increase and the protein at 21 days, which falls right in the middle of where Heino (Diringer) is not detecting the protein but is detecting infectivity by bioassay.

Diringer: For this reason you should also do an i.p. experiment. In i.c. inoculations with brain material you have to calculate very carefully how much SAF protein you inject into the animal in relation to the sensitivity of your immunoanalysis—if you inject too much it may stay there and you find it as injected SAF protein not newly formed SAF protein when you assay the samples.

Bolton: We have looked at 1 day, 7 days and 14 days and the infectivity titres are all low and the protein is below detectable limits.

Diringer: Our experimental design allows us to assay SAF protein quantitatively over a range of 3-4 logs, better than any other analysis. So I think it's quite sensitive and good.

Gabizon: But the infectivity range is over nine logs and you cannot correlate that with the protein because the sensitivity of protein measurement has a range of only a few logs.

Diringer: Stan, how sensitive is the measurement of incubation period?

Prusiner: If you really want to be sure of a measurement, you want a two log change.

Diringer: We all have to ask ourselves whether a test which cannot differentiate between less than two logs is a useful test. So far we had considered a loss of infectivity of one log (an increase in incubation period of at least 10 days) to be significant. But anyway—a change of infectivity of two logs in the final stage of virus replication in the hamster brain represents an increase from 10^7 to 10^9 infectious units per hamster brain. If SAF protein (PrP^{Sc}) and infectivity were correlated, we should be able to detect SAF in any animal that has infectivity titres that high in its brain, because the sensitivity of our test for this protein covers a range of at least three logs. In the earlier part of the i.p. kinetics (Czub et al 1986b), between 65–80 days, several animals were negative for SAF protein although infectivity had already reached these titres in the brain.

Bolton: You are comparing non-equivalent samples: for the bioassay you are using a homogenate of brain and for protein detection a purified fraction. The ability to purify this protein from the brain changes as the pathology progresses during the course of the disease, it is not a constant feature.

Chesebro: To me that observation implies that SAF or PrP may not be the agent.

McKinley: Perhaps the agent is changing throughout the life of the infected animal. More plausible is that the brain is maturing and changing, so a purification protocol applied to brain extracted from neonates may not readily apply to an animal that's two or three months old: development of the brain is an ongoing event.

Gabizon: Before this protein can aggregate, its concentration has to reach a critical amount. So at the time when you first measure the titre of infectivity, you are losing the protein because it's still in solution. You cannot purify the protein by that method. There are other ways of purifying the protein from supernatant, which may be the way to do it in your case, Heino. If you take a supernatant after precipitation of rods, even in the cases of higher infectivity you will still have some protein, a very small amount, left in solution, which has not been aggregated.

Diringer: I don't doubt that. Nevertheless, we know exactly why we did this experiment this way; we know the reliability of our way of looking for this protein in the purified fraction. This method is more sensitive and more specific than looking in the crude fraction. We are confident and Steve DeArmond's data confirm our beliefs.

Dickinson: If there is a true break in the correlation between data from different labs that would be important and it could occur if people were using different materials—so we should state in all these comparisons which strain of scrapie was used and which strain of hamster.

Diringer: We used scrapie strain 263K for hamster and 139A in mice. Hamsters were inbred CLAC hamsters in the i.c. experiment and outbred AURA hamsters in the i.p. kinetic experiment.

Dickinson: That is one difference because nobody else is using those hamsters.

Diringer: We also used randomly bred Swiss mice in the spleen experiment.

Merz: Rubenstein used 139A and 22L strains of scrapie and the reported results were ME7 in C57BL mice, but the procedure used was not a purification of SAF (Rubenstein et al 1986).

Tateishi: Shinagawa et al (1986) used a primary isolate of scrapie from sheep, infected into mice.

Dickinson: We have been trying to compare cheese and chalk. The criticism that three other groups disagree with Heino Diringer loses its force in the light of these differences.

Diringer: Our hypothesis of a virus-induced organ-specific amyloidosis of the

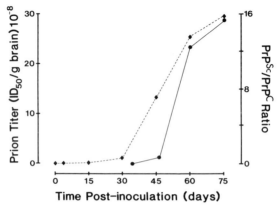

Fig. 1 (*DeArmond*) Double orthographic plot of scrapie infectivity titre and the PrP^{Sc}/PrP^C ratio as a function of time.

central nervous system makes sense to me as a virologist. It leads me to do new experiments—I have to look again for the virus (however horrible this may be because we thought we had it), on the other hand I can investigate the interesting biochemical question of why this amyloidosis occurs.

DeArmond: I took the raw data that was published in the Oesch (1985) paper and instead of plotting it logarithmically I plotted it orthographically. There is a problem of interpretation created when a logarithmic plot and orthographic plots are placed on the same graph. Log plots are very spread out and they rise very quickly. If both ordinates (infectivity and SAF in Dr Diringer's study) are made orthographic and equal in height, the two functions flow right next to each other. We have made a double orthographic plot of infectivity titre and the PrP^{Sc}/PrP^C ratio as a function of time. Even with problems of purification and detection of PrP protein, the two come much closer together than suggested by Dr Diringer's graph (Fig. 1).

*Paul Brown:*Despite the fact that the lines are closer, infectivity is temporally in advance of protein accumulation. However, the difference is only 0.1 log— earlier Stan Prusiner said that to be really sure about a point you need a difference of two logs.

*Diringer:*Steve, you reported that the titre of infectivity has increased after 40 days; this is very similar to our data. We think it is a little bit earlier because we say that the sensitivity of the infectivity assay is one log. The increase in SAF occurs much later.

F. Brown: But this is the same point–sensitivity of detection of the protein compared with detection of infectivity.

Diringer: 10^9 infectious units are equivalent to 25 µg of the SAF protein. The limit of detection by immunoblotting is about 10–20 ng, which is about 1000-fold less (Czub et al 1986b). If infectivity and SAF protein really correlate quantitatively, then we should be able to find the protein in a sample that contains 10^6 infectious units, but we don't. At the early time, when infectivity is up to at least 10^8 infectious units, we still do not find the SAF protein in some animals. There is only one possible reason, if this protein is an essential part of infectivity, when the increase in infectivity ceases, the production of SAF protein might continue as a kind of overproduction of a viral constituent which, although not infectious itself, could constitute part of the infectivity.

F. Brown: You mean that after infectivity reaches a certain level, protein apparently continues to be produced. When foot-and-mouth disease virus is grown in tissue culture, where there are no host immune responses involved, the infectivity titre first increases, then stays constant but the amount of virus protein continues to increase. This is because, although more virus particles are being produced, infectious particles are being inactivated at the same time.

Almond: In infections of tissue culture with many viruses, for example hepatitis A, high multiplicity infection of previously uninfected cells gives rise to accumulation of empty virus particles, so the particle:infectivity ratio becomes very high late in infection.

Diringer: This argument I accept as a possibility.

Kimberlin: The way I see it, your data show that the time when most of the protein is being made is after the time when most of the infectivity has built up. That says nothing about the relationship between protein and infectivity at earlier times.

Bolton: The most important aspect of this is that we are measuring two different fractions which are not directly related. When the experiment is done so that we measure the two different things in one fraction, then we can talk about the interpretation of the data.

References

Czub M, Braig HR, Blode H, Diringer H 1986a The major protein of SAF is absent from spleen and thus not an essential part of the scrapie agent. Arch Virol 91:383–386

Czub M, Braig HR, Diringer H 1986b Pathogenesis of scrapie: study on the temporal development of clinical symptoms, of infectivity titres and scrapie-associated fibrils in brains of hamsters infected intraperitoneally. J Gen Virol 67:2005–2009

Oesch B, Westaway D, Wälchli M et al 1985 A cellular gene encodes scrapie PrP 27–30 protein. Cell 40:735–746

Rubenstein R, Kascsak RJ, Merz PA et al 1986 Detection of scrapie associated fibril (SAF proteins using anti-SAF antibody in non-purified tissue preparations. J Gen Virol 67:671–681

Shinagawa M, Munekata E, Doi S, Takahashi K, Goto H et al 1986 Immunoreactivity of a synthetic pentadecapeptide corresponding to the N-terminal region of the scrapie prion protein. J Gen Virol 67:1745–1750

Scrapie-associated fibrils, PrP protein and the *Sinc* gene

James Hope and Nora Hunter

AFRC & MRC Neuropathogenesis Unit, West Mains Road, Edinburgh, EH9 3JF, UK

Abstract. Scrapie-associated fibrils (SAF) are disease-specific structures found in extracts of the brains of animals affected with scrapie. These structures are pathological aggregates of a normal host protein called PrP. In collaboration with Konrad Beyreuther (Heidelberg), we have characterized the multiple forms of PrP found in SAF fractions from mouse brain affected by the ME7 strain of scrapie. There is no *in vivo* N-terminal cleavage of the most abundant forms of PrP. However, N-terminal cleavage of some minor forms of PrP does occur *in vivo* within a domain of repetitive sequences at sites similar to but distinct from those cut by proteinase K *in vitro*. We suggest that such covalently modified forms of PrP may be the result of enzymic degradation occurring as a consequence rather than as a cause of disease. We also found a novel, as yet unidentified, amino acid derivative of the arginine residue at position 3 in both hamster and mouse PrP 33–35, which may predispose PrP to form SAF. Carlson and colleagues have discovered a linkage between the PrP gene and the murine gene provisionally called *Prn-i* which, from the work of Carp and coworkers, appears identical to the *Sinc* gene. The *Sinc* gene is the major gene determining the incubation period of all strains of scrapie in mice. We have evidence for a linkage of the PrP gene and *Sinc* using inbred mice of known *Sinc* genotype, including VM(*Sinc*[p7]) and VM(*Sinc*[s7]) congenic mice. PrP may even be the protein product of the *Sinc* gene.

1988 Novel infectious agents and the central nervous system. Wiley, Chichester (Ciba Foundation Symposium 135) p 146–163

Unconventional viral (UCV) infections produce a slow, but inexorable, degeneration of the central nervous system. Diagnosis of UCV infection is based on clinical symptoms and on the histopathological lesions seen in affected brain. Recently, a UCV-specific change was discovered in the physical and chemical properties of a neuronal sialoglycoprotein, PrP, and this has provided an additional marker for these infections.

PrP has the structure and biochemical properties of a transmembrane protein (Oesch et al 1985, Meyer et al 1986). In UCV-affected brain, most PrP can be sedimented from detergent-solubilized membranes in a fibrillar form (Diringer et al 1983, Meyer et al 1986, Hope et al 1988b). These fibrils were originally described as scrapie-associated fibrils (SAF), but they are common to all UCV infections including Creutzfeldt-Jakob disease of humans (Merz et al 1981, 1984). The aggregation of PrP into fibrils partially protects the protein from proteolysis; it was originally purified as a 27 000–30 000 Da polypeptide using detergents and proteinase K (Bolton et al 1982, McKinley et al 1983). Under these conditions, which were designed to purify scrapie infectivity, PrP in uninfected brain can be solubilized from membranes and completely hydrolysed (Oesch et al 1985, Kascsak et al 1986, Manuelidis et al 1985, Meyer et al 1986). The protease-resistant core structure of PrP in SAF was called PrP 27–30. Since this protein was not found in similar fractions purified from uninfected brain and the cyanogen bromide cleavage pattern of PrP 27–30 was different from that of proteins of the same molecular weight in uninfected brain, it was concluded that PrP was not a conformational isomer of a normal host protein but a protein unique to scrapie-affected brain. The co-purification of SAF, PrP and infectivity, and their comparable insensitivities to proteinase K led to the idea that PrP was a component of the scrapie infectious particle (Bolton et al 1982, Prusiner 1982, Diringer et al 1983, McKinley et al 1983). No scrapie-specific nucleic acid was identified in SAF fractions and it was speculated that PrP 27–30 alone was responsible for UCV infections (Prusiner et al 1982, McKinley et al 1983). However, further investigation of the molecular biology of PrP (see below), coupled with abundant evidence for the existence of many different strains of scrapie (Dickinson et al 1984), made this unlikely.

The N-terminal sequence of PrP 27–30 was determined by gas-phase protein sequencing and found to be heterogeneous, a so-called ragged-ended protein. However, sufficient sequence was obtained to predict the sequence of the mRNA. Complementary oligonucleotides were synthesized and used to isolate cDNA clones of PrP mRNA from scrapie-infected hamster brain (Oesch et al 1985). With these cDNAs it was discovered that PrP was coded for by a highly conserved host gene (Oesch et al 1985, Robakis et al 1986, Locht et al 1986, Basler et al 1986, Westaway & Prusiner 1986), which was expressed almost exclusively in neurons (Kretzschmar et al 1986). The molecular weight of non-glycosylated PrP was predicted to be about 25 000 Da. Immunoblotting using antisera to PrP 27–30 detected PrP in detergent extracts of uninfected, as well as scrapie-affected, brain and its apparent molecular weight was 33 000–35 000 Da (PrP 33–35) (Oesch et al 1985, Manuelidis et al 1985, Kascsak et al 1986, Hope et al 1988b). Lower molecular weight forms of PrP were found only in extracts of scrapie-affected brain (Fig. 1a).

Since the amounts of total PrP mRNA in whole hamster brain did not change during the course of the disease (Oesch et al 1985), it was important to know why a pathological aggregate of PrP was a specific by-product of unconventional viral infections. Braig and Diringer (1985) suggested that scrapie was a viral-induced amyloidosis of the brain. SAF share some of the structural and physicochemical properties of amyloid fibrils and scrapie infection might prevent the catabolism of PrP, resulting in its accumulation, by mechanisms similar to those proposed for the formation of other amyloids. For example, proteolysis appears to be involved in the deposition of the A4 peptide as cerebral amyloid in the brains of patients with Alzheimer's disease (Kang et al 1987). Although this human dementia is not known to be infectious, it has certain histopathological characteristics in common with some mouse scrapie models, including the formation of amyloid-containing neuritic plaques. Alternatively, some post-translational change(s) other than proteolytic cleavage might be the crucial factor causing the different properties of PrP in uninfected and infected brain.

This paper reviews our search for such changes and describes the molecular pathology of PrP in scrapie-affected mouse and hamster brain. We also report on studies of restriction fragment length polymorphisms in the region of the murine PrP gene and speculate that PrP might be the protein product of a gene (*Sinc*) which controls scrapie incubation period in mice.

SAF protein and normal brain PrP

To evaluate ideas that abnormal post-translational processing of PrP underlies its aberrant properties in scrapie-affected brain, we tried to define the structural relationship between PrP 33–35 in scrapie-affected and normal brain, and also between PrP 33–35 and PrP 27–30. We adapted methods for the purification of SAF by omitting proteinase K and taking steps to minimize exogenous proteolysis. Using an antiserum raised against hamster PrP 27–30, we looked at the molecular weight and distribution of PrP-related proteins at successive stages in this purification procedure applied to scrapie-infected and uninfected hamster brain. We found that the major polypeptide of the SAF fraction has the same molecular weight as the normal protein but can be sedimented (with SAF) under conditions which keep the normal protein in solution (Hope et al 1988b).

Purified hamster SAF proteins were analysed by two-dimensional electrophoresis (non-equilibrium pH gradient gel electrophesis, NEPHGE and SDS-PAGE) (Fig. 1c). An immunoblot of a detergent extract of non-infected brain showed that the normal, cellular PrP had the same molecular weight as the major SAF protein and a similar charge distribution (Fig. 1d). The PrP 33–35 protein of SAF and normal brain could be seen as a diffuse smear extending from pI 5 to pI 9 under the conditions of our analysis (Fig. 1c,d) (Hope et al 1986).

We sequenced the N-terminal amino acids of SAF PrP 33–35 from 263K-affected hamsters. The sequence was K^1-K-R-P-K-P-G-G- (Hope et al 1986), exactly that predicted to be the N-terminal sequence of the normal, cellular PrP of hamster brain after cleavage of a signal peptide (Basler et al 1986,

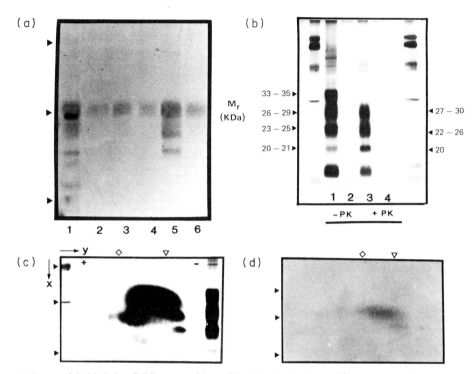

FIG. 1.   (a) SDS-PAGE/immunoblot of PrP in brain from different combinations of agent strain and mouse strain. 1, 87V scrapie in MB mouse; 2, uninfected MB mouse; 3, 87V scrapie in IM mouse; 4, uninfected IM mouse; 5, ME7 scrapie in RIII mouse; 6, uninfected RIII mouse. (b) SDS-PAGE/silver stain of PrP proteins extracted from SAF or the corresponding fraction of uninfected mouse brain. Purified without (−PK) or with (+PK) proteinase K. 1, 22L scrapie in VM mouse (−PK); 2, VM mouse (−PK); 3, 22L scrapie in VM mouse (+PK); 4, VM mouse (+PK). (c) 2-D gel analysis/silver stain of 263K/hamster SAF proteins. Hamster SAF proteins were purified without proteinase K and compared to M_r standards (M) or PrP-related proteins purified from the 22L/VM mouse model (VM). Note the lower M_r forms of PrP are more abundant in SAF from this particular mouse model than in SAF from 263K-infected hamster brain. (d) The immunoreactive PrP-related proteins in the 215 000 g supernatant of a detergent extract of uninfected hamster brain. (a, c and d) ▶ denotes M_r standards (top to bottom) ovalbumin (45 kDa), carbonic anhydrase (30 kDa), myoglobin (17 kDa). ◊ ▽ markers to align these gels in NEPHGE. Each 2-D gel analysis represents the equivalent of 0.1 hamster brain. +, position of sample loading. → y, direction in which proteins migrate in NEPHGE. → x, direction in which proteins migrate in SDS-PAGE.

Robakis et al 1986). We concluded that the major hamster SAF protein and its normal, cellular homologue are indistinguishable in size, charge distribution and N-terminal sequence and may have the same covalent structure (Hope et al 1986). Proof of this idea requires the structural analysis of both SAF protein and normal PrP. If they are the same protein, the different physicochemical properties of PrP 33–35 in scrapie-infected and normal brain could be due to purely conformational differences. Their relationship might be that of a native protein to an alternatively folded form which displays irreversible aggregation.

Models for the pathogenesis of SAF

To account for our observation that most 263K-infected hamster SAF protein is indistinguishable from the normal brain PrP, we suggested that PrP might function *in vivo* as part of an oligomeric structure in cellular membranes (Hope et al 1986, 1988b). Scrapie infection might then perturb the environment of this complex, perhaps by changing ion balance, pH or lipid integrity, and so initiate an alteration in its conformation (Fig. 2a). More provocatively, a conformational change could be induced by direct binding of scrapie agent (or one of its components, such as the putative nucleic acid genome) to PrP (Fig. 2b), so that the turnover of this altered complex differed from that of its normal counterpart. The accumulation of PrP, perhaps coupled with covalent modification of some PrP molecules (see below), could then lead to the pathological aggregation of the PrP oligomer and the formation of SAF, either *in vivo* or *in vitro* (Fig. 2a,b). If the 'agent receptor' model for the formation of SAF proposed in Fig. 2b were correct, then it would provide an explanation for the specificity of these abnormal fibrils to UCV-infected brains and for their association with infectivity.

The molecular pathology of mouse SAF protein

Although most SAF protein from 263K-affected hamster brain was indistinguishable from its normal cellular form, certain combinations of scrapie strain and mouse genotype yielded lower molecular weight forms of PrP which were present in abundance in association with SAF. To assess any role of proteolysis in the formation of these lower molecular weight forms (and SAF), we determined the N-terminal sequence of each variant of PrP in SAF purified from ME7-affected RIII or VL mouse brain. This enabled us to define the proteolytic changes in PrP occurring *in vivo* and to compare these changes with those produced by proteinase K *in vitro* (Hope et al 1988a).

The major immunoreactive form of PrP in brain homogenates from normal and from scrapie-affected mouse brain had an apparent molecular weight of 33 000–35 000 Da (PrP 33–35, Fig. 1a). The lower molecular weight forms, PrP 26–29 (M_r 26 000–29 000), PrP 23–25 (M_r 23 000–25 000) and PrP 20–21 (M_r 20 000–21 000) were found only in the homogenate of scrapie-affected brain (Fig. 1a), and co-purified with both PrP 33–35 and SAF (Fig. 1b, lane 1). PrP does not sediment in the corresponding fraction of normal brain (Fig. 1b, lane 2). The size variants of PrP were purified by SDS-PAGE and electroelution from gel slices, and their N-terminals were sequenced. PrP

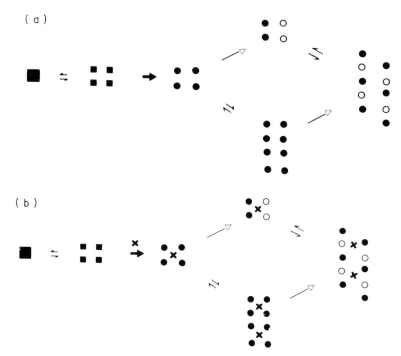

FIG. 2. Theoretical models of DIRECT or INDIRECT effects of scrapie on the aggregation of PrP. ■, the normal cellular PrP protein, which functions as part of an oligomeric complex in membranes; ●, conformational isomer(s) of PrP; ○, covalently modified forms of PrP; ⟶, irreversible event initiated directly or indirectly by scrapie infection; ⇌ , equilibrium between monomeric and oligomeric forms of PrP ×, the scrapie agent; ⟶▷, covalent modification of PrP. (a) the INDIRECT effect : SAF are produced without the need for a molecular interaction between PrP and a scrapie agent. In this case, any co-purification of infectivity with these structures would result from chance association. (b) the DIRECT effect : SAF are a specific consequence of the binding of infectious scrapie agent (or putative scrapie nucleic acid which alone is probably not infectious) to PrP. In this case, the altered membrane-bound proto-fibril ( ) and SAF could be regarded as forms of the infectious agent and could be resistant to hydrolysis by proteinase K. (From Hope et al 1988b.)

33–35, PrP 26–29 and PrP 23–25 had a major sequence of K^1 K R P K P G G, the same as that found for hamster SAF protein, and that which had been inferred from the cDNA sequence of mouse PrP mRNA. PrP 26–29 and PrP 23–25 contained additional minor sequences starting $S^{49,57}$ W G Q P H G G, which located their N-terminals in the octapeptide repeat segments of the protein. PrP 20–21 gave multiple signals resembling those predicted to flank a putative transmembrane region of the protein (Fig. 3). These results indicate that the enzyme(s) responsible for *in vivo* cleavage specifically cleave a GG $\downarrow$ X sequence and suggest a rationale for the design of compounds which might inhibit this process. Drugs such as amphotericin B which influence the incubation time of the disease (Pocchiari et al 1987) may do so via a membrane-related inhibition of this proteolysis.

The proteinase K-resistant structures of PrP in SAF had molecular weights of 27 000–30 000 Da (PrP 27–30), 22 000–26 000 Da (PrP 22–26) and 20 000 Da (PrP 20) (Fig. 1b, lane 3). PrP 27–30 and PrP 22–26 had the ragged N-terminal structures originally described for the 263K/hamster PrP 27–30 protein (Oesch et al 1985, Multhaup et al 1985). The major sequence of these molecular weight variants was G^{63} Q G P H G G G, similar but not identical to the sequences detected in the minor components of PrP 26–29 and PrP 23–25 (Hope et al 1988a). These data differ slightly from those reported for hamster PrP 27–30, where G^{68} (equivalent to residue 67 of mouse PrP) was the primary N-terminal amino acid. This may be due to the sequence variation between hamster and mouse PrP (Locht et al 1986) or to differences in the procedures for preparing proteinase-K digested SAF. PrP 20 gave similar results to those obtained for PrP 20–21, consistent with their near identity on one-dimensional gel analysis (Fig. 1b).

Non-proteolytic modification of SAF protein

The surprising result of sequencing hamster and mouse SAF protein was that their lower molecular weight forms of PrP contained predominantly the K^1 K R P K sequence (Hope et al 1986, 1988a). Hence the size diversity of PrP in SAF was not due primarily to N-terminal proteolysis. This diversity must be due to other pathological changes in the structure of PrP 33–35 or interference in its biosynthesis. For example, lectin binding (Manuelidis et al 1985) and amino-sugar analyses (Multhaup et al 1985) have provided evidence for differences in the number and type of carbohydrate chains attached to hamster SAF protein.

The low yield of tryptophan at residue 9 when sequencing hamster PrP 33–35 led us to speculate that *in vivo* oxidation of this amino acid might be involved in the pathogenesis of SAF (Hope et al 1986). Further work has shown that this was due to inappropriate purification methods (Hope et al 1988a). Some of the arginine residues at positions 3 and 15 of hamster and mouse SAF are covalently modified (Hope et al 1988a). The nature or significance of this post-translational modification is not known, although it might affect the location and topography of the protein in the cell membrane, and perhaps predispose PrP to form SAF.

Protein topography

The sites of *in vivo* and *in vitro* proteolysis of PrP help to map the domain structure of this protein in SAF and/or in its proto-fibrillar form (Hope et al 1988a, 1988b; Fig. 3). Their similarity suggests that the topography of the protein

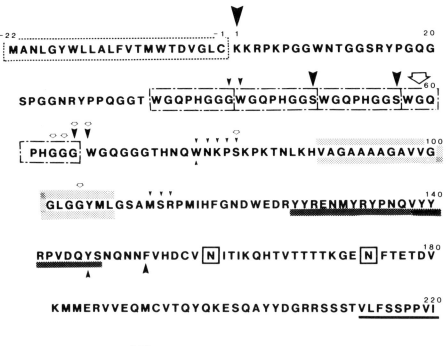

FIG. 3. Domain structure of mouse PrP based on the sequence derived by Locht and colleagues in relation to the cleavage pattern defined by amino acid sequencing of SAF protein prepared with (⟳) or without (▼) proteinase K. ⟦ ⟧, the sequence of the first 22 amino acids of PrP resembles that of a signal peptide involved in protein transport across membranes; ⟦ ⟧, a series of four octapeptide repeat sequences similar to those seen in the epidermal keratins; ▒, a possible membrane-spanning region with a high proportion of glycine and alanine residues; ▬, a second possible transmembrane region similar to that in hamster PrP which has been proposed to serve as part of a hydrophilic membrane channel (Hay et al 1987). [N], sites for asparagine-linked glycosylation; ▬▬, hydrophobic C-terminal region which may act as a membrane anchor sequence. The arrows denote the first amino acid of protein fragments found in the molecular weight variants of mouse SAF protein (similar to those in Fig. 1b) : ▼ ME7/VL(non-proteinase K); ⟳ ME7/VL(proteinase K). The relative abundance of each sequence varied depending on which size variant was analysed but the size of the arrow indicates the ranking of abundance of these individual sequences in total SAF protein. (From Hope et al 1988a.)

or its accessibility to proteinases is essentially equivalent *in vivo* and *in vitro* and that its conformation does not change significantly during purification or, in the case of proto-fibrils, on further aggregation into fibrils. In addition to those sites of cleavage identified in the repetitive domain of PrP, we found others which delineate regions predicted to lie within the cell membrane by modelling of its secondary structure (Bazan et al 1987) or inferred from experiments on its *in vitro* biogenesis (Hay et al 1987). For example, PrP 20–21 contains polypeptides with N-terminal sequences equivalent to segments of PrP on either side of a putative transmembrane region, and in total SAF protein from ME7-affected RIII mouse brain we found fragments of PrP starting F^{152} V H D X V (Hope et al 1988a). Interestingly, *in vitro* biogenesis studies have implied that this latter site is the point where the protein emerges from the membrane into the extracellular space, and that the segment of the protein which immediately precedes it may form part of a hydrophilic channel (Hay et al 1987). This fits with our idea that the protein may function in normal cells as a subunit in a membrane-bound oligomeric complex (Hope et al 1986, 1988a), similar to a membrane receptor or channel pore subunit. Alternatively, the limited proteolysis sites may reflect the folded structure of PrP monomer or oligomer in scrapie-affected brain; in addition, the partial protection of fragments of PrP starting around F^{152} may be afforded by nearby oligosaccharide chains at N^{158} and/or N^{174}, rather than by insertion of the polypeptide chain into membranes.

Linkage of PrP gene and the Sinc gene

Interest in the role of PrP in the pathogenesis of scrapie has been stimulated by the discovery of a linkage between the PrP gene and the murine gene provisionally called *Prn-i* (Carlson et al 1986) which appears to be identical to the *Sinc* gene (Carp et al 1987). *Sinc* controls the incubation period of all strains of scrapie in mice and has two known alleles (Dickinson et al 1984). Most laboratory mouse strains are *Sinc*[s7] and have a relatively short incubation period for the ME7 group of scrapie strains. Until recently, VM mice and lines derived from this stock were the only known source of the *Sinc*[p7] allele, which produces a longer incubation period for the ME7 group strains relative to their incubation periods in *Sinc*[s7] mice. In contrast, members of the 22A group of scrapie strains have longer incubation times in s7 than p7 mice. I ('I/LnJ') mice are another mouse strain homozygous for the p7 allele of *Sinc* (Carp et al 1987). Carlson and co-workers recently described a restriction fragment length polymorphism (RFLP) linked to the *Sinc* gene, which they designated *Prn-i*. The RFLP was found using the restriction endonuclease *Xba*I and a nucleic acid probe specific for the coding region of the PrP gene (now provisionally called *Prn-p*) (Carlson et al 1986).

We have confirmed this finding using the congenic mouse strains VM(*Sinc*[p7]) and VM(*Sinc*[s7]) (Hunter et al 1987). VM(*Sinc*[s7]) congenics were produced by 19 generations of backcrossing to VM mice the progeny of an original VM × C57BL(*Sinc*[s7]) cross, with selection at each generation on the basis of scrapie incubation times. High molecular weight DNA was extracted from the livers of normal, uninfected mice, digested with *Xba*I and subjected

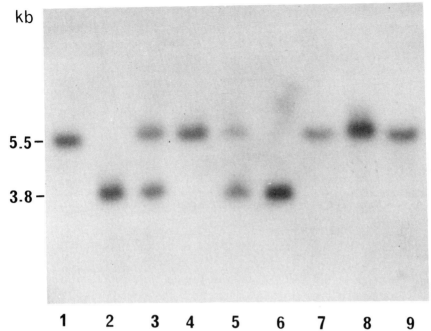

FIG. 4.   Southern analysis of normal mouse DNA digested with *Xba*I and hybridized to ³²P-labelled pEA974. The mouse strains were : track 1, RIII; 2, VM (*Sinc*ˢ⁷) congenics; 3, VM × VM (*Sinc*ˢ⁷) congenics F1; 4, VM; 5, VM × C57BL F1; 6, C57BL; 7, IM; 8, VL, 9, MB. (From Hunter et al 1987.)

to Southern analysis using a cDNA probe, pEA974, made to hamster PrP mRNA (Robakis et al 1986). This cDNA hybridized to a 5.5 kb *Xba*I fragment in VM DNA and to a 3.8 kb fragment in VM(*Sinc*ˢ⁷) congenics (Fig. 4). These results are similar to those previously described (Carlson et al 1986), except that we used congenic mice which differ at the *Sinc* locus and at regions linked to *Sinc*. VM × VM(*Sinc*ˢ⁷) congenic F1 mice had both the 5.5 kb and the 3.8 kb fragments. The mouse strain which donated the s7 allele to the congenics also had the 3.8 kb fragment and other *Sinc*ᵖ⁷ inbred mice (IM and MB, which were derived from VM crosses) had the 5.5 kb *Xba*I fragment. No such RFLP has been shown with several other enzymes (*Bam*HI, *Pvu*II, *Hin*dIII, *Eco*RI, *Pst*I, *Kpn*I, *Sst*I). On this evidence the two genes PrP and *Sinc* appear to be closely linked and could even be the same gene.

However, the 5.5 kb fragment is not a definitive marker for the p7 allele because two unrelated mouse strains, RIII and VL, both homozygous for *Sinc*ˢ⁷, possessed the 5.5 kb *Xba*I fragment. A restriction map constructed from our data placed the polymorphic *Xba*I site in the 3' flanking region of the mouse PrP gene (Hunter et al 1987).

TABLE 1   Linkage of SAF protein (PrP) gene and Sinc

Mouse strain	Sinc genotype	Restriction fragments hybridizing to PrP cDNA		
		XbaI	TaqI	HhaI
VM	p7	5.5 kb[a]	8.1 kb	20 kb[a]
VM(Sinc[s7]) congenics	s7	3.8 kb[a]	9.6 kb	>30 kb[a]
C57BL	s7	3.8 kb	9.6 kb	>30 kb[a]
RIII	s7	5.5 kb[a]	9.6 kb	20 kb, 9.4 kb[b]

[a] liver and brain DNA
[b] signal at 9.4 kb stronger in liver than brain

In a search for other RFLPs, the enzymes TaqI and HhaI revealed differences amongst the Sinc genotypes. Because of the sensitivity of HhaI to methylation of the internal cytosine in its recognition sequence (GCGC), we think it likely that the RFLP seen with this enzyme reflects differences in methylation rather than sequence. This possibility was supported by evidence that in RIII brain DNA, the pattern of hybridization to HhaI fragments differed consistently from that seen in RIII liver DNA. In the congenic mice, VM(Sinc[p7]) and VM(Sinc[s7]), no difference was seen in HhaI digests of liver and brain DNA. Therefore, we were able to divide the mice used in our study into three groups based on hybridization of different restriction fragments to the hamster PrP cDNA clone (pEA974) (Table 1) (Hunter et al 1987).

The functional significance of these observations and their relationship, if any, to the action of the Sinc gene have yet to be established. However, even if PrP is the protein product of the Sinc gene, the difference between the s7 and p7 alleles that accounts for their profound effect on scrapie incubation period may be discerned only by nucleotide sequencing of the genes themselves.

Conclusion

Scrapie-associated fibrils and PrP have provided exciting fodder for molecular biologists in the past few years, although as yet their relationship to infectivity is still controversial. This controversy may only be resolved by the in vitro synthesis and assembly of an infectious particle, be it protein or a composite of protein and nucleic acid. Optimistically, the continuing study of SAF and PrP will provide insight into the molecular processes of UCV disease and yield clues to two outstanding problems in UCV research: 1) the molecular basis of UCV strain variation and infectivity, and 2) the molecular mechanism of control of scrapie replication, and hence incubation period, by the alleles of the Sinc gene.

Acknowledgements

Our protein sequencing work was achieved in collaboration with Professor K. Beyreuther and Dr G. Multhaup (Cologne/Heidelberg). We thank Professor H. Diringer (Berlin) and Dr R. Kascsak (New York) for generous gifts of antisera to hamster and mouse PrP 27–30, and Dr N. Robakis (New York) for pEA974. This work benefited by the award of a NATO collaborative research grant (No. 86/0112) to J.H. and Professor Beyreuther.

References

Basler K, Oesch B, Scott M et al 1986 Scrapie and cellular PrP isoforms are encoded by the same chromosomal gene. Cell 46:417–428

Bazan JF, Fletterick RJ, McKinley MP, Prusiner SB 1987 Predicted secondary structure and membrane topology of the scrapie prion protein. Protein Eng 1:125–135

Bolton DC, McKinley MP, Prusiner SB 1982 Identification of a protein that purifies with the scrapie prion. Science (Wash DC) 218:1309–1311

Braig HR, Diringer H 1985 Scrapie: concept of a virus-induced amyloidosis of the brain. EMBO (Eur Mol Biol Organ) J 4:2309–2312

Carlson GA, Kingsbury DT, Goodman PA et al 1986 Linkage of prion protein and scrapie incubation time genes. Cell 46:503–511

Carp RI, Moretz RC, Natelli M, Dickinson AG 1987 Genetic control of scrapie: incubation period and plaque formation in I mice. J Gen Virol 68:401–407

Dickinson AG, Bruce ME, Outram GW, Kimberlin RH 1984 Scrapie strain differences: the implications of stability and mutation. In: Tateishi J (ed) Proc Workshop on slow transmissable diseases, Tokyo. Jpn Min Health & Welfare Publ, p 105–118

Diringer H, Gelderblom H, Hilmert H, Ozel M, Edelbluth C, Kimberlin RH 1983 Scrapie infectivity, fibrils and low molecular weight protein. Nature (Lond) 306:376–478

Hay B, Barry RA, Lieberburg I, Prusiner SB, Vishwanath VR 1987 Biogenesis and transmembrane orientation of the cellular isoform of the scrapie prion protein. Mol Cell Biol 7:914–920

Hope J, Morton LJD, Farquhar CF, Multhaup G, Beyreuther K, Kimberlin RH 1986 The major protein of scrapie-associated fibrils (SAF) has the same size, charge distribution and N-terminal protein sequence as predicted for the normal brain protein (PrP). EMBO (Eur Mol Biol Organ) J 5:2591–2597

Hope J, Multhaup G, Reekie LJD, Kimberlin RH, Beyreuther K 1988a Molecular pathology of scrapie-associated fibril protein (PrP) in mouse brain affected by the ME7 strain of scrapie. Eur J Biochem, in press

Hope J, Reekie LJD, Gibson PH 1988b On the pathogenesis of SAF. In: Court LA et al (eds) Unconventional viruses and central nervous system diseases. Atelier d'Arts Graphiques, Abbaye de Melleray, in press

Hunter N, Hope J, McConnell I, Dickinson AG 1987 Linkage of the SAF protein (PrP) gene and Sinc using congenic mice and restriction fragment length polymorphism analysis. J Gen Virol 68:2711–2716

Kang J, Lemaire H-G, Unterbeck A et al 1987 The precursor of Alzheimer's disease amyloid A4 protein resembles a cell-surface receptor. Nature (Lond) 325:733–736

Kascsak RJ, Rubenstein R, Merz PA et al 1986 Immunological comparison of scrapie-associated fibrils isolated from animals infected with four different scrapie strains. J Virol 59:676–683

Kretzschmar HA, Prusiner SB, Stowring LE, DeArmond SJ 1986 Scrapie prion proteins are synthesized in neurones. Am J Pathol 122:1–5

Locht C, Chesebro B, Race R, Keith JM 1986 Molecular cloning and complete sequence of prion protein cDNA from mouse brain infected by the scrapie agent. Proc Natl Acad Sci USA 83:6372–6376

McKinley MP, Bolton DC, Prusiner SB 1983 A protease-resistant protein is a structural component of the scrapie prion. Cell 35:57–62

Manuelidis L, Valley S, Manuelidis EE 1985 Specific proteins associated with Creutzfeldt-Jakob disease and scrapie share antigenic and carbohydrate determinants. Proc Natl Acad Sci USA 82:4263–4267

Merz PA, Somerville RA, Wisniewski HM, Iqbal K 1981 Abnormal fibrils from scrapie-infected brain. Acta Neuropathol 65:63–74

Merz PA, Rowher RG, Kascsak R et al 1984 Infection-specific particle from the unconventional slow virus diseases. Science (Wash DC) 225:437–440

Meyer RK, McKinley MP, Bowman KA, Braunfeld MB, Barry RA, Prusiner SB 1986 Separation and properties of cellular and scrapie prion proteins. Proc Natl Acad Sci USA 83:2310–2314

Multhaup G, Diringer H, Hilmert H, Prinz H, Heukeshoven J, Beyreuther K 1985 The protein component of scrapie associated fibrils is a glycosylated low molecular weight protein. EMBO (Eur Mol Biol Organ) J 4:1495–1501

Oesch B, Westaway D, Wälchli M et al 1985 A cellular gene encodes scrapie PrP 27–30 protein. Cell 40:735–746

Pocchiari M, Schmittinger S, Masullo C 1987 Amphotericin B delays the incubation period of scrapie in intracerebrally inoculated hamsters. J Gen Virol 68:219–223

Prusiner SB 1982 Novel proteinaceous infectious particles cause scrapie. Science (Wash DC) 216:136–144

Robakis NK, Sawh PR, Wolfe GC, Rubenstein R, Carp RI, Innis MA 1986 Isolation of a cDNA clone encoding the leader peptide of prion protein and expression of the homologous gene in various tissues. Proc Natl Acad Sci USA 83:6377–6381

Westaway D, Prusiner SB 1986 Conservation of the cellular gene encoding the scrapie prion protein PrP 27–30. Nucl Acids Res 14:2035–2044

DISCUSSION

Stahl: Do you find this post-translational modification of arginine in hamster PrP^{Sc}?

Hope: Yes.

Stahl: If PrP 27-30 is responsible for infectivity, then this modified arginine cannot be involved because PrP 27-30 doesn't have it.

Hope: We're looking for a post-translational modification of PrP in SAF, which might produce the different physicochemical properties observed in some molecules of this protein in scrapie-affected brain. Perhaps, but not necessarily, this will tell us about infectivity.

Stahl: Properties such as protease resistance?

Hope: I think protease resistance is due to the aggregation of PrP into an abnormal multimer in scrapie-infected brain. The protein itself, when dissociated from this multimer (SAF or proto-fibril), is proteinase K sensitive.

Stahl: PrP 27-30 can form aggregates, so the modified arginines that you have found are not responsible for the aggregation.

Hope: PrP 27-30 is not present in scrapie-affected brain; it is an artifact produced by using proteinase K. Most PrP in 263K-affected hamster brain has a relative molecular weight of 33 000-35 000 (PrP 33-35) (Hope et al 1986). Unlike PrP in normal brain, this protein can be pelleted from detergent extracts of scrapie-affected brain. PrP33-35 does contain the modified arginine residues in question, and so the altered properties of PrP in scrapie-affected brain may be due to this post-translational modification. We need to know if PrP in uninfected brain has this same modification and what it is before we can assess its significance.

Stahl: There are several different bands on a gel after SDS-PAGE of the PrP 33-35^{Sc} reaction and you have shown convincingly that the majority of them have the same N terminus and therefore they probably differ because of post-translational modification or differences at the C-terminus.

Hope: Or incomplete biosynthesis; it could be that the protein never gets fully processed as it would do in an uninfected brain.

Prusiner: In Meyer's studies (Meyer et al 1986), we concluded that the prion rods are an artifact of detergent extraction and showed that the scrapie form of the prion protein was resistant to proteinase K. PrP 27-30 was produced when we treated the membranes with proteinase K. A rod-shaped structure is not essential for protease resistance.

Hope: I would get round that by saying that PrP is in a proto-fibrillar form.

Gabizon: Can you elaborate, what is the meaning of this?

Hope: We would say the altered oligomeric complex of our model for the formation of SAF — this proto-fibril, abnormal multimer or aggregate of PrP — has the proteinase K resistance of the full SAF structure, even though the proto-fibril might consist of only a few molecules.

Gabizon: How many?

Hope: Who knows? Two, four, whatever molecular assembly is necessary to have some resistance to proteinase K hydrolysis.

Almond: When you run the normal PrP protein from an uninfected brain on a 2D gel is there any heterogeneity or is there a single spot? In other words is there any post-translational modification of the normal form?

Hope: The normal PrP protein from uninfected brain has a relative molecular weight of 33 000-35 000 and a charge distribution between pI 5 and 9. We see another variant, molecular weight about 30 000 and charge distribution pI 7 to 9.5, by 2D Western analysis of a detergent extract of uninfected hamster brain (Fig. 1d, Hope & Hunter, this volume). This may be a desialylated form of the normal PrP molecule.

Stahl: Do you get the same result on a Western blot?

Hope: So far we've seen normal PrP by Western blotting alone. We use silver staining to look at PrP in SAF as, in our hands, it is a more sensitive technique for looking at the molecular heterogeneity of this protein.

Manuelidis: Do you find the same pattern on 2D gels of protein from CJD-infected brain?

Hope: We have not looked at CJD-affected brain.

Manuelidis: We have shown that in CJD there are multiple spots with multiple sialic acid residues using specific sugar cleavage enzymes (Sklaviadis et al 1986, Manuelidis et al 1988).

Hope: The three more basic protein groupings of PrP variants which we see by 2D gel analysis correspond to PrP molecules with their N-terminal region intact; that is, they have the K^1 K R P K N-terminal sequence and do not resolve into discrete spots. Those more acidic groupings of PrP, which we have corre-lated with proteolysis products (Hope et al 1988), do resolve into several well defined spots. As you point out, differences in sialic acid content may be an additional reason for the charge/size heterogeneity we see on this 2D gel analysis of PrP in SAF.

Oesch: Jim, by Western blotting, when you use crude brain extracts without purification, do you find the same heterogeneity? I would say that these lower molecular weight products in the purified preparation are artifacts of the preparation procedure, because you don't see them in the original extract.

Hope: They are present in the crude extracts (Fig. 1a, lanes 1 and 5); the reason you can't see them in some cases (Fig. 1a, lane 3) is a problem of detection in the presence of a large excess of other protein. It relates to what I was saying to Mike (McKinley) yesterday, that there is so much protein present in the crude homogenate that it (non-specifically) blocks detection of PrP, by silver staining or by immunoblotting.

McKinley: When you purify your crude fraction it appears as though the concentration of the contaminating bands has increased to a much greater extent than the concentration of PrP 33-35.

Hope: Yes, that's correct. In lanes 1, 3 and 5 (Fig. 1a), the PrP 33-35 signal is a composite of what is found in scrapie-affected and normal brain. Lower molecular weight variants are only seen in scrapie-affected brain homogenates; these smaller variants co-purify with SAF. Since only the scrapie-affected fraction of PrP 33-35 co-purifies with SAF, there is an enrichment of the lower molecular weight forms relative to PrP 33-35 in the SAF fraction (Fig. 1b, lane 1).

Manuelidis: It looks like you are still getting protein breakdown. In CJD-infected hamster brain fractions, we get spots in material that is at least 95% PrP 33-35 (Gp 34) and the breakdown products are very minor.

Hope: The pattern of size/charge variants of PrP in 263K-induced SAF shows a similar high proportion of PrP 33-35 (Fig. 1c). This pattern depends on the particular scrapie strain/host model used as source of affected brain: in some mouse models PrP 33-35 represents a much lower fraction of the total PrP protein in SAF (22L in VM mice, Fig. 1b).

Manuelidis: Maybe because there's more proteolysis during the preparation.

Hope: Or in the brain during the course of the disease.

Manuelidis: When you run on a gel the same amount of material from your purified scrapie preparation, you have the breakdown products which you didn't have in the initial infectious material. If preparative procedures alone lead to the proteolysis, you should see at least a faint signal in the uninfected brain extract in the low molecular weight regions. The proteolysis therefore appears to be related to the disease process.

Stahl: You propose that cellular protein hinders detection of the PrP heterogeneity by Western blotting of crude homogenates. This could be tested by a mixing experiment; take your purified material, mix it back with crude extract and see if you can detect the original band.

Hope: Yes. So far what we have done is to look at the effects on the size and charge heterogeneity of SAF protein of various protease inhibitors specific for each of four groups of protease (serine, S, aspartate, D, cysteine, C, or metallo, X^+, endopeptidases). We used three scrapie models: 263K in hamsters; ME7 in the VL mice and 87V in IM mice; and the following inhibitors (final concentrations in the initial homogenate): N-α-rhamnopyranosyloxy hydroxyphosphinyl)-L-leucyl-tryptophan (type X^+), 0.01 mM; leupeptin (type C), 0.2 mM; pepstatin A (type D), 0.2 mM; 1,10-phenanthroline (type X^+), 2mM; ethylene glycol bis (β-amino-ethyl-ether) N,N,N',N'-tetraacetic acid (type X^+), 2 mM, in addition to a standard cocktail of serine protease inhibitors (phenyl methyl sulphonyl chloride, 1 mM; diisopropyl fluorophosphate, 0.1 mM) and the cysteine-protease inhibitor, N-ethyl maleimide, 1 mM. No effect was noted on the 1D or 2D gel patterns of SAF protein prepared using these various inhibitors. If proteases are degrading the protein during the purification of SAF, then they are not inhibited by the concentrations and types of inhibitors we have tested.

*Beyreuther:*We have sequenced isolates of CJD amyloid, of kuru amyloid and GSS amyloid prepared according to the SAF protocol published by Dr Diringer. This was done in collaboration with Paul Brown. We have also sequenced amyloid of plaque cores prepared from the same GSS case that Paul Brown used to prepare SAF. The plaque cores were prepared by Colin Masters using the procedure that he used for preparing plaque cores from post-mortem brains of patients with Alzheimer's disease. All different isolates give different sequences but all isolates were found to be PrP fragments and unrelated to the A4 amyloid protein of Alzheimer's disease. The SAF procedure yielded material which was heterogeneous in molecular weight and N-terminal sequences. The N-termini are similar to those proteins you described as proteinase K-digested PrP fragments. However, the cleavage sites are different. Kuru PrP proteins have different N-termini from CJD or GSS proteins. The major protein component of the plaque core preparation from the GSS case is a very small peptide, 10 kDa, some 80 residues, starting at the proteinase K site but stopping before the carbohydrate attachment site. This peptide is seen in crude homogenates. Obviously, the degree of proteolysis and where proteolysis occurs depends on the agent that infected the brain. Whether additional proteolysis occurs during preparation is unclear but that doesn't eliminate the characteristic differences. The latter are seen as different N-terminal sequences for the isolates from CJD, GSS and kuru cases.

Prusiner: In your initial sequencing studies on PrP, you showed that the 'SAF protein' is 55 amino acids in length (Multhaup et al 1985) but you now believe that that was due to extensive proteolysis during the preparation of the protein; is that right?

Beyreuther: This work was done with a specific hamster strain, inbred strain CLAC. We repeated this work with outbred AURA hamsters using the same procedure for deglycosylation (treatment with HF) and we get 19 kDa and 14 kDa PrP fragments. PrP from CLAC strains infected with the 263K strain of scrapie agent consistently gave a 5-8 kDa peptide after deglycosylation treatment with HF.

Prusiner: So you now don't believe it's proteolysis.

Beyreuther: I don't know what it is. It could be strain specificity.

Oesch: Did you prepare Western blots?

Beyreuther: Yes, the deglycosylated PrP proteins did not react with polyclonal antibodies directed against glycosylated PrP (the antisera were obtained from Heino Diringer).

Bolton: But you do treat with proteinase K during preparation?

Beyreuther: Yes.

Prusiner: That may mean that the post-translational modifications as well as the protein conformation are different and this determines the protease sensitivity of PrP^{Sc}.

Beyreuther: I agree, these differences seen by sequencing may reflect different folding patterns of the protein.

References

Hope J, Morton LJD, Farquhar CF, Multhaup G, Beyreuther K, Kimberlin RH 1986 The major protein of scrapie-associated fibrils (SAF) has the same size, charge distribution and N-terminal protein sequence as predicted for the normal brain protein (PrP). EMBO (Eur Mol Biol Organ) J 5:2591–2597

Hope J, Multhaup G, Reekie LJD, Kimberlin RH, Beyreuther K 1988 Molecular pathology of scrapie-associated fibril protein (PrP) in mouse brain affected by the ME7 strain of scrapie. Eur J Biochem, in press

Manuelidis L, Sklaviadis T, Manuelidis EE 1988 On the origin and formation of SAF. In: Court L et al (eds) Unconventional viruses and central nervous system diseases. Atelier d'Arts Graphiques, Abbaye de Melleray, in press

Meyer RK, McKinley MP, Bowman KA, Barry RA, Prusiner SB 1986 Separation and properties of cellular and scrapie prion proteins. Proc Natl Acad Sci USA 83:2310–2314

Multhaup G, Diringer H, Hilmert H, Prinz H, Heukeshoven J, Beyreuther K 1985 The protein component of scrapie-associated fibrils is a glycosylated low molecular weight protein. EMBO (Eur Mol Biol Organ) J 4:1495–1501

Sklaviadis T, Manuelidis L, Manuelidis EE 1986 Characterization of major peptides in Creutzfeldt-Jakob disease and scrapie. Proc Natl Acad Sci USA 83:6146–6150

A modified host protein model of scrapie

David C. Bolton* and Paul E. Bendheim†

*Departments of * Molecular Biology and † Pathological Neurobiology, Institute for Basic Research, New York State Office of Mental Retardation and Developmental Disabilities, 1050 Forest Hill Road, Staten Island, NY 10314, USA*

Abstract. The scrapie agent is still not completely characterized biochemically and ultrastructurally, but its requirement for a functional protein has been established. Purification of the scrapie agent by methods using digestion with proteinase K yields a glycoprotein with an apparent mass of 27–30 kDa (PrP 27–30). In contrast, a 33–37 kDa glycoprotein, called Sp33–37, is the major protein component isolated from scrapie-affected brain when protease digestion is not used. Sp33–37 is the product of a normal host gene and is a larger form of PrP 27–30. We propose a model in which Sp33–37, a modified host protein, is the critical component of the scrapie agent; a non-host nucleic acid is not part of the agent. We postulate that Sp33–37, perhaps in concert with other unidentified host components, is capable of inducing the disease and directing the production of more of itself by acting on the normal protein directly or by affecting one of the steps in protein processing. Agent replication requires that: 1) a constant supply of the substrate protein Cp33–37 is available, 2) aggregates of Sp33–37 are resistant to degradation and accumulate in cells or cell membranes, and 3) membrane damage and cell death facilitate spread to adjacent cells. The model predicts that disease can be transmitted by the scrapie agent or initiated by a spontaneous metabolic error resulting in accumulation of the abnormal protein.

1988 Novel infectious agents and the central nervous system. Wiley, Chichester (Ciba Foundation Symposium 135) p 164–181

The biochemical composition and ultrastructure of the scrapie agent remain controversial, despite recent advances in its characterization. Based on the unusual properties of the scrapie agent inferred from its partial characterization, numerous hypotheses for its nature have been proposed (reviewed by Prusiner 1982, Carp et al 1985). Many of the proposed structures can now be excluded. The scrapie agent is not a viroid (Diener et al 1982) and its physical and chemical properties are unlike those of any known single family of viruses (Gajdusek 1977, Prusiner 1982).

Three theoretical models are currently supported: the virus, virino and modified host protein models. The virus model proposes that the scrapie agent is a virus with 'unconventional' properties (Rohwer 1984a,b, Czub et al

1986, Manuelidis et al 1987). The virino model proposes a pathogen-specific nucleic acid protected by a host protein coat (Dickinson & Outram 1979). We have proposed a modified host protein model of scrapie (Bendheim & Bolton 1986), in which a particle containing a modified host protein, but devoid of a specific foreign nucleic acid, is the scrapie agent.

The virus model is attractive for historical and biological reasons: viruses cause some diseases with scrapie-like features, the scrapie agent exhibits several virus-like properties, and the apparent existence of scrapie agent strains is easily explained by the virus model. Upon closer examination the virus model fails to account for several other features of scrapie, most notably: lack of a host immune response to the agent, extreme resistance of the agent to ultrasonic disruption or ultraviolet and ionizing radiation, and failure to identify a viral genome in diseased tissues or fractions highly enriched for biological activity.

The other two scrapie agent models are consistent with the existing data, but have no precedents in microbiology. The virino model fills a niche between viruses and viroids by placing a renegade pathogenic nucleic acid in a coat made of host protein (Dickinson & Outram 1979, Carp et al 1985). The host protein coat protects the scrapie agent nucleic acid from degradation and subverts the host immune response because the protein is seen as 'self'. The virino model is intellectually intriguing and can explain scrapie agent strains by variation in nucleotide sequence. However, the putative virino nucleic acid has not been identified and physical or chemical evidence for its presence is lacking.

The modified host protein model presents the most radical deviation from known microbiological systems. In essence the model proposes that an abnormally modified protein, perhaps in concert with other unidentified host components, is capable of inducing the disease and directing the manufacture of more of the abnormal protein (Oesch et al 1985, Carp et al 1985, Bendheim & Bolton 1986, Meyer et al 1986, Brown et al 1987). The model satisfies the absence of an immune response (the protein is 'self') and the apparent lack of a specific nucleic acid. Explaining scrapie agent strains with this model is more complex; we postulate that strain 'information' is stored and transmitted in the form of protein modifications.

These models attempt to explain the major features of scrapie and present testable hypotheses. As more data are gathered the models will be refined, revised or eliminated. In this report we outline the critical observations that must be explained by any model (Table 1) and develop further our interpretation of the modified host protein model.

Unusual aspects of scrapie

Scrapie-affected animals and humans with Creutzfeldt-Jakob disease (CJD), kuru and Gerstmann-Sträussler syndrome have normal haematological and

TABLE 1   Parameters that restrict models of the scrapie agent

Unusual aspects of scrapie disease
    Lack of immune or inflammatory response
    Prolonged incubation period and slow disease course
    Sporadic cases occur without obvious transmission

Physical, chemical and molecular properties of the agent
    Agent contains an essential protein
    Sp33–37 copurifies with agent and appears to be the essential protein
    Sp33–37 is an abnormal form of a cellular protein, Cp33–37
    Unusual resistance to physical and chemical inactivation
    No evidence for nucleic acid in the agent particle

Scrapie agent strains
    Two distinct groups of agent strains occur in mice
    Strains of agent produce distinct pathology
    Scrapie agents vary in their biological stability
    Adaptation to a new host may require several passages
    Competition between strains for reproduction

Host genotype
    Host genotype influences incubation period and pathology
    Sinc and *Prn*[i] genes are probably identical
    Cp33–37 gene (*Prn*[p]) and *Prn*[i] gene are closely linked and may be identical
    Two alleles of Cp33–37 gene and *Sinc/Prn*[i] gene are known
    Long incubation periods generally correlate with amyloid plaque production
    F1 heterozygotes can have longer incubation than homozygous parental
        strains

cerebrospinal fluid profiles. At no time during the disease are humoral or cellular immune responses against the causative agent detected. Tissues from affected animals and individuals show no evidence of inflammation. Pathology is limited to the central nervous system and consists of astrocytosis, vacuolation, and neuronal depletion. Amyloid plaque formation is widespread in some cases. A hallmark of these diseases is the prolonged asymptomatic period from inoculation to onset of clinical disease. In CJD, and perhaps in natural cases of scrapie, sporadic disease appears without obvious transmission.

Physical, chemical and molecular properties of the agent

Diverse approaches in several laboratories have documented that the scrapie agent contains an essential protein component. A method for purifying the scrapie agent that included proteinase K digestion led to identification in hamsters of a size-heterogeneous, protease-resistant sialoglycoprotein (M_r 27 000–30 000) (Bolton et al 1982, 1985, Prusiner et al 1982). The protein was unique to fractions from scrapie-diseased brain. We denote this protease-resistant scrapie protein by the term PrP 27–30. Many studies have shown that this protein purifies with the protease-treated scrapie agent and that its properties are entirely consistent with the properties predicted for the scrapie agent protein. Similar proteins are found in substantially purified, protease-treated preparations of murine scrapie agents (Bolton et al 1984, Kascsak et al 1985) and in analogous fractions enriched for Creutzfeldt-Jakob disease agents from human brain or mouse brain (Bendheim et al 1985, Bockman et al 1985, Manuelidis et al 1985).

Subsequent studies have demonstrated that a larger form of this protein (33–37 kDa) is obtained when the scrapie agent is purified in the absence of protease digestion (Bolton et al 1986, 1987, Hope et al 1986). We denote this scrapie agent protein as Sp33–37. Gene cloning studies have shown that this protein is derived from the product of a normal host gene (Oesch et al 1985, Chesebro et al 1985, Basler et al 1986, Robakis et al 1986). The scrapie protein Sp33–37 can be distinguished from its normal cellular form (Cp33–37) by physical separation methods and resistance to proteolysis (Meyer et al 1986, Bolton et al 1987). However, both Sp33–37 and CP33–37 are heterogeneous in charge and size and have many isomers in common. Thus, it appears that the scrapie agent protein is an abnormally modified host protein.

The scrapie agent is unique among microbial pathogens in the scope of its resistance to physical and chemical inactivation. The agent resists inactivation by heat, formaldehyde, ultrasonic disruption, ultraviolet and ionizing radiation, nucleases and psoralens. Resistance to procedures that inactivate nucleic acids and the apparent absence of a scrapie-specific nucleic acid in scrapie-enriched fractions support the modified host protein model for the agent.

Effects of the host genotype

Host genotype plays a major role in determining the rate at which scrapie develops in mice and the type and distribution of pathology. A single agent, for example ME7, will produce disease in one host strain (C57/BL) in a much shorter period of time (180 days) than it will in a second host strain (VM mice, 350 days) at the same dose of agent (Dickinson & Outram 1979). The gene controlling this phenotype, called *Sinc*, has two known alleles in mice. Mouse strains of the *Sinc*^{s7s7} genotype have short incubation periods with the ME7 group of agents; *Sinc*^{p7p7} mice have prolonged incubation periods with these agents.

Recently, a gene on mouse chromosome 2 was described which also plays a major role in determining incubation periods (Carlson et al 1986). This gene, *Prn*^{i}, is closely linked to the gene coding for Cp33–37 (the *Prn*^{p} gene), and these may actually be identical. *Prn*^{i} and *Sinc* show the same segregation properties in the mouse strains examined so far and have the same biological effects on scrapie incubation periods. It is likely that *Prn*^{i} and *Sinc* are the same gene. Therefore, *Sinc*, *Prn*[i] and *Prn*[p] probably represent three descriptions of a single gene (or gene complex), i.e. the gene coding for Cp33–37. Other genes not yet identified are known to have minor effects on scrapie incubation period and pathology.

The phenomenon of overdominance in scrapie refers to the observation that incubation periods of some agents are longer in heterozygous F1 mice (*Sinc*[s7p7]) than in either homozygous parental strain. It has been postulated that this occurs because each host possesses only a limited number of 'replication sites' that are controlled by the *Sinc* gene (Dickinson & Outram 1979). It was proposed that these sites consist of multimers of the *Sinc* gene product (Cp 33–35) and that heterogeneous multimers are less efficient in supporting agent replication than are homomultimers.

Effects of scrapie agent strains

The primary characteristics that distinguish strains of the scrapie agent are summarized in Table 2. Two major groups of mouse scrapie agent strains are known. The ME7 group has short incubation periods in *Sinc*[s7s7] mice and long incubation periods in *Sinc*[p7p7] mice. In contrast, the 22A group has long incubation periods in *Sinc*[s7s7] mice and shorter incubation periods in *Sinc*[p7p7] mice. In addition to incubation period, some scrapie agent strains can be distinguished by the pathology they produce.

Apart from strain variation as described above, the biological properties of a scrapie agent strain can change as it is passaged. This phenomenon has been used to classify scrapie agent strains into three 'biological stability types' (Bruce & Dickinson 1979). Type I agents are stable when propagated in any host strain. The ME7 agent is the prototype and its properties do not change when passaged in *Sinc*[s7s7] or *Sinc*[p7p7] mice. Type II agents are stable in the host strain in which they are normally propagated, but are unstable when passaged in a host of different *Sinc* genotype. The biological characteristics change on passage in the other host and after several passages a new strain is obtained. The 22A scrapie agent is an example of this type. Crossing species barriers represents an extreme example of this process. Passage of the Chandler

TABLE 2 Scrapie agent strain characteristics

Biological	*Physical, chemical, immunological*
Host range	Charge and size variants
Incubation period	Resistance to proteolysis
Pathology	Antigenic variation
Biological stability type I, II or III	

mouse agent (139A) into hamsters yielded two isolates; one of these lost its ability to replicate in mice (Kimberlin & Walker 1978). Type III agents are unstable in either host, especially when passaged at high concentration. Scrapie agent 87A is an example. When passaged at high concentration, conversion to 7D (an ME7-like agent) occurs.

Competition between strains in a single host is termed 'blocking' (Dickinson & Outram 1979). This occurs after an animal is inoculated first with a long incubation period agent then with a short incubation period agent 100–200 days later. The onset of disease occurs at the time predicted for replication of the long incubation period agent alone; this is significantly later than that predicted if the short incubation agent had been inoculated alone. The pathology is characteristic of the long incubation period agent. The blocking phenomenon appears to demonstrate that the presence of the first agent precludes replication of the second.

These results are summarized by several important points that form the basis of the model we discuss below. 1) Long incubation period, absence of an immune response and sporadic occurrence are features of the spongiform encephalopathies. 2) The biophysical properties of the agent are unique. 3) A scrapie-specific nucleic acid has not been identified. 4) A modified host protein, Sp33–37, is a scrapie agent component. 5) The gene(s) controlling incubation period in mice is linked to or is identical with the Cp33–37 gene. 6) The interaction between the scrapie agent and the *Sinc/Prn*[i] gene(s) or *Sinc/Prn*[i] gene product(s) is the major determinant of incubation period and pathological profile. 7) Other host genes have a minor influence on incubation period and disease.

The modified host protein model

This model proposes that the critical component of the scrapie agent is a degradation-resistant modified host protein (Table 3). Any other components are host derived; a non-host nucleic acid is excluded. We postulate that the disease is a neurotoxic disorder induced by the abnormal protein. The modified host protein initiates its reproduction by acting on the normal protein directly or by affecting one of the steps in protein processing. Interaction between the host and scrapie agent determines the replication efficiency and disease characteristics. Aggregation of the protein into dimers or higher order multimers increases its resistance to degradation and is integral to disease production. Disease can be transmitted by the scrapie agent or initiated by a spontaneous metabolic error resulting in accumulation of the abnormal protein.

The specific protein modification may be either covalent or non-covalent. Some of the possibilities are listed in Table 4. Fig. 1 shows in schematic form the processing of Cp33–37 in the normal and scrapie-diseased cell. In the

TABLE 3   Modified host protein model of scrapie

Scrapie agent components
    Modified host protein is essential (Sp33–37)
    Sp33–37 is resistant to degradation
    Any other components are host derived
    Non-host nucleic acid is excluded

Disease initiation
    Transmission of scrapie agent
    Spontaneous metabolic error

Scrapie agent strains
    Specific protein modification is directed by agent strain
    Host limits possible modifications

Host/agent strain interaction defines disease characteristics

Host-specified	Agent-specified
Ability to degrade modified protein	Affinity for replication site
Ability to neutralize neurotoxic effect	Efficiency at promoting modification
Fidelity of post-translational modification system	Resistance to degradation
Biosynthetic rate for Cp33–37	

Efficiency of transmission

Interspecies	Intraspecies
Species variation in amino acid sequence	Protein modification can be major determinant of strain characteristics
Species-specific processing of Cp33–37	High homology of amino acid sequence
Abnormal modification to Sp33–37	Protein modification is independent of *Sinc* genotype

healthy cell, normal transcription, translation and post-translational processing produce balanced biosynthesis and degradation of Cp33–37; if Sp33–37 is produced by abnormal processing, it is rapidly degraded. Disease occurs when the cell loses its ability to process Cp33–37 correctly or to degrade Cp33–37 or Sp33–37. As noted above, the process can be initiated by exogenous Sp33–37 or triggered *de novo* by a rare metabolic error.

Application of the model

The modified host protein model can explain several features of scrapie: 1) replication of the agent by propagation of specific protein modifications, 2) host species barrier, and 3) agent strains and their biological stability.

Agent replication and protein modifications

The principal requirement of this model is that the scrapie agent directs specific modification(s) of a normal host protein. The nature of the

A

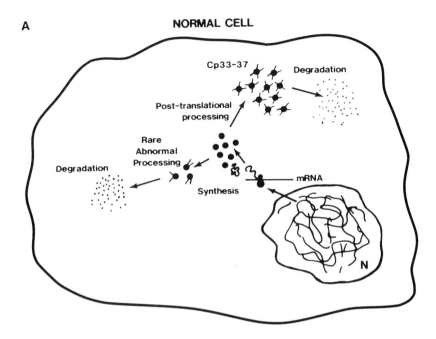

B

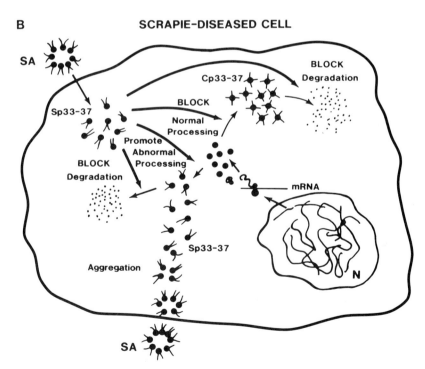

FIG. 1.   Protein processing in the normal and scrapie-diseased cell. (a) Normal cell,
(b) scrapie-diseased cell. SA, scrapie agent. See text for details.

TABLE 4   Possible protein modifications

Covalent	Non-covalent
Glycosylation	Aggregation
Phosphorylation	Denaturation or refolding
Partial proteolysis	Alteration of cellular compartment
Acylation with fatty acids	Binding of a co-factor
Cross-linking	
Other side chain modifications	
Amino- or carboxy-terminal blocking	

modification(s) is not known at this time. Table 4 lists the main possibilities. An example of covalent modification would be disruption of the glycosylation pathway of Cp33–37 by the modified protein. If Sp33–37 inhibited a step in the normal glycosylation sequence, the cellular protein would be incompletely processed. This could cause it to be directed to the wrong cellular compartment or shunted to a different modification pathway. The abnormal protein would then accumulate and aggregate into a degradation-resistant, neurotoxic form.

An example of reproduction of non-covalent modifications is shown schematically in Fig. 2. Membrane-bound Cp33–37 combines with the abnormal form, Sp33–37, which directs an abnormal refolding event in the cellular protein. Alternatively, if the degradation of Cp33–37 is blocked by Sp33–37, its increased concentration could produce the same effect. The Sp33–37 dimer formed can dissociate into two monomers to repeat the process (replication) or assemble into larger aggregates. Once a threshold concentration is reached, membrane damage results from the effect of Sp33–37 dimers or larger aggregates. Aggregation of Sp33–37 increases its resistance to proteolysis. Amyloid fibrils may form and be deposited extracellularly as plaques. Vacuolation, cell dysfunction and cell death lead to clinical disease.

In these examples the process is driven by three factors: 1) a constant supply of the substrate protein, Cp33–37, is available throughout the incubation period, 2) dimers and higher-order aggregates (including fibrils) are stable and act as a sink for the modified protein; re-incorporation of protein from fibrils into the membrane is an unfavourable process, and 3) membrane damage and cell death facilitate spread to adjacent cells.

Host species barrier

Efficiency of transmission between species is governed by the affinity of the agent for the replication site in the new host and the ability of the new host to degrade or neutralize the agent. In the new host, the scrapie agent protein is likely to be recognized as abnormal or foreign because of species-specific

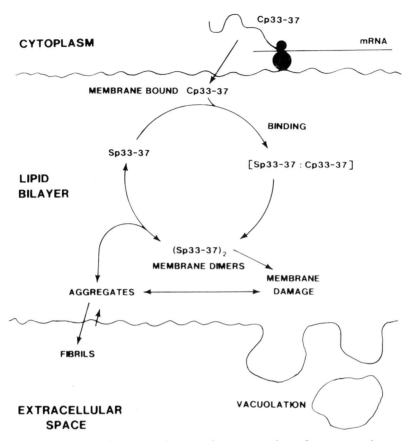

FIG. 2.   Replication of the scrapie agent by propagation of a non-covalent protein modification. The figure depicts the abnormal processing events occurring within a membrane. Cp33–37 is synthesized on membrane-bound ribosomes and inserted into the membrane. Vacuoles and fibrils are depicted as extracellular.

differences in amino acid sequence and post-translational processing. Once the protein is recognized as abnormal, the host attempts to degrade or neutralize it. If the scrapie protein is not degraded, it can initiate reproduction by acting on the normal protein directly or by interfering with processing of the normal protein. The efficiency of reproduction is a function of the affinity of the abnormal protein for the specific host components involved; an agent that has a high affinity for components of one species may have a low affinity for the analogous components in another species.

Agent strains and stability

Within a single host species, differences in amino acid sequence of Cp33–37

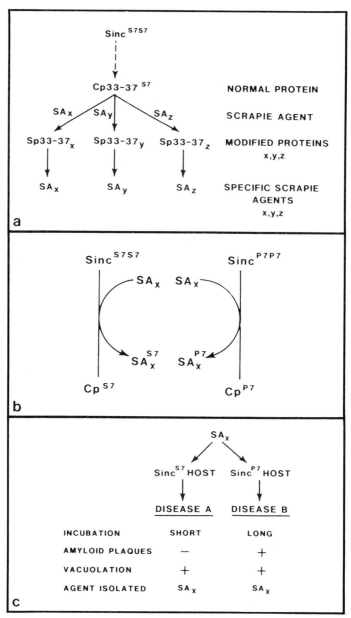

FIG. 3. Scrapie agent strains and biological stability. (a) One host, three agents. $Sinc^{s7s7}$ genotype produces Cp33–37^{s7}. This protein can be modified by SA$_x$, producing Sp33–37$_x$ and more SA$_x$. SA$_y$ produces Sp33–37$_y$, replicating more SA$_y$, and so on. (b) Two host strains, one agent. In a $Sinc^{s7s7}$ host SA$_x$ modifies Cp33–37^{s7} to produce Sp33–37$_x$ and more SA$_x$. This modification can also be produced in $Sinc^{p7p7}$ hosts under direction of SA$_x$. (c) One agent, two hosts, two diseases. SA$_x$ produces different diseases in $Sinc^{s7s7}$ or $Sinc^{p7p7}$ hosts.

due to allelic polymorphism and differences in normal protein processing are less pronounced than those between species. In this case, specific protein modifications are a major determinant of strain differences. Amino acid sequence and normal processing play a minor role. Scrapie agent protein modifications are independent of the $Sinc/Prn^i$ genotype to the extent that Cp33–37^{s7} and Cp33–37^{p7} can undergo the same modification to give Sp33–37^{s7} and Sp33–37^{p7} (Fig. 3).

Biologically stable agents (Type I) are reproduced faithfully in all host strains. In this case, the specific modification of Cp33–37 by scrapie agent strain$_x$ (SA$_x$) produces Sp33–37$_x$ (Fig. 3A). Sp33–37$_x$ is distinct from Sp33–37$_y$ that is produced by modification of Cp33–37 by scrapie agent strain$_y$ (SA$_y$). The specific modification is independent of $Sinc$ genotype, so either host protein (Cp33–37^{s7} or Cp33–37^{p7}) can be altered to Sp33–37$_x$ by SA$_x$ or to Sp33–37$_y$ by SA$_y$ (Fig. 3B). Since disease characteristics are determined by the interaction between SA$_x$ and the host, distinct disease variants are produced when one agent is inoculated into hosts of two different $Sinc$ genotypes (Fig. 3C).

Agents having Type II 'biological stability' have a single protein modification (or a mixture of protein modifications in a fixed ratio) that is reproduced faithfully in one host strain but not the other. For example, a processing step that is efficiently altered by SA$_x$ in one host strain might not be affected to the same degree in the second host. During several passages in the second host a gradual shift occurs to produce a new agent strain, SA$_z$, by a different protein modification.

This model predicts that scrapie strains of Type III stability occur because two types of modification can be produced: a 'slow' agent modification (Sp33–37$_{slow}$) and a 'fast' agent modification (Sp33–37$_{fast}$). During routine passage the slow agent is present in vast excess and induces the cell to produce Sp33–37$_{slow}$ efficiently, giving rise to more of the slow agent. At a low frequency the cell also produces the Sp33–37$_{fast}$ modification, even when slow agent alone is inoculated. This can give rise to some of the fast agent at any passage. The anatomical site (type of neuron) where the agent replicates may have a substantial influence on which modification predominates. When Type III agents are passaged at high concentration, enough of the fast agent is present to replicate and produce disease.

Summary

The modified host protein model presents a testable alternative to the virus and virino models of scrapie. Regardless of which model proves correct, progress made on scrapie will further our understanding of the analogous human spongiform encephalopathies.

Acknowledgements

Supported in part by United States Public Health Service Grant NS 23948 (DCB) and the American Federation for Aging Research (PEB). Dr Anna Potempska, Alan D. Marmorstein and Teresa Angus-Rooss performed much of the experimental work in our laboratories that contributed to the development of this model. We thank Drs Henryk M. Wisniewski, Richard I. Carp, David L. Miller, Anna Potempska, Julia Currie and Nikoloas K, Robakis for helpful discussions. The illustrations were produced by the Biomedical Photography department under the direction of Mr Richard Weed.

References

Basler K, Oesch B, Scott M et al 1986 Scrapie and cellular PrP isoforms are encoded by the same chromosomal gene. Cell 46:417–428

Bendheim PE, Bolton DC 1986 A 54 k-Da normal cellular protein may be the precursor of the scrapie agent protease-resistant protein. Proc Natl Acad Sci USA 83:2214–2218

Bendheim PE, Bockman JM, McKinley MP, Kingsbury DT, Prusiner SB 1985 Scrapie and Creutzfeldt-Jakob disease prion proteins share physical properties and antigenic determinants. Proc Natl Acad Sci USA 82:997–1001

Bockman JM, Kingsbury DT, McKinley MP, Bendheim PE, Prusiner SB 1985 Creutzfeldt-Jakob disease prion proteins in human brains. N Engl J Med 312:73–78

Bolton DC, McKinley MP, Prusiner SB 1982 Identification of a protein that purifies with the scrapie agent. Science (Wash DC) 218:1309–1311

Bolton DC, McKinley MP, Prusiner SB 1984 Molecular characteristics of the major scrapie prion protein. Biochemistry 23:5898–5906

Bolton DC, Meyer RK, Prusiner SB 1985 Scrapie PrP 27–30 is a sialoglycoprotein. J Virol 53:596–606

Bolton DC, Bendheim PE, Marmorstein AD, Potempska A, Scala L, Carp RI 1986 Purification and N-terminal sequencing of the intact scrapie agent protein, PrP 35–38. Neurology 36 (Suppl 1):222–223

Bolton DC, Bendheim PE, Marmorstein AD, Potempska A 1987 Isolation and structural studies of the intact scrapie agent protein. Arch Biochem Biophys 258:579–590

Brown P, Cathala F, Raubertas RF, Gajdusek DC, Castaigne P 1987 The epidemiology of Creutzfeldt-Jakob disease: Conclusion of a 15-year investigation in France and review of the world literature. Neurology 37:895–904

Bruce ME, Dickinson AG 1979 Biological stability of different classes of scrapie agent. In: Prusiner SB, Hadlow WJ (eds) Slow transmissible diseases of the nervous system. Academic Press, New York, vol 2:71–86

Carlson GA, Kingsbury DT, Goodman PA et al 1986 Linkage of prion protein and scrapie incubation time genes. Cell 46:503–511

Carp RI, Merz PA, Kascsak RJ, Merz GS, Wisniewski HM 1985 Nature of the scrapie agent: current status of facts and hypotheses. J Gen Virol 66:1357–1368

Chesebro B, Race R, Wehrly K et al 1985 Identification of scrapie prion protein-specific mRNA in scrapie-infected and uninfected brain. Nature (Lond) 315:331–333

Czub M, Braig HR, Diringer H 1986 Pathogenesis of scrapie: Study of the temporal development of clinical symptoms, of infectivity titres and scrapie-associated fibrils in brains of hamsters infected intraperitoneally. J Gen Virol 67:2005–2009

Dickinson AG, Outram G 1979 The scrapie replication-site hypothesis and its implications for pathogenesis. In: Prusiner SB, Hadlow WJ (eds) Slow transmissible diseases of the nervous system. Academic Press, New York, vol 1:367–385

Diener TO, McKinley MP, Prusiner SB 1982 Viroids and prions. Proc Natl Acad Sci USA 79:5220–5224

Gajdusek DC 1977 Unconventional viruses and the origin and disappearance of kuru. Science (Wash DC) 197:943–960

Hope J. Morton LJD, Farquhar CF, Multhaup G, Beyreuther K, Kimberlin RH 1986 The major polypeptide of scrapie-associated fibrils (SAF) has the same size, charge distribution and N-terminal protein sequence as predicted for the normal brain protein (PrP). EMBO (Eur Mol Biol Organ) J 5:2591–2597

Kascsak RJ, Rubenstein R, Merz PA, Carp RI, Wisniewski HM, Diringer H 1985 Biological diversity of scrapie agents supported by biochemical differences among SAF. J Gen Virol 66:1715–1722

Kimberlin RH, Walker CA 1978 Evidence that the transmission of one source of scrapie agent to hamsters involves separation of agent strains from a mixture. J Gen Virol 39:487–496

Manuelidis L, Valley S, Manuelidis EE 1985 Specific proteins in Creutzfeldt-Jakob disease and scrapie share antigenic and carbohydrate determinants. Proc Natl Acad Sci USA 82:4263–4267

Manuelidis L, Sklaviadis T, Manuelidis EE 1987 Evidence suggesting that PrP is not the infectious agent in Creutzfeldt-Jakob disease. EMBO (Eur Mol Biol Organ) J 6:341–347

Meyer RK, McKinley MP, Bowman KA, Braunfeld MB, Barry RA, Prusiner SB 1986 Separation and properties of cellular and scrapie prion proteins. Proc Natl Acad Sci USA 83:2310–2314

Oesch B, Westaway D, Wälchli M et al 1985. A cellular gene encodes scrapie PrP 27–30 protein. Cell 40:735–746

Prusiner SB 1982 Novel proteinaceous infectious particles cause scrapie. Science (Wash DC) 216:136–144

Prusiner SB, Bolton DC, Groth DF, Bowman KA, Cochran SP, McKinley MP 1982 Further purification and characterization of scrapie prions. Biochemistry 21:6942–6950

Robakis NK, Sawh PR, Wolfe GC, Rubenstein R, Carp RI, Innis MA 1986 Isolation of a cDNA clone encoding the leader peptide of prion protein and expression of the homologous gene in various tissues. Proc Natl Acad Sci USA 83:6377–6381

Rohwer RG 1984a Scrapie infectious agent is virus-like in size and susceptibility to inactivation. Nature (Lond) 308:658–662

Rohwer RG 1984b Virus-like sensitivity of the scrapie agent to heat inactivation. Science (Wash DC) 223:600–602

DISCUSSION

P. Brown: One of the problems with post-translational modification (especially in the context of, for example, the RNA ribosomal modification kind of scheme), is that of all the cell constituents, the ribosomes themselves are virtually free of scrapie infectivity.

Bolton: Yes, I would expect that. In our model the key factor is the modification of the protein after it has been translated and inserted into the cell membrane.

Diringer: You propose that this modified protein is itself infectious. PrP mRNA is found in the spleen, in heart, in lung and in brain–what about the infectivity in all of these organs? Why do you only get disease-specific changes in the brain?

Bolton: The simplest explanation is that all organs are not the same. The environment in the brain is different from that in the spleen. An abnormally modified protein may accumulate in the brain because the brain is not able to remove it or degrade it, whereas in the spleen it may be recognized as an abnormal form and rapidly degraded. It is interesting that in the brain, in contrast to the general situation, cells are able to pull this protein out of membranes and deposit it as amyloid. In general, the plaque-forming animal models live longer than those animals that don't form plaques. That does not prove a causal relationship between plaque formation and prolonged incubation but it is interesting that animals that make plaques can live longer.

Dickinson: Animals that live longer have more opportunity to make plaques.

F. Brown: How many of your hypotheses (Tables 3 and 4) can be tested experimentally?

Bolton: I wanted to present these hypotheses here so that we can get some good ideas about how to test them. I believe most, if not all, possible modifications can be detected.

Dickinson: I agree that the onus is on us to use more purified fractions and prove that the strain differences still exist. An alternative is to ask, how harshly can we treat crude homogenates and still preserve the exact strain differences. Many strain differences have withstood dry heating in an oven for an hour at 160°C, 3.8. megarads, or a fortnight's treatment with ethanol. We haven't found a strain difference that disappears with any of these treatments.

Stahl: David, can you explain how you think a strain could selectively perpetuate itself according to your model?

Bolton: The model is necessarily vague—we don't know what the post-translational modification would be. Phosphorylation is one candidate; you can phosphorylate a protein and alter its characteristics; and sometimes a phosphorylated protein will increase or decrease phosphorylation of other proteins. So, for example, if the normal protein is phosphorylated at site A but abnormally it is phosphorylated at site B, then phosphorylation at site B may block the ability of the host to phosphorylate the protein at site A. For example, the B phosphorylated form could be an inhibitor of that protein kinase. Then, assuming that the B site protein kinase is also present in the cell, the cell would have an opportunity to phosphorylate that protein at the B site. Over a period of time, more of the B phosphorylated form accumulates, inhibits phosphorylation at site A and a system of positive feedback develops.

Stahl: I agree that this model could explain the existence of three or four strains but it becomes more difficult if there is a large variety of strains.

Bolton: My perspective on the mouse data is that there are two distinct groups of agents. How many different variants there are within those groups, I am not sure. We need to look at purified agents within those groups, to find out how many of the biological properties are due to contaminants within the preparation, within that large group, as opposed to real, different strain characteristics.

Almond: The crucial support for this hypothesis would be the establishment of infectivity from material derived from the expressed cDNA clone of PrP. Has anyone investigated what modifications occur in cells expressing that protein? Can any further modifications be seen after superinfecting cells in which the cDNA is being expressed with the scrapie agent?

Bolton: We haven't tried those exact experiments. We are comparing scrapie and normal forms of the protein. The scrapie and normal forms of the protein have a number of different isoforms. HaSp 33–37 has at least nine or 10 isoforms and there may be 15 to 20.

Almond: When you look at different strains of scrapie, do you see different ratios of those various isoforms?

Bolton: We have not looked at that.

Hope: The impression we have is that if you load the same amount of protein on a polyacrylamide gel, then you see equivalent patterns after silver staining. That's not to say that you get the same amount of SAF protein from brain infected with one strain compared to another.

Bolton: In 1D gels there are clear differences in the protein profiles of different agents isolated from the same strain of mouse.

Carp: However, the same strain of scrapie gives similar protein patterns in two different *Sinc* genotype hosts. For example, the pattern that ME7 gives in *Sinc* ^{s7s7} mice is the same as that which it gives in *Sinc* ^{p7p7} mice. 139A produces a different pattern from ME7, but it is the same pattern in either host *Sinc* genotype.

Merz: But it differs in the hamster.

Lectin binding is also strain specific: in the same strain of mouse infected with different strains of scrapie, the proteins isolated show different lectin-binding affinities (Kascsak et al 1986).

Beyreuther: There is accumulating evidence from protein sequencing that all these different protein fragments start near this 'keratin' site. Computer searches show that this repeated site has homology to RNA binding proteins, proteins which are part of hnRNP particles. Can you accommodate this in your model?

Bolton: I think it's too early yet. You can look at different regions of a protein, take the predicted secondary structure and find homologies to all kinds of proteins. There may be a nucleotide binding site in Cp 33-37, but the evidence argues against a specific normal function of this protein as a nucleic acid binding protein.

Beyreuther: But it is interesting that precisely this region is found in all these breakdown products.

Bolton: Sp 33–37 has a predicted secondary structure that is rather extended and we would predict it to be in the extracellular space, which one would expect to be a good site for non-specific proteolytic cleavage.

Beyreuther: Such a model would predict proteolysis to occur at these sites. But, we do not find cleavage at that site. This sequence is still found included in the proteins constituting the fibrils and is protected against proteolysis. Whether this protection is due to the aggregation resulting in fibril formation is not known.

*Dormont:*By immunoblotting, we detected different reactivities in normal and scrapie material against a small RNA-associated protein, 'p27'.

Almond: If one adds highly labelled exogenous RNA to scrapie brain material, then takes it through the SAF preparation, can you detect any label in the SAF?

Gabizon: No, we have done that.

Diringer: On the contrary I think one can. We radioactively labelled RNA *in vivo*, then ran our general purification scheme for SAF and tried to find radioactivity in the purified SAF fraction. This way we still find a very little amount of labelled nucleic acid; we also find nucleic acid in this fraction by electron microscopy.

Gabizon: After RNAse or DNAse treatment can you still find it?

Diringer: Yes, nucleic acid protected by protein.

*Wisniewski:*Mutation can be considered an act of *creation*—new gene, new product, sometimes new disease. As we know, genetically inherited diseases are not infectious. Infection, by definition, means invasion of the body by pathogenic microorganisms, which reproduce in the host body. If a sporadic case of CJD is considered the result of gene mutation, how can one reconcile this with the fact that CJD can be transmitted experimentally to animals?

Bolton: Superficially that sounds like a refutation of this type of model—I don't think that's the case. The rare instances of CJD that occur, not necessarily through mutation but possibly through environmental insult, would require a genetic background that is marginally able to regulate the metabolism of this protein. For example, in Alzheimer's disease an individual may be marginally able to regulate the metabolism of the Alzheimer's amyloid core protein. When you take some of the abnormal form of the scrapie protein which has built up to tremendous amounts in the brain and inoculate it into a hamster, that abnormal form compromises the ability of the new host (which has a different genetic background and normally would not develop this disease) to process or degrade this protein. That sets the process in motion again, produces more protein, then the disease. I don't think you need to invoke a mutation at the nucleic acid level of the host at all.

Dickinson: It worries me when people start speculating about spontaneous generation within the system because there are plenty of hard facts still to be explained which are much more important. There could be very mundane explanations, for example, if exposure to these kinds of agent was much more common then we are aware of, that would immediately change the whole picture.

References

Kascsak RJ, Rubenstein R, Merz PA et al 1986 Immunological analysis of scrapie associated fibrils isolated from four different scrapie agents. J Virol 59:676–683

Properties of scrapie prion proteins in liposomes and amyloid rods

Ruth Gabizon, Michael P. McKinley and Stanley B. Prusiner†

Departments of Neurology and †Biochemistry and Biophysics, University of California, San Francisco, California 94143, USA

Abstract. The scrapie prion protein (PrP 27–30) has been demonstrated to be required for infectivity. Aggregates of PrP 27–30 form insoluble amyloid rods which resist dissociation by non-denaturing detergents. Mixtures of the detergent cholate and phospholipids were found to solubilize PrP 27–30 with full retention of scrapie prion infectivity. No evidence for a prion-associated nucleic acid could be found when the phospholipid vesicles with PrP 27–30 were digested with nucleases and Zn^{2+}. Under digestion conditions which allowed hydrolysis of exogenous nucleic acids, no diminution of prion infectivity was observed. Tobacco mosaic virions added to the liposomes at a concentration 100 times lower than the scrapie prion titre could be seen by electron microscopy. These studies indicate that there is no subpopulation of filamentous scrapie viruses hidden amongst the prion rods — indeed, they would have been observed among the liposomes. The partitioning of PrP 27–30 and scrapie infectivity into phospholipid vesicles argues for a central role of PrP 27–30 in scrapie pathogenesis and establishes that the prion amyloid rods are not essential for infectivity.

1988 Novel infectious agents and the central nervous system. Wiley, Chichester (Ciba Foundation Symposium 135) p 182–196

Antibodies raised against PrP 27–30 and a synthetic peptide corresponding to its N-terminus have been used to demonstrate that a proportion of the scrapie prion proteins aggregate into filamentous polymers during scrapie infection and these extracellular filaments coalesce to form amyloid plaques (Bendheim et al 1984, DeArmond et al 1985, Barry et al 1986). Similarly, Creutzfeldt-Jakob disease (a human disease which resembles scrapie) prion proteins aggregate into amyloid rods in purified preparations (Bendheim et al 1985, Bockman et al 1985) and polymerize into filaments which form amyloid plaques in diseased brains (Kitamoto et al 1986).

The aggregation of PrP 27–30 into prion amyloid rods, together with its protease resistance, permitted the development of a purification procedure which yields large quantities of highly purified prions (Prusiner et al 1983). However, the formation of the rods created another problem; they could not be solubilized in non-denaturing detergent. Only boiling in the presence of sodium dodecyl sulphate (SDS) could dissociate the rod structure and solubilize the protein (Bolton et al 1984, Prusiner et al 1983, McKinley et al 1986). The denaturation of PrP 27–30 resulted in the loss of scrapie prion infectivity and rendered the protein sensitive to proteolytic digestion (Bolton et al 1984, Prusiner et al 1983). Subsequent studies showed that PrP 27–30 is derived from a larger protein of 33–35 kDa, designated PrP^{Sc} (Oesch et al 1985, Barry & Prusiner 1986).

Discovering conditions for the solubilization of PrP 27–30 with retention of scrapie prion infectivity has greatly facilitated studies defining the molecular structure of the infectious particle (Gabizon et al 1987). While prion amyloid rods cannot be dissociated by non-denaturing detergent alone, a mixture of phospholipids and non-denaturing detergent is capable of dissociating the rods to form detergent-lipid-protein complexes (DLPC). These DLPC exhibit full retention of scrapie infectivity.

As shown in Fig. 1, PrP 27–30 which had polymerized into rods was sedimented completely by low-speed centrifugation even in the presence of detergent. In contrast, most of the PrP 27–30 did not sediment in the presence of phosphatidylcholine (PC) even with ultracentrifugation at 170 000 g for 30 min. A protein which does not sediment at this centrifugation rate is considered to be soluble under these conditions. In fact, even the protein which remains in the pellet under these conditions is not in rods. We attribute the small amount of PrP 27–30 found in this fraction to large lipid/protein aggregates that sediment even though the rods are fully disrupted. When we removed most of the detergent by dialysis, we obtained liposomes in which PrP 27–30 is probably in the lipid phase.

Electron micrographs of prion rods and PrP 27–30 liposomes reveal striking differences in structure and size, yet both are associated with high levels of infectivity (Fig. 2). The rods measure 10 to 20 nm in diameter and 100 to 200 nm in length; the average diameter of the liposomes is about 20 nm. Laser light-scattering measurements of particle size confirmed those calculated from electron microscopy. To determine the average number of PrP 27–30 molecules in a liposome, we calculated the number of PC molecules per 20 nm liposome. Based on published data (Hauser et al 1973), there are approximately 4000 PC molecules per liposome. Phospholipids were measured by the ammonium ferrothyiocyanate method (Charles & Stewart 1980) and protein by the bicinchoninic acid (BCA) procedure (Smith et al 1985). We estimate the phospholipid:protein ratio to be between 1000:1 and 2000:1; thus, the average number of PrP 27–30 molecules per liposome is between two and 4. This estimate of between 2 and 4 PrP 27–30 molecules per liposome agrees with earlier ionizing radiation and size exclusion chromatography studies suggesting that the smallest infectious unit of the scrapie agent has a relative molecular weight less than 10^5 (Alper et al 1966, Prusiner 1982).

The rods reappeared after chloroform/methanol extraction of the lipo-

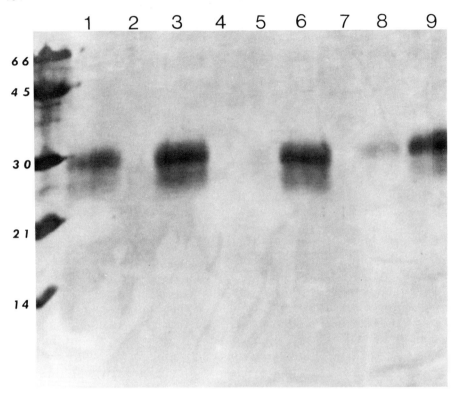

FIG. 1.   Solubilization of PrP 27–30 in the presence of PC. 10 ml of purified PrP
27–30 (30 µg/ml) in sucrose (50%) were concentrated by methanol precipitation. The
precipitate was dried and resuspended in 4 ml of buffer containing 10 mM Na HEPES,
pH 7.4, and 100 mM NaCl. The solution was divided into 4 equal aliquots. Sample A
was the control and received no further treatment. Sample B received Na cholate to a
final concentration of 2%, pH 7.4. Sample C received Na cholate and then was added
to a glass test-tube containing 30 mg of PC. The tube was vortexed for 10 s (or until no
more lipid was observed on the test-tube wall) and then sonicated in a cylindrical bath
sonicator until the solution was transparent (around 15 min). These 3 samples were
centrifuged at 21 000 g for 25 min. Sample D was prepared as sample C except that the
supernatant of the 21 000 g centrifugation was centrifuged at 170 000 g for 30 min. All
the samples were chloroform:methanol (1:2) precipitated and boiled in a buffer
containing 1% SDS, 5% β-mercaptoethanol and bromophenol blue, and electrophoresed on an SDS-polyacrylamide gel (Laemmli 1970). The gel was developed by
silver stain. Lane 1, sample A, pellet; lane 2, sample A, supernatant; lane 3, sample B,
pellet; lane 4, sample B, supernatant; lane 5, sample C, pellet; lane 6, sample C,
supernatant; lane 7, sample D, pellet; lane 8, pellet from sample D supernatant
centrifuged at 170 000 g for 30 min; lane 9, supernatant from lane 8. Molecular
weights in kDa.

somes containing PrP 27–30 (not shown). This treatment extracts the lipids
resulting in the reaggregation of PrP 27–30. Additionally, we found that the

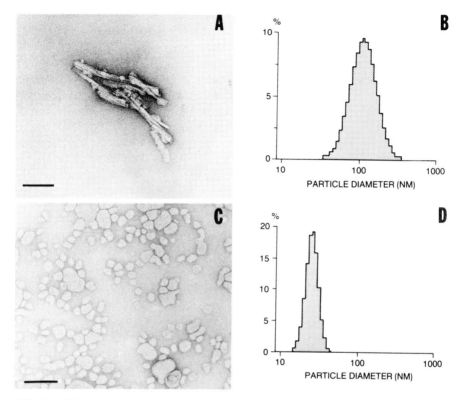

FIG. 2.   Electron microscopy and dynamic light-scattering of rods and liposomes. (A) Typical prion rods negatively stained with uranyl formate. Bar = 100 nm. (B) Light-scattering profile of rods determined with laser particle analyser (Model NY, Coulter Electronics). (C) Negatively stained liposomes containing PrP 27–30. (D) Light-scattering profile of liposomes.

rods are not a necessary precursor for the introduction of PrP 27–30 into liposomes, since liposome-associated PrP[Sc] can be formed directly from scrapie-infected brain microsomes (not shown).

Bioassays in hamsters demonstrate that scrapie prion infectivity is retained when amyloid rods composed of PrP 27–30 dissociate and the protein is incorporated into phospholipid vesicles (Table 1). We have frequently observed that prion titres rise at least 10-fold when PrP 27–30 is dispersed into liposomes. Presumably, this increase in prion titre reflects dissociation of PrP 27–30 rod-shaped aggregates.

TABLE 1   Scrapie prion infectivity in phospholipid vesicles

	Experiment 1	Experiment 2	Experiment 3
		Log titre ($ID_{50}/ml \pm SE$)	
Rods	7.7 ± 0.3	6.6 ± 0.3	7.9 ± 0.2
DLPC	8.7 ± 0.1	7.8 ± 0.1	8.9 ± 0.2
Liposomes	9.0 ± 0.8	7.1 ± 0.2	8.7 ± 0.1

Purified prions from sucrose gradient fractions (30 μg/ml) were methanol precipitated and re-suspended to a final protein concentration of 50 μg/ml in a buffer containing 10 mM Na HEPES, pH 7.4, and 100 mM NaCl. The only protein identifiable by silver staining of SDS-polyacry-lamide gel electrophoresis was PrP 27–30 (Fig. 1, lane 1) which was polymerized into rods (Fig. 2A). The resuspended rods (100 μg of protein) were mixed with 2% (w/v) Na cholate, pH 7.4, then added to a Corex glass 30 ml test-tube containing dried PC (10 mg). The sample was vortexed, sonicated and centrifuged at 31 000 *g* for 25 min as in Fig. 1. This sample was called DLPC (detergent-lipid-protein complex). Liposomes were formed from the DLPC by dialysis against detergent-free buffer. The protein concentrations for the rods, DLPC and liposomes were 25, 12 and 18 μg/ml, respectively. Inocula for bioassay were prepared by diluting 10 μl of the above preparations into 0.99 ml of phosphate-buffered saline containing 9.5% bovine serum albumin. Bioassays were then performed as previously described (Prusiner et al 1982b).

The transfer of scrapie prion infectivity from rods to liposomes provided a new method by which we could search for a hidden or cryptic nucleic acid within the prion. Treatment of DLPC and liposomes with nucleases or Zn^{2+} failed to alter scrapie infectivity (Table 2). Control experiments with exo-

TABLE 2   Resistance of scrapie prion infectivity in phospholipid vesicles to inactivation by nucleases or Zn^{2+}

	Rods	DLPC	Liposomes
	Log titre ($ID_{50}/ml \pm SE$)		
Control	7.7 ± 0.3	8.7 ± 0.1	9.0 ± 0.8
DNase I (100 μg/ml)	7.2 ± 0.2	8.8 ± 0.2	8.9 ± 0.2
RNase A (100 μg/ml)	7.4 ± 0.3	9.5 ± 0.2	8.7 ± 0.2
Micrococcal nuclease (12.5 u/ml)	7.8 ± 0.3	8.8 ± 0.3	8.7 ± 0.1
Zn^{2+} (2 mM)	7.8 ± 0.2	8.6 ± 0.2	8.5 ± 0.2

Fractions were prepared and bioassayed as described in Table 1. These were digested with nucleases for 24 h at 37°C or incubated with $ZnSO_4$ for 24 h at 65°C. In control experiments, exogenous nucleic acids were added at concentrations of one molecule per ID_{50} in order to establish that the nucleases and Zn^{2+} hydrolysed these molecules in the presence of DLPC. [^{32}P]-labelled PrP cDNA probes were used to assay the degradation of exogenously added PrP cDNA or poly(A)$^+$ mRNA using slot blots as previously described (Oesch et al 1985). After nuclease or Zn^{2+}-catalysed hydrolysis of the nucleic acid, less than 5% of the exogenously added nucleic acid could be detected by hybridization.

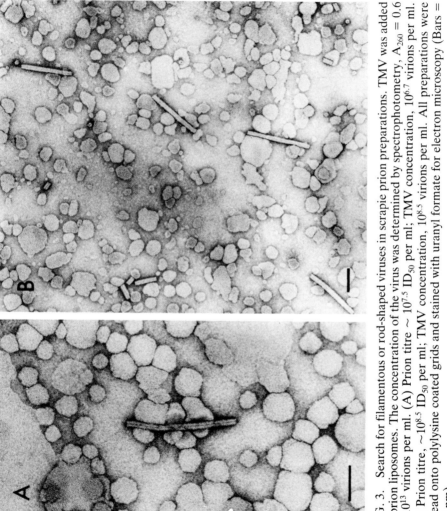

FIG. 3. Search for filamentous or rod-shaped viruses in scrapie prion preparations. TMV was added to prion liposomes. The concentration of the virus was determined by spectrophotometry, $A_{260} = 0.6 \times 10^{13}$ virions per ml. (A) Prion titre $\sim 10^{7.5}$ ID_{50} per ml; TMV concentration, $10^{6.7}$ virions per ml. (B) Prion titre, $\sim 10^{8.5}$ ID_{50} per ml; TMV concentration, $10^{8.5}$ virions per ml. All preparations were spread onto polylysine coated grids and stained with uranyl formate for electron microscopy (Bars = 100 nm).

genously added nucleic acid demonstrated that under the conditions of our experiments nucleases or Zn^{2+} degraded DNA or RNA. In contrast to the hydrophobic prion protein, polynucleotides are water soluble and would be expected to be excluded, largely if not entirely, from the phospholipid bilayer; thus, they should be accessible to nuclease or Zn^{2+}-catalysed hydrolysis. This was the case when exogenous nucleic acids were added to our preparations (Table 2). While liposomes have been used to protect nucleic acids by entrapping them within vesicles, this is not the case in the presence of detergent, where DLPC or fragments of vesicles are formed. These results agree with those of earlier studies, all of which have failed to provide evidence for a nucleic acid moiety within the infectious prion particle (Alper et al 1967, Diener et al 1982, Prusiner 1982, McKinley et al 1983b). Some investigators continue to argue that prions must possess intrinsic nucleic acids (Merz et al 1984, Rohwer 1984, Braig & Diringer 1985, Brown et al 1986) while others suggest that they may be devoid of nucleic acid but prefer to label them viruses (Gajdusek 1986).

We have considered the possibility that a small virus having a particle-to-infectivity ratio of unity is hiding in our preparations and that most or even all of the PrP 27–30 is not associated with the virus. Let us assume that a filamentous virus is responsible for scrapie infectivity and it is hidden amongst the PrP 27–30 amyloid rods. Then, upon dissolving the rods into liposomes, we would expect to see the putative filamentous 'scrapie virus'; however, no elongated particles were found. As a control, tobacco mosaic virus (TMV) at a concentration of $10^{6.7}$ virions per ml was added to prion liposomes with infectivity titres of approximately $10^{7.5}$ or $10^{8.5}$ ID_{50} per ml. The TMV was visible by electron microscopy but no other elongated structures were seen (Fig. 3A). The efficacy of TMV binding to electron microscope grids was the same whether it was performed in the presence or absence of liposomes containing PrP 27–30 molecules. If a filamentous or rod-shaped 'scrapie virus' were hidden amongst the prion amyloid rods, then at least one of these putative virions would be present for each prion ID_{50} unit — i.e., a particle-to-infectivity ratio of unity. Numerous TMV were seen amongst the liposomes when added at a concentration of $10^{8.5}$ virions per ml — i.e., one virion per prion ID_{50} unit (Fig. 3B). Our experimental results show that scrapie infectivity does not require a filamentous or rod-shaped particle.

The incorporation of PrP 27–30 into DLPC and liposomes provided an opportunity to examine the protease resistance of the scrapie prion infectivity and PrP 27–30. Incubation of DLPC or liposomes with proteinase K (100 µg/ml) for 30 or 120 min did not alter the scrapie infectivity. This is consistent with earlier results which showed the formation of PrP 27–30 in microsomal membranes on digestion with proteinase K (Meyer et al 1986). These studies clearly demonstrate that the protease resistance of PrP 27–30 is not a consequence of amyloid rod formation.

The incorporation of PrP 27–30 and scrapie prion infectivity into phospho-lipid vesicles provides an important and compelling line of evidence for PrP 27–30 being a component of the infectious scrapie prion. The results from five different experimental approaches, including the studies described here, con-tend that PrP 27–30 is required for scrapie infectivity. First, PrP 27–30 is the most abundant macromolecule in purified prion preparations (Prusiner et al 1983, 1984). Second, the concentration of PrP 27–30 is proportional to scrapie prion titre (Prusiner et al 1982a, 1983, McKinley et al 1983a). Third, hydro-lysis or denaturation of PrP 27–30 results in a diminution of prion titre (McKinley et al 1983a, Bolton et al 1984). Fourth, the murine PrP gene (*Prn-p*) on chromosome 2 (Sparkes et al 1986) is linked to a gene (*Prn-i*) controlling the length of the scrapie incubation time (Carlson et al 1986). Prolonged incubation periods are a cardinal feature of scrapie infection. Fifth, the studies reported here establish that PrP 27–30 and scrapie prion infectivity are inseparable — both may exist as rods, DLPC and liposomes. Other studies have shown that the rods may be disrupted into spherical particles composed of PrP 27–30 with retention of infectivity (McKinley et al 1986, McKinley & Prusiner 1987).

Recent molecular cloning studies have shown that the prion protein is encoded by a cellular gene and not by a nucleic acid within the infectious particle (Oesch et al 1985, Basler et al 1986). Dissociation of the rods with retention of infectivity allowed us to extend our search for a prion nucleic acid, however, no evidence for a polynucleotide could be found by digesting phospholipid vesicles containing PrP 27–30 with nucleases or Zn^{2+} (Table 2). While it can be argued that the putative prion nucleic acid remains protected from nucleases and Zn^{2+} even during the transfer of PrP 27–30 and infectivity from rods to phospholipid vesicles, it seems more likely that prions are composed solely of PrP^{Sc} molecules.

The partitioning of PrP 27–30 and scrapie prion infectivity into phospho-lipid vesicles establishes that prion amyloid rods are not essential for infec-tivity. Solubilization of membrane proteins in the presence of detergent/lipid mixtures (Poste & Nicolson 1982) has been useful in the study of transport and receptor mechanisms as well as membrane enzymes. Moreover, lipo-somes have been widely used for delivery of macromolecules, such as proteins and nucleic acids, into cells. Prion liposomes open new avenues of scrapie research; being able to study PrP^{Sc} in a functionally soluble form will allow many studies not possible previously.

Acknowledgements

The authors thank J. Valletta and M. Braunfeld for technical assistance as well as L. Gallagher for document production assistance. R.G. was supported by Chaim Weiz-mann Postdoctoral Fellowship for Scientific Research. S.B.P. was supported by re-search grants from the National Institutes of Health (AG02132 and NS14069) and a

Senator Jacob Javits Center of Excellence in Neuroscience (NS22786) as well as gifts from Sherman Fairchild Foundation and RJR-Nabisco, Inc.

References

Alper T, Haig DA, Clarke MC 1966 The exceptionally small size of the scrapie agent. Biochem Biophys Res Commun 22:278–284

Alper T, Cramp WA, Haig DA, Clarke MC 1967 Does the agent of scrapie replicate without nucleic acid? Nature (Lond) 214:764–766

Barry RA, Prusiner SB 1986 Monoclonal antibodies to the cellular and scrapie prion protein. J Infect Dis 154:518–521

Barry RA, Kent SBH, McKinley MP et al 1986 Scrapie and cellular prion proteins share polypeptide epitopes. J Infect Dis 153:848–854

Basler K, Oesch B, Scott M et al 1986 Scrapie and cellular PrP isoforms are encoded by the same chromosomal gene. Cell 46:417–428

Bendheim PE, Barry RA, DeArmond SJ, Stites DP, Prusiner SB 1984 Antibodies to a scrapie prion protein. Nature (Lond) 310:418–421

Bendheim PE, Bockman JM, McKinley MP, Kingsbury DT, Prusiner SB 1985 Scrapie and Creutzfeldt-Jakob disease prion protein share physical properties and antigenic determinants. Proc Natl Acad Sci USA 82:997–1001

Bockman JM, Kingsbury DT, McKinley MP, Bendheim PE, Prusiner SB 1985 Creutzfeldt-Jakob disease prion proteins in human brains. N Engl J Med 312:73–78

Bolton DC, McKinley MP, Prusiner SB 1984 Molecular characteristics of the major scrapie prion protein. Biochemistry 23:5898–5905

Braig H, Diringer H 1985 Scrapie: concept of a virus-induced amyloidosis of the brain. EMBO (Eur Mol Biol Organ) J 4:2309–2312

Brown P, Coker-Vann M, Pomeroy K et al 1986 Diagnosis of Creutzfeldt-Jakob disease by Western blot identification of marker protein in human brain tissue. N Engl J Med 314:547–551

Carlson GA, Kingsbury DT, Goodman P et al 1986 Linkage of prion protein and scrapie incubation time genes. Cell 46:503–511

Charles S, Stewart M 1980 Colorimetric determination of phospholipids with ammonium ferrothiocyanate. Anal Biochem 104:10–14

DeArmond SJ, McKinley MP, Barry RA, Braunfeld MB, McColloch JR, Prusiner SB 1985 Identification of prion amyloid filaments in scrapie-infected brain. Cell 41:221–235

Diener TO, McKinley MP, Prusiner SB 1982 Viroids and prions. Proc Natl Acad Sci USA 79:5220–5224

Gabizon R, McKinley MP, Prusiner SB 1987 Purified prion proteins and scrapie infectivity copartition into liposomes. Proc Natl Acad Sci USA 84:4017–4021

Gadjusek DC 1986 Chronic dementia caused by small unconventional viruses apparently containing no nucleic acid. In: Scheibel AB et al (eds) The biological substrates of alzheimer's disease (UCLA Forum in Medical Sciences, No 27). Academic Press, Orlando, p 33–54

Hauser H, Oldani D, Phillips MD 1973 Mechanisms of ion escape from phosphatidylcholine and phosphatidylserine single bilayer vesicles. Biochemistry 12:4507–4517

Kitamoto T, Tateishi J, Tashima T, Takeshita I, Barry RA, DeArmond SJ, Prusiner SB 1986 Amyloid plaques in Creutzfeldt-Jakob disease stain with prion protein antibodies. Ann Neurol 20:204–208

Laemmli UA 1970 Cleavage of structural proteins during the assembly of the head of bacteriophage T-4. Nature (Lond) 227:680–685

McKinley MP, Prusiner SB 1987 Scrapie prions, amyloid plaques, and a possible link with Alzheimer's disease. In: Bradley RJ (ed) Alzheimer's disease and dementia. Plenum Press, New York, in press

McKinley MP, Bolton DC, Prusiner SB 1983a A protease-resistant protein is a structural component of the scrapie prion. Cell 35:57–62

McKinley MP, Masiarz FR, Isaacs ST, Hearst JE, Prusiner SB 1983b Resistance of the scrapie agent to inactivation by psoralens. Photochem Photobiol 37:539–545

McKinley MP, Braunfeld MB, Bellinger CG, Prusiner SB 1986 Molecular characteristics of prion rods purified from scrapie-infected hamster brains. J Infect Dis 154:110–120

Merz PA, Rohwer RG, Kascsak R et al 1984 Infection-specific particle from the unconventional slow virus diseases. Science (Wash DC) 225:437–440

Meyer RK, McKinley MP, Bowman KA, Barry RA, Prusiner SB 1986 Separation and properties of cellular and scrapie prion proteins. Proc Natl Acad Sci USA 83:2310–2314

Oesch B, Westaway D, Wälchli M et al 1985 A cellular gene encodes scrapie PrP 27–30 protein. Cell 40:735–746

Poste B, Nicolson GL (eds) 1982 Membrane reconstitution. (Cell Surface Reviews vol 8) Elsevier Biomedical Press, Amsterdam

Prusiner SB 1982 Novel proteinaceous infectious particles cause scrapie. Science (Wash DC) 216:136–144

Prusiner SB, Bolton DC, Groth DF, Bowman KA, Cochran SP, McKinley MP 1982a Further purification and characterization of scrapie prions. Biochemistry 21:6942–6950

Prusiner SB, Cochran SP, Groth DF, Downey DE, Bowman KA, Martinez HM 1982b Measurement of the scrapie agent using an incubation time interval assay. Ann Neurol 11:353–358

Prusiner SB, McKinley MP, Bowman KA et al 1983 Scrapie prions aggregate to form amyloid-like birefringent rods. Cell 35:349–358

Prusiner SB, McKinley MP, Bolton DC et al 1984 Prions: methods for assay, purification and characterization. In: Maramorosch K, Koprowski H (eds) Methods in virology. Academic Press, New York, vol 8:293–345

Rohwer RG 1984 Scrapie infectious agent is virus-like in size and susceptibility to inactivation. Nature (Lond) 308:658–662

Smith PK, Krohn RI, Hermanson GT et al 1985 Measurement of protein using bicinchoninic acid. Anal Biochem 150:76–85

Sparkes RS, Simon M, Cohn VH et al 1986 Assignment of the human and mouse prion protein genes to homologous chromosomes. Proc Natl Acad Sci USA 83:7358–7362

DISCUSSION

Hope: Ruth, what are the operational constraints on your system, because they are important when you make statements about solubilization? Would you say that a dimer of the protein comes under the definition of insoluble in your system?

Gabizon: No.

Hope: But that is an aggregated form of PrP.

Gabizon: I am using the membrane biology definition of solubilization i.e., the protein stays in solution after centrifugation at $100000g$ for an hour.

Hope: That is a functional definition. You said, 'every other aggregated form is not needed', and the operational constraint does not allow you to say that.

Gabizon: From measurements we have done, we know that we can have between 2–4 molecules of PrP in a liposome and it stays in solution.

Prusiner: Jim, I would differ with your definition of aggregates. When one talks about multimeric enzymes, they are not called aggregates of the enzyme, they are called oligomers or multimers. Glutamine synthetase has 12 subunits but it is not called an aggregate—if you have many glutamine synthetase molecules all aggregated together, for example in the presence of zinc ions, then that is an aggregate. Ruth is saying that when you have large structures with hundreds of PrP molecules, that's an aggregate.

Hope: OK, I was trying to relate Ruth's work to the proto-fibril model that we have proposed for the change in properties of PrP induced during scrapie infection (Hope et al 1988, Hope & Hunter, this volume). In that model, we considered that an abnormal multimer (or aggregate) of PrP, which did not have a fibril shape, might consist of only two or four molecules of PrP but possess the partial proteinase K resistance which characterizes some PrP molecules in scrapie-affected brain.

Manuelidis: Ruth, you have anti-PrP antibodies bound on a Sepharose column and you elute the binding material, which contains PrP, at pH 9.5–11.0. Why don't you use more standard conditions for antigen elution, such as acetic acid which may be more compatible with the preservation of infectivity?

Gabizon: The optimum pH for elution is 11.5 but I knew that high pH was supposed to diminish scrapie infectivity. I thought the best way to do it was to start as low as possible, which is pH 9.2.

Manuelidis: Have you tried acid elution followed by neutralization?

Gabizon: This is the best method for this specific system.

Beyreuther: Can you separate those liposomes which carry the protein from those which don't carry the protein? And have you compared them with regard to infectivity?

Gabizon: We can separate them but we have not studied that.

Stahl: The problem is that the protein is going to be aligned in one direction or the other in equal amounts. An immunoaffinity column would select out the liposomes that had the antigen binding site facing outwards, but the 50% of liposomes with the binding site towards the interior of the liposomes would remain, so there could still be infectivity.

Gabizon: Even if the purification is very good (80–90%) there is still the problem of measuring this by bioassay. In principle it can be done but because we measure the difference in logs, it is very difficult to get a big numerical difference.

Chesebro: If you can get a 95% separation with affinity columns you are doing very well.

Beyreuther: If you add protease to these liposomes you should be able to degrade the protein in both orientations. Could you then do the infectivity assay?

Gabizon: But that returns to this point–I need 99.9% purification to get three logs difference and this is very difficult to achieve.

Diringer: You add a virus and you can see the virus by electron microscopy. You add some nucleic acid to your starting material but at the end it's gone. What about adding a very small virus such as poliovirus, in which the nucleic acid is protected within a protein shell so you won't be able to destroy it by treatment with proteases, do exactly the same experiment and then, where your liposomal prion protein is, check for polio infectivity.

McKinley: We have done that experiment with the rods (i.e., addition of rod-shaped or spherical viruses as a control) and the same experiment using the liposomes is in progress.

Carp: Have you looked with the electron microscope at the material in which poliovirus has been mixed with liposomes?

Gabizon: The problem is that you want to look for a little round thing between a lot of little round things under the microscope–you need to stay there for hours and look at every window in the microscope!

Chesebro: You should add antibodies to poliovirus, then you will see them— it will increase your sensitivity at least 100-fold by aggregating the virus particles.

Stahl: That is cheating! The point of the experiment was to show that an *unidentified* spherical virus could be detected among the rods, and that a fibrillar virus could be detected among the liposomes.

Chesebro: You can just use it to increase the sensitivity of the final readout.

Diringer: It would be very interesting to know where the infectivity of a conventional virus would go to—whether it would disappear from this liposome fraction, which I doubt.

Prusiner: I don't think that if you add RNase to the poliovirus/liposome mixture it will do anything to the poliovirus, but that's not the issue, that's not why we added the tobacco mosaic virus (TMV). We added TMV as a morphological marker. Similarly, with the poliovirus we have only used it as a morphological marker to ask whether we can see the poliovirus and distinguish it from liposomes. Poliovirus cannot be easily distinguished from small liposomes by electron microscopy; thus, I am not convinced that we can get any useful information from the poliovirus experiments.

Diringer: What is the diameter of the liposomes?

Gabizon: About 20 nm.

Prusiner: Poliovirus has no distinctive substructure that you can readily identify in the electron microscope, it's just a little 20 nm sphere.

Almond: It's 30 nm (Hogle et al 1985).

Diringer: You could have the virus surrounded by a double layer of lipid—to exclude this and thus prove that scrapie agent according to your liposome technique is smaller than a conventional virus you have to test your preparation not only for scrapie infectivity as you did, but also for infectivity of a conventional virus run through this procedure.

McKinley: The point of this experiment was to look at samples in which we had a 2–3 log greater amount of scrapie infectivity compared to the number of added viral particles. We would then hope that we were able to see the virus. The first experiment was done with a rod-shaped virus, TMV. In order to see your proposed virus/lipid structure you have to observe the samples at 50 000-fold magnification. But it is not feasible to look at 400 or 500 windows on one grid at 50000-fold magnification. With TMV we can look at 5000–6000-fold magnification and detect the TMV with one or two scans per grid window. In the middle of a field of the liposomes the TMV stands out because it is a rod. Now you say, let's do the same thing with poliovirus, but instead of preliminary scanning at 5000-fold magnification I must scan the grids at a much greater magnification. You are looking for a little round object in the middle of millions of little round objects. You have to look at very high magnification and then perhaps the one poliovirus is sitting underneath a liposome so you miss it.

Diringer: You don't look under the electron microscope at all, you put your liposome fraction on a dish of susceptible tissue culture cells and see whether infectivity is there.

Merz: The point is whether or not the poliovirus nucleic acid will go into the liposome and retain infectivity, and whether or not under the conditions Ruth described, she will have destroyed the infectivity and the nucleic acid of that poliovirus. It's a perfect control for these experiments.

Gabizon: What about the UV?

Almond: You would expect to destroy polio infectivity by UV irradiation: the lipid bilayer would not protect it.

Gabizon: Or ionizing radiation.

Diringer: Why don't you do the simplest experiment? Put your sample on susceptible tissue culture cells.

Gabizon: Because I am not here to prove anything negative. If I do that that you will say, OK it doesn't work for polio but scrapie is different.

Diringer: If you prove it's negative, then you are really great!

Prusiner: They are saying, take poliovirus and carry it through your preparation procedure. I am saying that in the treatments we have used, poliovirus will resist the nuclease digestions but poliovirus at 65 °C will fall apart: it won't survive the zinc digestion but that is peculiar to poliovirus, if you take another virus it will. That's not what we are trying to show here. The caveat in this experiment is that there may be a small nucleic acid, it may remain protected between this dimer of two proteins, and we cannot say unequivocally that there is no nucleic acid. All we say is that under the conditions of our experiment, if there is a nucleic acid that was made accessible by the transformation of the rod into the detergent-lipid-protein complex, then our nuclease and ion treatments would have attacked it.

Gabizon: I just say that from the UV and ionizing radiation experiment I can predict the maximum possible size for the nucleic acid which could be there and it is too small to be biologically significant.

Chesebro: Doesn't adding exogenous labelled nucleic acid have the same sort of shielding problem?

Prusiner: That is the caveat of the experiment.

Almond: Could you enhance the infectivity of the liposomes by incorporating a virus envelope protein, like an influenza virus HA or the HN from Sendai virus or, better still, the G protein from rabies virus?

Gabizon: I cannot see any way of increasing the infectivity of the scrapie agent by this kind of procedure.

Dickinson: It could easily be the issue of initial presentation to a cell. You are automatically liable to change that by anything you do chemically to the infective preparations.

Gabizon: But you said that this is very mathematical, that by two weeks in alcohol you cannot change the properties.

Dickinson: The logic has to be understood: it is the difference between all that we have ever done in genetic and strain-typing approaches, and all that the biochemists do. When a biochemist makes any treatment the comparison is with the status before the treatment or with some other treatment. The geneticist has two starting points (i.e. separate inocula) and one recipient, or one starting point into two types of recipient: there are many unknowns present in the system, but the unknowns balance out on both sides of the equation because there are no differences in treatment of the inocula. I then make statements about relative differences in the face of equal unknowns. The logical status is different between the biochemical statements and the genetic ones, because the unknowns balance out in the latter case but not in the former.

Chesebro: Regarding the increase in infectivity, how does that compare with what Mike (McKinley) found when he sonicated the rods?

Gabizon: It's very different. We use very mild sonication so it does not denature the protein–we don't think it does but maybe this is why we get an increase of only one or two logs, not four or five.

Chesebro: But you just saw a plateau, no detectable change.

McKinley: We saw no change in infectivity after sonication for 16–20 minutes.

Chesebro: You also had pretty big particles, big enough to see by electron microscopy. I guess we would all agree that they were aggregates even though we don't know how big they are.

Wisniewski: We all agree that the nature of the infectious agents in scrapie,

CJD, kuru and GSS is unknown. Therefore, we should not apply a name, such as virino or prion, until the informational molecule in the infectious agent is determined.

Gabizon: I don't care what these things are called! The name is not important. We have PrP protein, we inject it into brains of animals and they get an infectious disease. What I am trying to do is to narrow the possibilities. We have these big aggregates of PrP protein and maybe something else. We solubilize the aggregates and get this supernatant after ultracentrifugation for two hours. We inject it into the brain and the mouse gets sick. I am trying to eliminate the things which are not important and be left with the things that are most important.

References

Hogle JM, Chow M, Filman DJ 1985 The three-dimensional structure of poliovirus at 2.9 Å resolution. Science (Wash DC) 229:1358–1365

Hope J, Hunter N 1988 Scrapie-associated fibrils, PrP protein and the Sinc gene. In: Novel infectious agents and the central nervous system. Wiley, Chichester (Ciba Found Symp 135) p 146–163

Hope J, Reekie LJD, Gibson PH 1988 On the pathogenesis of SAF. In: Court LA et al (eds) Unconventional viruses and central nervous system diseases. Atelier d'Arts Graphiques, Abbaye de Melleray, in press

In vitro expression of cloned PrP cDNA derived from scrapie-infected mouse brain: lack of transmission of scrapie infectivity

Byron Caughey, Richard Race, Mari Vogel, Michael Buchmeier* and Bruce Chesebro

*Laboratory of Persistent Viral Diseases, NIAID, NIH, Rocky Mountain Laboratories, Hamilton, Montana 59840, and *Department of Immunology, Scripps Clinic and Research Foundation, La Jolla, California, USA*

Abstract. A cDNA for the prion protein (PrP) derived from scrapie-infected mouse brain was expressed in C127 mouse cells *in vitro* under the control of the mouse metallothionein promoter. PrP synthesis was detected by immunoprecipitation using a rabbit antibody specific for a 15 amino acid PrP peptide. Homogenates of cells expressing the cloned PrP cDNA inoculated into weanling mice failed to induce clinical scrapie during 190 days of observation. We conclude that either PrP is not the transmissible agent of scrapie or the PrP is not processed appropriately in this cell system to create the infectious agent.

1988 Novel infectious agents and the central nervous system. Wiley, Chichester (Ciba Foundation Symposium 135) p 197–208

Scrapie is a disease of sheep and goats which has also been transmitted experimentally to rodents and subhuman primates. Based on the neuropathology and properties of the transmissible agent, scrapie appears to be similar to human spongiform encephalopathies. The nature of the agent is still unknown but its resistance to inactivation by X- and UV-irradiation and by treatment with formaldehyde suggests that it might differ considerably from previously recognized infectious agents.

Early studies of partially purified infectious fractions detected unusual macroscopic scrapie-associated fibrils (SAF) in scrapie-infected tissues (Merz et al 1981, Diringer et al 1983, Prusiner et al 1983). Further biochemical purification indicated the presence of a predominant protein species, called prion protein or PrP (Bolton et al 1982, McKinley et al 1983). Since no nucleic acid was detected in these fractions, it was suggested that the agent might be devoid of nucleic acid. After a partial N-terminal amino acid sequence of PrP had been obtained (Prusiner et al 1984), cloning of the PrP cDNA from hamster and mouse scrapie-infected brain was carried out. This cDNA was used to show that PrP mRNA transcripts were expressed in brain and other tissues at equal levels in both normal and scrapie-infected animals (Oesch et al 1985, Chesebro et al 1985, Robakis et al 1986). Thus, the PrP gene was an endogenous gene rather than an exogenous gene associated with an infectious agent. However, it remained possible that either the PrP gene or the PrP protein product might have different structures in normal and scrapie-infected animals. This idea was supported by the observation that PrP from scrapie brain was unusually resistant to digestion by proteinase K (Meyer et al 1986). It remains unclear whether this alteration is secondary to scrapie disease or whether it represents a structural change which is sufficient to both initiate and transmit scrapie pathogenesis (Czub et al 1986).

Because of the uncertainty over the role of PrP in scrapie induction, we decided to express the mouse PrP cDNA derived from scrapie-infected brain in eukaryotic cells in order to test directly whether this PrP product was capable of transmitting scrapie disease. The results presented here indicate that the cloned PrP cDNA was expressed in mouse cells but extracts of these cells failed to cause scrapie when they were inoculated into susceptible mice.

Methods

DNA constructions and transfection of C127 cells.   The 1.3 kb insert of mouse PrP clone 7 described previously (Locht et al 1986) was excised from the plasmid pEMBL8 with *Eco*RI and purified on a low melting agarose gel. The ends were blunted by Klenow enzyme and *Bgl*II linkers were added. Following digestion with *Bgl*II, the fragment was inserted into the *Bgl*II site of plasmid p341–1, kindly provided by Dr Peter Howley (Eiden et al 1985). After transformation of JM109 cells with this construct, recombinants containing the insert in the correct orientation were selected, the DNA was cut with *Bam*HI and the entire bovine papilloma virus genome, derived from *Bam*HI digestion of plasmid p142–6, was inserted (Sarver et al 1982). Appropriate recombinants were selected and the DNA was transfected into mouse C127 cells (Lowy et al 1978). Morphologically transformed colonies were visible after about two weeks; these were picked and amplified. Southern blot analysis of DNA from these cells indicated that the PrP and BPV inserts remained intact and were present in an episomal form. As a control, a similar construct lacking the PrP insert was made and control C127 transformants obtained with this BPV construct were also analysed.

Immunoprecipitation.   Rabbit anti-PrP serum was raised in the laboratory of Dr M. Buchmeier (Wiley et al 1987). In brief, a 16 amino acid peptide was synthesized, starting with an N-terminal cysteine and followed by the first 15 amino acids of the original PrP 27–30 sequence (Prusiner et al 1984). This peptide was coupled by the sulphydryl group of the cysteine to keyhole limpet haemocyanin and the complex was used to immunize rabbits.

C127 cells transformed with a PrP-BPV plasmid or with a control BPV plasmid were labelled for between 15 minutes and four hours with [^{35}S]methionine at 100 μCi/ml. After labelling, cells were lysed with triple detergent (0.5% NP40, 0.5% deoxycholate and 0.1% SDS in 0.01 M Tris HC1, pH 7.2, 0.14 M NaC1). Lysates were precleared by incubation for several hours with normal rabbit serum and Sepharose-Protein A, followed by ultracentrifugation or microfuging. Aliquots of precleared lysate containing 2.5 × 10^5 cell equivalents were incubated with 2 μl rabbit anti-PrP peptide antiserum followed by Sepharose-Protein A. Sepharose beads were pelleted and washed three times with triple detergent, then boiled in SDS-PAGE eluting buffer; eluates were analysed by SDS-PAGE on 8.5% gels.

Analysis of scrapie infectivity.   Tissue culture cells were processed by freezing and thawing and sonicating before dilution and inoculation into susceptible RML mice as previously described (Race et al 1987). As controls, mouse neuroblastoma cells carrying scrapie infectivity and extracts of mouse scrapie brain were used.

Results

Construction of a PrP expression vector

To express the mouse PrP gene in a eukaryotic cell line, a 1.3 kb fragment of a cDNA clone containing the entire open reading frame of PrP derived from scrapie-infected mouse brain was used. This fragment was ligated into the *Bgl*II site downstream from the metallothionein promoter in plasmid p341–1. Following selection of a clone containing the PrP insert in the correct orientation, the plasmid was cut at the single *Bam*HI site and the 7.9 kb genome of bovine papilloma virus (BPV) was inserted. The final construction was transfected into the mouse cell line, C127, and colonies were selected 14 days later, based on their loss of contact inhibition.

Immunoprecipitation of mouse PrP

To identify PrP, a C127 line (clone 2P) transformed with pPrP-BPV was labelled with [^{35}S]methionine and cell lysates were immunoprecipitated with a rabbit anti-PrP peptide serum. Lysates from cells labelled for different amounts of time showed different PrP bands (Fig. 1). After 15 minutes of labelling, major bands were detected at 37 and 33 kDa. Minor bands were also seen at 31, 29, 27 and 23 kDa. After one and four hour labelling periods, the 37 kDa band remained equal in intensity but the 33 kDa band was

15m 1h 4h

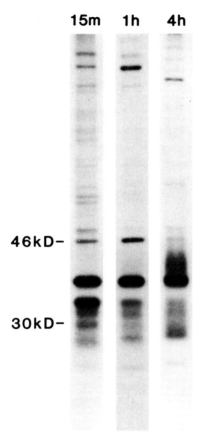

46kD–

30kD–

FIG. 1. Immunoprecipitation with anti-PrP peptide antiserum. Mouse C127 cells transformed with a PrP-BPV plasmid shuttle vector were labelled with [^{35}S]methionine for various times. Detergent lysates were immunoprecipitated with rabbit anti-PrP peptide antiserum and analysed by SDS-PAGE. Molecular weight markers indicated were ovalbumin (46 kDa) and carbonic anhydrase (30 kDa).

diminished; after four hours a new, broad band appeared between 35 and 41 kDa.

PrP bands were also detected in a C127 cell line (clone 1A) transformed with a control BPV plasmid lacking the PrP insert (data not shown). However, the intensity of these PrP bands was 10 to 20-fold less than those seen in clone 2P. The apparent molecular weights of those bands were 31, 27 and 23 kDa, and they were identical to bands detected in clone 2P cells.

To confirm the PrP specificity of the bands observed in both clones, immunoprecipitation was performed in the presence of excess PrP peptide to competitively inhibit the anti-PrP serum. In all cases, precipitation of the bands described above was blocked by the presence of the PrP peptide (data

TABLE 1   Lack of transmission of clinical scrapie to mice using C127 cells expressing a cloned mouse PrP cDNA

Cell equivalents inoculated	Scrapie-positive/Total		
	PrP–BPV C127 cells (Clone 2P)	Scrapie-infected mouse neuroblastoma cells	Scrapie brain homogenate
3×10^6	0/10	10/10	10/10
3×10^5	0/10	10/10	10/10
3×10^4	0/10	5/10	10/10
3×10^3	0/10	1/10	10/10
3×10^2	nt	0/10	10/10
3×10^1	nt	0/10	10/10

Data shown are from 190 days after intracerebral inoculation of RML mice. nt, not tested

not shown). Thus, the bands contained antigens present in the PrP peptide.

Assay of scrapie infectivity in cells expressing cloned PrP

Because of the interest in the possibility that PrP might be the agent of scrapie infectivity (Prusiner 1982), clone 2P cells expressing the PrP cDNA cloned from mouse scrapie brain were tested for infectivity in mice. Clone 2P cells were counted and homogenized in a manner similar to that used for scrapie-infected tissue culture cells (Race et al 1987). Dilutions corresponding to given numbers of cell equivalents were inoculated intracerebrally into mice, which were then observed for clinical signs of scrapie. Results at 190 days after infection indicated that no scrapie was transmitted by homogenates of clone 2P cells (Table 1). In contrast, control scrapie-infected tissue culture cells and scrapie-infected brain homogenates at high dilutions both induced disease by this time.

Discussion

These results demonstrate the expression of a PrP cDNA cloned from mouse scrapie brain in mouse C127 cells. Although some endogenous PrP was detected in cells transformed with the PrP-negative BPV construct, the PrP levels were much higher in cells containing the PrP-BPV construct. Either the high copy number of this episomal DNA and/or the activity of the strong metallothionein promoter might be responsible for the increased PrP expression. The fact that some additional PrP-specific bands were seen in these cells compared to controls suggested that these bands were expressed from the transferred PrP rather than the endogenous gene.

Attempts to transmit scrapie disease using extracts of cells expressing cloned PrP were not successful. The nature of this result is such that we cannot conclude whether PrP is either necessary or sufficient for the transmission of scrapie. There are several less definitive interpretations. First, if both normal and abnormal, i.e. scrapie-associated, PrP genes exist, then our cloned PrP cDNA might be from the normal rather than the abnormal gene. However, at present there is no evidence for two distinct genes. Second, even if there is only one PrP gene, its product might be processed differently under different circumstances. The distinct PrP bands seen in our two C127 clones support this possibility: one can easily imagine that different cell types could markedly influence processing. Furthermore, it is unclear whether scrapie agent infectivity is capable of replicating in C127 cells. Thus, there are many possible explanations for a negative outcome in these experiments. However, in the altered processing hypothesis, ways by which the agent might be changed from its endogenous form to an activated, disease-transmitting form remain speculative.

We would like to consider an alternative explanation, which we currently favour: that PrP is not the scrapie agent but a normal protein which aggregates and accumulates in a protease-resistant form in brain and perhaps other tissues secondary to scrapie pathogenesis. The accumulation of SAF or PrP during the course of disease might itself contribute to and accelerate the pathogenic process. If so, this might explain the apparent linkage between scrapie incubation period and a genetic marker close to the PrP gene in some mouse strains (Carlson et al 1986). Concerning the biochemical association of PrP with scrapie infectivity, one can only speculate that aggregated PrP might bind non-specifically to the infectious agent, since PrP was found by differential centrifugation to bind to cellular components of various sizes (Prusiner et al 1978). This might occur to such an extent that the biophysical properties of the agent are altered, further confusing the issue.

The present results have failed to confirm PrP as the agent of scrapie. Future efforts should be focused on expressing PrP in cells capable of replicating the infectious agent, to resolve the problem of altered PrP processing in different cells. In addition, it would be desirable to take a fresh look at the 'agent' controversy and perhaps use new biochemical approaches to isolate the agent from different sources. This might eliminate systematic pitfalls or artifacts associated with fractionation of a single tissue source such as brain.

References

Bolton DC, McKinley MP, Prusiner SB 1982 Identification of a protein that purifies with the scrapie prion. Science (Wash DC) 218:1309–1311

Carlson GA, Kingsbury DT, Goodman PA et al 1986 Linkage of prion protein and scrapie incubation time genes. Cell 46:503–511

Chesebro B, Race RE, Wehrly K et al 1985 Identification of scrapie prion protein-specific mRNA in scrapie-infected and uninfected brain. Nature (Lond) 315:331–333

Czub M, Braig HR, Diringer H 1986 Pathogenesis of scrapie: study of the temporal development of clinical symptoms, of infectivity titres and scrapie-associated fibrils in brains of hamsters infected intraperitoneally. J Gen Virol 67:2005–2009

Diringer H, Gelderblom H, Hilmert H, Ozel M, Edelbluth C, Kimberlin RH 1983 Scrapie infectivity, fibrils, and low molecular weight protein. Nature (Lond) 306:476–478

Eiden M, Newman M, Fisher AG, Mann DL, Howley PM, Reitz MS 1985 Type 1 human T-cell leukemia virus small envelope protein expressed in mouse cells by using a bovine papilloma virus-derived shuttle vector. Mol Cell Biol 5:3320–3324

Locht C, Chesebro B, Race R, Keith JM 1986 Molecular cloning and complete sequence of prion protein cDNA from mouse brain infected with the scrapie agent. Proc Natl Acad Sci USA 83:6372–6376

Lowy DR, Rands E, Scolnick EM 1978 Helper-independent transformation by unintegrated Harvey sarcoma virus DNA. J Virol 26:291–298

McKinley MP, Bolton DC, Prusiner SB 1983 A protease-resistant protein is a structural component of the scrapie prion. Cell 35:57–62

Merz PA, Somerville RA, Wisniewski HM, Iqbal K 1981 Abnormal fibrils from scrapie-infected brain. Acta Neuropathol 54:63–74

Meyer RK, McKinley MP, Bowman KA, Braunfeld MB, Barry RA, Prusiner SB 1986 Separation and properties of cellular and scrapie prion proteins. Proc Natl Acad Sci USA 83:2310–2314

Oesch B, Westaway D, Wälchli M et al 1985 A cellular gene encodes scrapie PrP 27–30 protein. Cell 40:735–746

Prusiner SB 1982 Novel proteinaceous infectious particles cause scrapie. Science (Wash DC) 216:136–144

Prusiner SB, Hadlow WJ, Eklund CM, Race RE, Cochran SP 1978 Sedimentation characteristics of the scrapie agent from murine spleen and brain. Biochemistry 17:4987–4992

Prusiner SB, McKinley MP, Bowman KA et al 1983 Scrapie prions aggregate to form amyloid-like birefringent rods. Cell 35:349–358

Prusiner SB, Groth DF, Bolton DC, Kent SB, Hood LE 1984 Purification and structural studies of a major scrapie prion protein. Cell 38:127–134

Race RE, Fadness LH, Chesebro B 1987 Characterization of scrapie infection in mouse neuroblastoma cells. J Gen Virol, in press

Robakis NK, Sawh PR, Wolfe GC, Rubenstein R, Carp RI, Innis MA 1986 Isolation of a cDNA clone encoding the leader peptide of prion protein and expression of the homologous gene in various tissues. Proc Natl Acad Sci USA 83:6377–6381

Sarver N, Byrne JC, Howley PM 1982 Transformation and replication in mouse cells of a bovine papilloma virus-pML2 plasmid vector that can be rescued in bacteria. Proc Natl Acad Sci USA 79:7147–7151

Wiley CA, Burrola PG, Buchmeier MJ et al 1987 Immuno-gold localization of prion filaments in scrapie-infected hamster brains. Lab Invest 57:

DISCUSSION

Gabizon: Surely you don't expect to produce infectious particles in this system? We have shown that you need the proteinase K resistant form of PrP, at least as a marker.

Chesebro: We don't know which variables are really necessary. All we know is that we need brain from scrapie-infected animals, from which we get something that causes infectivity.

Gabizon: We all agree that the proteinase K-resistant form of PrP is present in scrapie-infected brains and we know that there is a normal homologue. This protein that you have tested is not proteinase K resistant, so obviously it is not like the marker for scrapie infectivity.

Chesebro: We are testing its resistance to proteinase K. I think there are possible situations, such as in the spleen, where the PrP will not be proteinase K resistant but the infectivity will still be there *in vivo*.

Gabizon: We don't know about the spleen, we don't have any evidence either way.

Chesebro: That's the problem–somebody should look at spleen because there may be such a situation in the spleen. We have to look a this with an open mind, a year ago we thought that aggregation was essential, now your data suggest that aggregation is not essential. Proteinase K resistance may not be essential but a secondary factor. Our experiment is an independent test of whether PrP expressed from cDNA cloned from scrapie brain can cause clinical scrapie: apparently it cannot.

Carlson: Did you look at PrP protein in the tissue culture cell lines where the mRNA for PrP was present?

Chesebro: No; not yet.

Kimberlin: You raised the issue of species barriers when discussing evolutionary aspects of sequence differences of PrP in different species. We have studied in detail the transmission of scrapie between species. Sometimes there is a big species barrier effect and sometimes none at all. Sometimes the greatly lengthened incubation period occurs only at the first passage in the new host, which might suggest modification of pathogenesis, just at that first passage. On other occasions the 'adaptation' (as you call it) takes several passages before average incubation periods settle down to a constant value. In this situation, we have evidence that what is happening is the gradual selection of a mutant strain or perhaps of a single strain from a pre-existing mixture (Kimberlin et al 1987). I think this kind of process is somewhat different to what you had in mind.

Chesebro: I was just hoping that perhaps from some of those different situations one might be able to identify molecular events associated with the various shifts.

Dickinson: The word adaptation is very vague, when you can be highly specific. For example, we have shown that it is possible to exclude information—we would refer to it as removing one strain from a mixture of strains—and it doesn't reappear. This example is directly relevant because it can occur at the crossing of species barriers in serial passage of scrapie through sheep, goats and mice. We have found that two strains of scrapie, 22C and 22H (or a precursor they share) can pass these three species barriers, yet in mice of different *Sinc* genotypes one or other of them can be excluded. Also, 22C can be excluded from the mixture by microbiological cloning without changing the *Sinc* genotype used for passage (Dickinson et al 1988).

Chesebro: So we may be cloning when we adapt, or mutating, or selecting; one can't tell the difference.

Merz: We have been tracking PrP by Western blotting and isolation of PrP from one strain of agent that has been passaged in multiple strains of mice, rats and hamsters; it is only the host protein that is detected.

Almond: You talked about using the wrong PrP gene, would you elaborate on there only being one gene (of course it is diploid, so there are two)? You mentioned this amino acid difference between the two clones as possibly a result of reverse transcription error, it could also be due to two different messenger RNAs from the different alleles. Therefore, you may have chosen the wrong one and the other allele would have been infectious.

Chesebro: We should ligate the other clone into the expression vector and test it. With regard to whether or not there are multiple genes, I think we have to sequence the endogenous DNA and Stan's (Prusiner) group has done that, at least for hamster.

Prusiner: We think it is a single copy gene.

Chesebro: There do not seem to be different multiple splicing patterns, so we have no positive evidence to suggest that there are different genes.

DeArmond: Alleles have not been looked for yet, have they?

Almond: That was my point. But these are inbred mice, you wouldn't expect there to be much difference between the two alleles.

Chesebro: Ours are not inbred mice. Therefore it is still theoretically possible that there are two different normal PrP alleles in any single outbred mouse.

Almond: Have you looked at your product on a 2D gel and if so, do you see the spread of spots that Jim Hope showed on his 2D gels, suggesting heterogeneity or post-translational processing?

Chesebro: We haven't looked at 2D gels, that is something worth doing. One beneficial aspect of this system is that it may provide a good background against which to compare other post-translational modifications, for instance, of PrP lipid. Our system provides a source of PrP that is not compromised by having been through the extraction procedure.

Hope: It's interesting that, superficially at least, the multiple forms of the artificially expressed protein look like what we see in a non-proteinase K-treated aggregate. It could be a way of determining whether those forms are biosynthetic intermediates, produced when biosynthesis of the protein is inhibited, or whether they are degradation products. If structural analysis shows that your proteins are the same as ours, then pulse–chase experiments could show whether yours were biosynthetic intermediates or degradation products; that would give us clue about what might be happening in the brain.

Chesebro: It has been difficult to get pulse–chase experiments to work, because of certain technical problems that we have had.

Hope: If you have these different forms, it may be that they form a metabolically stable multimer, from which the labelled protein cannot be chased.

Chesebro: It's possible. The nearest thing we have to a pulse–chase is the extended labelling, where there seems to be a progressive appearance of higher molecular weight forms of PrP, but we haven't been able to chase radioactive counts from the early labelling material into that late form of the protein.

Prusiner: Do you have any estimate of the number of nanograms of PrP produced per cell?

Chesebro: No, you can't get that from [^{35} S] methionine-labelling experiments because we don't know the pool size of methionine in the cell. A Western blot is a better way to get that information. Rick Race is running Western blots now, but I don't think there is much protein present.

Gabizon: So your expression system would not be a useful source of large amounts of PrP.

Prusiner: There is an important point with respect to infectivity, i.e. that one needs to calculate the number of PrP molecules in an experiment. With our recombinant baculovirus constructs, Michael Scott produced approximately 10^{12} molecules of recombinant hamster PrP and inoculated these PrP molecules into hamsters. After 150 days none of the hamsters developed scrapie.

F. Brown: But only one viral protein, that of hepatitis B virus, when expressed in an artificial system has proved to be immunogenic and that was one which aggregated. So there may be something subtle about the infectivity or biological activity of a protein produced artificially in that way.

Chesebro: I don't agree, I have been working with vaccinia constructs that make lots of different viral proteins and they are all immunogenic when expressed in vaccinia-infected cells and in tissue culture lines. This is also true for hepatitis B, herpes simplex and rabies viral proteins.

Merz: You tested the epithelial cell line that had been transformed by a papilloma virus containing the PrP insert for infectivity. Does that epithelial line support scrapie infectivity?

Chesebro: Rick Race is doing that at the moment. We are also trying to put these vectors into other cells that we know support scrapie infectivity.

Prusiner: The development of cell culture systems that can express reasonable levels of prion proteins or other molecules, if there are other molecules, that are important for infectivity is going to be one of the most important avenues of research in the future. The whole field has been thwarted for 35–40 years by not having a cell culture system. We are also trying to do this. We have very similar results with, for instance, the astrocytic cell lines—they do express PrP mRNA but they don't express the prion protein. Most cell lines that we have studied have detectable PrP mRNA but not the prion protein. The use of expression vectors will allow us to increase the amount of prion protein production in these cells.

Almond: Bruce, in the spleen and brain there is a higher level of expression than in other tissue types and this correlates with infectivity. It would be useful to make transgenic mice containing this gene linked to an insulin promoter, for example, and then seeing first, whether there is a higher level of expression in the pancreas of the transgenic animal, and second, whether this correlates with a high level of infectivity in the pancreas. Similarly, you could use the (corticosteroid-responsive) mouse mammary tumour virus long terminal repeat sequence and then look for infectivity in the mammary gland during lactation. Those sorts of experiments would provide a correlation between PrP gene expression and scrapie infectivity.

Chesebro: If PrP is the important disease-inducing protein, it doesn't have to be synthesized in the organs where infectivity is found. It's interesting, but not necessarily totally relevant, to look for PrP messenger RNA; we know from other virus systems that the proteins or viruses can be synthesized in one cell and transported to another cell where they accumulate.

Almond: Concerning the level of sequence divergence between the mouse and the hamster PrP genes: it was gratifying to see that based on comparison of nucleotide sequences these animals are separated by an estimated 25 000 000 years, which seems reasonable for the mouse and hamster. This observation argues that if there is a nucleic acid in the scrapie agent, then this nucleic acid cannot be anything to do with the PrP gene, because if there were replication of the nucleic acid it would have acquired far more mutations than those observed.

I was intrigued by the high level of conservation you reported in the 5' non-coding region, which is unusual in an ordinary messenger RNA. It is common in the picornaviruses.

Oesch: Usually non-coding sequences show more sequence divergence than the adjacent coding sequences but certain segments are conserved, for example, the polyadenylation site and the signal regulating the stability of the message, where similar sequences are found in the 3' untranslated region of various genes (Shaw & Kamen 1986).

Almond: But how large is that conserved sequence?

Oesch: It's about 60 nucleotides, but added together these sequences could form a much longer conserved region.

Almond: Bruce is talking about 150 nucleotides and 90% conservation. It is a higher level of conservation over a much larger region than anything I've come across before in a messenger RNA from two related animal species. This is fascinating and potentially significant. Have you removed the conserved sequence to see the effect this has on expression?

Prusiner: We have performed our expression studies in cultured cells without that 3' region, using an artificially constructed vector where we have removed that portion of the 3' sequence. Under these conditions, PrP is synthesized.

Chesebro: Our vector also has that sequence removed. We are thinking about putting it back on.

Almond: One thing that comes to mind is something like a *psi* sequence, the packaging signal in a retrovirus (Mann et al 1983). That again raises the notion of this RNA being packaged in the SAF but we have just discounted that by consideration of the level of sequence divergence.

References

Dickinson AG, Outram GW, Taylor DM, Foster JD 1988 Further evidence that scrapie agent has an independent genome. In: Court LA et al (eds) Unconventional viruses and central nervous system diseases. Atelier d'Arts Graphiques, Abbaye de Melleray, in press

Kimberlin RH, Cole S, Walker CA 1987 Temporary and permanent modifications to a single strain of mouse scrapie on transmission to rats and hamsters. J Gen Virol 68:1875–1881

Mann R, Mulligan RC, Baltimore DB 1983 Construction of a retrovirus packaging mutant and its use to produce helper-free defective retrovirus. Cell 33:153–159

Shaw G, Kamen R 1986 A conserved AU sequence from the 3' untranslated region of GM-CSF mRNA mediates selective mRNA degradation. Cell 46:659–667

Search for a scrapie-specific nucleic acid: a progress report

B. Oesch, D.F. Groth*, S.B. Prusiner* and C. Weissmann

*Institut für Molekulabiologie I, Universität Zürich, CH-8093 Zürich and *Department of Neurology and Biochemistry and Biophysics, University of California, San Francisco, CA 94143, USA*

Abstract. Scrapie agent contains a proteinaceous component as well as an 'informational' molecule (suggested by the existence of distinct strains of scrapie). These operationally defined entities may be the same molecule, an infectious protein, or distinct, in which case a nucleic acid might encode the genetic information. Purification of scrapie agent enriched a protein, PrP^{Sc}, by virtue of its relative protease resistance. There is only a single PrP gene and the primary translation product of PrP mRNA is the same in normal and scrapie-infected brain; therefore the normal PrP^C and the protease-resistant isoform, PrP^{Sc}, found in scrapie, probably result from different post-translational events.

To search for scrapie-specific nucleic acid, globin RNA made *in vitro* was added to highly purified infectious preparations at a ratio of 10^3 molecules per infectious unit, nucleic acids were isolated and denatured, and cDNA synthesized using random oligonucleotide primers. Clones containing globin-related sequences were identified by *in situ* hybridization. 150 plaques not hybridizing to the globin probe were isolated. Inserts larger than 50 base pairs were analysed. By hybridization to a globin probe at reduced stringency all but four clones were found to contain small globin related inserts; two of these hybridized to hamster repetitive sequences as shown by Southern blot analysis. The other clones not related to hamster nucleic acids may be derived from unknown sources of contamination or from scrapie-specific nucleic acids.

1988 Novel infectious agents and the central nervous system. Wiley, Chichester (Ciba Foundation Symposium 135) p 209–223

Hypotheses regarding the nature of the scrapie agent, also designated prion (Prusiner 1982), must take into account a number of observations reported in the literature.

(1)   Infectivity is inactivated by treatments or reagents which destroy or denature proteins, but not by nucleolytic agents (Prusiner 1982, Diener et al 1982), arguing that the infectious agent is not an unprotected, free nucleic acid, such as a viroid.

(2)   The target size of the scrapie agent, as determined by ionizing radiation, is small compared to conventional viruses; estimates range from 50–150 kDa (Alper et al 1966) to $0.5-2 \times 10^3$ kDa (Rohwer 1984).

(3) Purified preparations of infectious scrapie agent consist mainly of a single glycoprotein, PrP 27–30, which is derived from a larger molecule, PrP^{Sc}, by proteolysis during purification (McKinley et al 1983, Oesch et al 1985).

(4) Despite intensive efforts, it has not been possible to detect a defined nucleic acid in the most highly purified preparations (K. Gilles, D. Riesner, S.B. Prusiner, personal communication). However, it should be noted that such preparations contain about 10^8 infectious units per ml; for a nucleic acid with a relative molecular weight of 100 000 and a ratio of infectious to total particles of one, this corresponds to about 0.2–0.4 fmole or 20 pg nucleic acids per ml, an amount which is at the limit of detectability.

(5) PrP protein is encoded by a single chromosomal host gene (Oesch et al 1985, Chesebro et al 1985, Basler et al 1986, Westaway & Prusiner 1986). However, an episomal form of the PrP gene has not been searched for and may have escaped detection, particularly if it occurs in only a small proportion of brain cells.

(6) The gene is expressed to equal extents in normal and scrapie-infected animals (Oesch et al 1985, Chesebro et al 1985, Kretzschmar et al 1986, Robakis et al 1986), giving rise to the same primary translation product. The protein found in normal tissue (PrP^C) differs from PrP^{Sc} in its physical properties and its susceptibility to proteinase K, probably due to post-translational modifications (Oesch et al 1985, Basler et al 1986).

(7) The PrP gene is either closely linked or identical to a genetic locus, *Prn-i*, which controls the incubation time of scrapie (Carlson et al 1986). Other studies suggest that *Prn-i* and the previously described incubation time gene *Sinc* (Dickinson et al 1968) are the same locus (Carp et al 1987); close linkage between the PrP gene and *Sinc* has been reported by Hunter et al (1987).

(8) Distinct strains of scrapie agent breed true when in the same host strain (Bruce & Dickinson 1979, 1987, Dickinson & Fraser 1979). Bruce & Dickinson (1987) have reported scrapie strain conversion, which they attribute to mutational events. These results suggest that the infectious particle carries genetic information, which is replicated.

(9) Scrapie-infected animals show no immune response (McFarlin et al 1971, Kasper et al 1981).

Two main hypotheses are currently under discussion as regards the nature of the infectious agent, neither of which can be conclusively ruled out: (1) it is a protein or protein derivative, devoid of nucleic acid (Alper et al 1966, Gibbons & Hunter 1967, Prusiner 1982), or (2) it is a small, as yet unidentified, nucleic acid carrying at least part of the scrapie genetic information, enveloped by a protein which is encoded by the host genome (Kimberlin 1982, Prusiner 1982).

The 'protein only' hypothesis

So far, PrP^{Sc} is the only characterized macromolecule found in purified preparations of scrapie agent (McKinley et al 1983) and is the most likely candidate for the conjectured infectious protein. This implies that the introduction of PrP^{Sc} into a host both elicits the pathological processes characteristic for scrapie and gives rise to more PrP^{Sc} than the amount used for inoculation. Since there is only a single PrP gene in a homozygous animal, one has to conclude that host-encoded, non-pathogenic PrP^{C} or its precursor is converted into the modified, infectious form as a consequence of the introduction of PrP^{Sc} (or PrP 27–30) into the organism. How could this transformation be triggered? The action of PrP^{Sc} could be direct or indirect.

In the case of direct action, PrP^{Sc} might act like an enzyme, converting either PrP^{C} or its precursor into PrP^{Sc} which in turn would catalyse further conversion (Fig. 1A). As pointed out by Brunori & Talbot (1985), this process may be compared to the conversion of trypsinogen to trypsin. One may visualize this model by considering a hypothetical disease, 'trypsinosis', which would occur in an imaginary animal in whose blood a stable trypsinogen circulates. The trypsinogen would remain inactive and the animal healthy until it was inoculated with a trace of trypsin, whereupon trypsinogen would be activated to trypsin and autolysis would occur, leading to the animal's death. 'Trypsinosis' could be transmitted to other animals naturally, for example, by cannibalism, or experimentally, by inoculation with blood from a 'trypsinotic' animal. In due course, investigators would isolate trypsin and identify it as the infectious agent, by demonstrating that it conformed, *mutatis mutandis*, to Koch's four postulates. It should, however, be stressed that there is no evidence whatsoever that PrP^{Sc} arises from PrP^{C} by proteolytic cleavage.

In an indirect mode of action, conversion of PrP^{C} to PrP^{Sc} would be catalysed by a protein, distinct from PrP^{Sc}, encoded but not expressed in the uninfected cell. PrP^{Sc} would initiate synthesis of more PrP^{Sc} by inducing a conjectural 'Prp-converting enzyme' which acts at some post-transcriptional level (Fig. 1C). One might even envisage PrP^{Sc} initiating a cascade of events, which would ultimately lead to activation of the converting enzyme. It is interesting to note that 20 years ago Gibbons and Hunter (1967) suggested that the scrapie agent might be a polysaccharide or glycoprotein which induces the formation of a host-encoded 'polysaccharase' or 'transferase' that would generate more of the pathogenic polysaccharide or glycoprotein.

How can one account for distinct, stable strains of scrapie agent within the framework of the 'protein only' model? In the 'direct action' model, each strain of scrapie agent would be represented by a different variant of the PrP^{Sc} molecule. Each such variant would be able to modify the same precursor (there is evidence for only one PrP gene in homozygous animals!) such that

Figure 1

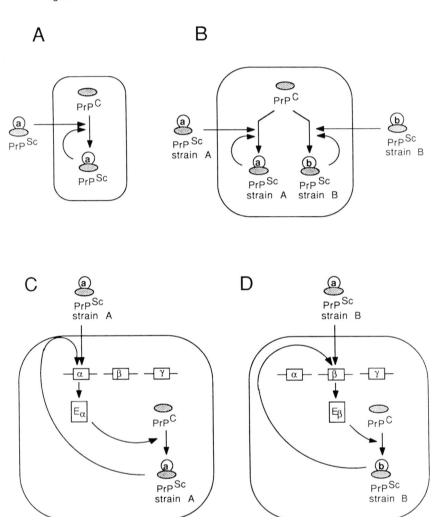

FIG. 1.   Models for the replication of scrapie agent without a nucleic acid component ('protein only'). PrP^{Sc} is the infectious agent. (A,B) 'Direct action' model. (A) On infection, PrP^{Sc} converts PrP^C (or its precursor) into PrP^{Sc}, which in turn leads to further modification of PrP^C. (B) The replication of different strains of PrP^{Sc} is explained by assuming that strain specificity resides in different modifications (a,b) which direct the conversion of PrP^C into PrP^{Sc} carrying the same modification as the infecting strain. (C,D) 'Indirect action' model. PrP^{Sc}, strain A, activates a cellular gene α, whose product, E$_α$, converts cellular PrP into PrP^{Sc}. To explain the propagation of different strains of PrP^{Sc} in a single host genotype, one would postulate the existence of a battery of such cellular genes, each encoding a differer.• 'PrP converting enzyme'.

the product resembles the incoming agent (Fig. 1B). It is difficult to imagine a molecular basis for this kind of specificity, and becomes more difficult the greater the number of discrete scrapie strains that can be stably transmitted by an inbred host. The conversion of one scrapie strain to another during passage in a different host could be accounted for by polymorphic variants of the PrP gene, if the incoming PrP^{Sc} of one type could convert the endogenous PrP precursor of another type, and if the same modification on a different PrP polypeptide gave rise to a new PrP strain.

Within the framework of the 'indirect action' model, the variety of scrapie species would have to be explained by a battery of distinct converting enzymes, each of which would convert the same PrP precursor to a different type of PrP^{Sc} and would be specifically activated by that particular type of PrP^{Sc} (Fig. 1C.D). Mutations in the converting enzyme genes could give rise to new, apparently mutated, strains of scrapie agent. Moreover, the set of converting enzymes could differ in different host species, accounting for the 'mutation' of some PrP strains on changing the host.

Models involving a nucleic acid as the inheritable informational molecule

The existence of distinct scrapie strains which undergo what appears to be mutation and selection (Bruce & Dickinson 1987) is conventionally explained by the assumption that the scrapie agent comprises a nucleic acid of some sort. It has been proposed that the scrapie agent might consist of a scrapie-specific nucleic acid coated by a host-encoded protein (Kimberlin 1982, Prusiner 1982) and that both components might contribute to the scrapie phenotype. PrP^{Sc} would be a likely candidate for such a host-specified coat protein (Oesch et al 1985) and this model would explain many properties of the scrapie agent. The existence of different strains and the occurrence of mutations could be ascribed to variations in the small nucleic acid, as for example, in viroids (Schnölzer et al 1985). Reproducible changes of scrapie agent strain on passage in a certain host could be explained by mutation followed by selection (Bruce & Dickinson 1987). Because PrP is a host-encoded protein, a scrapie-specific nucleic acid would not need to encode a coat protein and could be quite small. Finally, the striking finding that the scrapie agent is not immunogenic and that the disease is not accompanied by any inflammatory reactions (McFarlin et al 1971, Kasper et al 1981) is explained by the tolerance of the host to an only slightly modified host protein. Within the framework of this model the conversion of PrP^{C} to PrP^{Sc} could be associated with the recruitment of PrP from a host cell membrane into the infectious particle (Fig. 2).

A search for nucleic acids in infectious preparations by a molecular cloning strategy

Although no nucleic acid has been detected in purified infectious

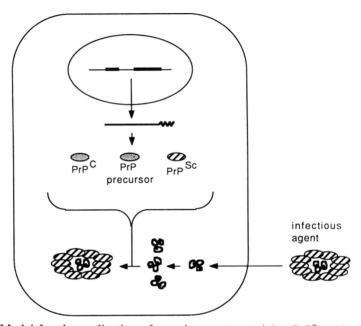

FIG. 2.   Model for the replication of scrapie agent containing PrP^{Sc} and a nucleic acid. A nucleic acid with an envelope consisting of host-encoded PrP^{Sc} infects the cell. After replication of the nucleic acid, infectious particles are assembled from nucleic acid and PrP. In the most simple scenario, conversion of PrP^{C} to PrP^{Sc} is caused by the association with the nucleic acid. Alternatively, PrP^{C} or its precursor may be converted to PrP^{Sc}, which then coats the scrapie-specific nucleic acid.

preparations, the analytical methods may not have been sensitive enough to reveal a concentration as low as one copy of an essential nucleic acid per infectious unit. Nonetheless, it should be possible to detect such a nucleic acid by molecular cloning.

The most highly purified infectious preparations were used as starting material to minimize contamination with normal hamster nucleic acids. Because the type and higher order structure of the conjectured nucleic acid are unknown, heat denaturation of the preparation followed by synthesis of double-stranded cDNA with random oligonucleotides as primers was chosen as the most promising approach. By this strategy, linear and circular single-stranded RNA, as well as single-stranded and double-stranded linear DNA, should be converted into double-stranded linear DNA suitable for cloning. Other forms such as double-stranded RNA or double-stranded circular DNA may not be clonable by this procedure; double-stranded RNA might not denature under the conditions used and double-stranded circular DNA would yield Form IV DNA, a structure which might not permit reverse transcription.

Nucleic acids from 10^{8} infectious units of scrapie agent were deproteinized in the presence of 10^{11} molecules of β-globin RNA that had been added as a carrier and internal reference. The purified nucleic acids were reverse transcribed using random oligonucleotides as primers and cloned after *Eco*RI linker addition in the vector λgt11/amp3 (Kemp et al 1983), yielding approximately 10^6 independent recombinants. Assuming that the conjectured scrapie-related nucleic acid was cloned with the same efficiency as the β-globin RNA, the ratio of scrapie-specific to β-globin-related clones was expected to be at least $1:10^3$. Thirty thousand plaques were screened by *in situ* hybridization with the globin probe; 0.5% of these showed development of the blue colour indicative for an intact β-galactosidase gene and therefore represented clones without an insert. Of the colourless plaques, 99.9% gave a strong signal with a β-globin probe under stringent hybridization conditions; clones giving no clear signal contained either β-globin inserts too short to hybridize, *Eco*RI linkers or inserts derived from the infectious preparation. These clones were picked and 10 inserts of 50 base pairs (bp) to 900 bp were isolated and subcloned into plasmid vectors. Six of these inserts hybridized to a β-globin probe under less stringent conditions. The remaining four may be derived from contaminating nucleic acids such as hamster RNA or DNA from the purified PrP preparation, from traces of fungal or bacterial nucleic acid in enzyme preparations or buffers, or from the conjectured 'scrapie nucleic acid.'

Purified [^{32}P]-labelled inserts were hybridized to Southern blots of hamster genomic DNA. Two inserts of 900 bp and 200 bp, respectively, hybridized to repetitive sequences of the hamster genome. This shows that hamster-derived nucleic acids can be present in highly purified infectious preparations, although they were not detected by conventional methods (K. Gilles, D. Riesner, S.B. Prusiner, personal communication). Such hamster-specific DNA clones probably represent random contamination of the preparation with genomic DNA. However, at least formally, they may be derived from a 'scrapie nucleic acid' related to hamster DNA, just as retroviral DNA may be present integrated into the chromosomal DNA of a normal mouse.

If the putative 'scrapie' nucleic acid was cloned with the same efficiency as the control globin RNA, several related clones should be present in our cDNA library, while the probability that a random contaminant, even a fragment of middle repetitive hamster DNA, would be represented more than once is negligible. We are therefore monitoring the non-globin inserts isolated so far by hybridizing them to the cDNA library, in search of those that light up one or more additional plaques.

In conclusion, to reach a final decision between the two hypotheses formulated above one will have to either show that PrP^C (synthesized *in vitro* or purified from normal tissue) can be converted into infectious PrP^{Sc} *in vitro*, thereby proving the 'protein only' hypothesis, or isolate a scrapie-specific nucleic acid which can give rise to scrapie either by itself or in combination with PrP^{Sc} or some other protein.

References

Alper TA, Haig DA, Clarke MC 1966 The exceptionally small size of the scrapie agent. Biochem Biophys Res Commun 22:278–284

Basler K, Oesch B, Scott M et al 1986 Scrapie and cellular PrP isoforms are encoded by the same chromosomal gene. Cell 46:417–428

Bruce ME, Dickinson AG 1979 Biological stability of different classes of scrapie agent. In: Prusiner SB, Hadlow WJ (eds) Slow transmissible diseases of the nervous system: pathogenesis, immunology, virology & molecular biology of the spongiform encephalopathies, vol 2. Academic Press, New York & London, p 71–86

Bruce ME, Dickinson AG 1987 Biological evidence that scrapie agent has an independent genome. J Gen Virol 68:79–89

Brunori M, Talbot B 1985 A mechanism for prion replication. Nature (Lond) 314:676

Carlson GA, Kingsbury DT, Goodman P et al 1986 Linkage of prion protein and scrapie incubation time genes. Cell 46:503–511

Carp RI, Moretz RC, Natelli M, Dickinson AG 1987 Genetic control of scrapie: incubation period and plaque formation in I mice. J Gen Virol 68:401–407

Chesebro B, Race R, Wehrly K et al 1985 Identification of scrapie prion protein-specific mRNA in scrapie-infected and uninfected brain. Nature (Lond) 315:331–333

Dickinson AG, Fraser H 1979 An assessment of the genetics of scrapie in sheep and mice. In: Prusiner SB, Hadlow WJ (eds) Slow transmissible diseases of the nervous system: Clinical, epidemiological, genetic & pathological aspects of the spongiform encephalopathie, vol 1. Academic Press, New York & London, p 367–385

Dickinson AG, Meikle VMH, Fraser H 1968 Identification of a gene which controls the incubation period of some strains of scrapie agent in mice. J Comp Pathol 78:293–299

Diener TO, McKinley MP, Prusiner SB 1982 Viroids and prions. Proc Natl Acad Sci USA 79:5520–5224

Gibbons RA, Hunter GD 1967 Nature of the scrapie agent. Nature (Lond) 215:1041–1043

Hunter N, Hope J, McConnell I, Dickinson AG 1987 Linkage of the SAF protein (PrP) gene and Sinc using congenic mice and restriction fragment length polymorphism analysis. J Gen Virology 68:2711–2716

Kasper KC, Bowman K, Stites DP, Prusiner SB 1981 Toward development of assays for scrapie-specific antibodies. In: Streilein DA et al (eds) Hamster immune responses in infectious and oncologic diseases. Plenum, New York, p 401–413

Kemp DJ, Coppel RL, Cowman AF, Saint RB, Brown GV, Anders RF 1983 Expression of Plasmodium falciparum blood-stage antigens in Escherichia coli: detection with antibodies from immune humans. Proc Natl Acad Sci USA 80:3787–3791

Kimberlin RH 1982 Reflections on the nature of scrapie agent. Trends Biochem Sci 7:392–394

Kretzschmar HA, Prusiner SB, Stowring LE, DeArmond SJ 1986 Scrapie prion proteins are synthesized in neurons. Am J Pathol 122:1–5

McFarlin DE, Raff MC, Simpson E, Nehlsen S 1971 Scrapie in immunologically deficient mice. Nature (Lond) 233:336

McKinley MP, Bolton DC, Prusiner SB 1983 A protease-resistant protein is a structural component of the scrapie prion. Cell 35:57–62

Oesch B, Westaway D, Wälchli M et al 1985 A cellular gene encodes scrapie PrP 27–30 protein. Cell 40:735–746

Prusiner SB 1982 Novel proteinaceous infectious particles cause scrapie. Science (Wash DC) 216:136–144

Robakis NK, Sawh PR, Wolfe GC, Rubenstein R, Carp RI, Innis MA 1986 Isolation of a cDNA clone encoding the leader peptide of PrP protein and expression of the homologous gene in various tissues. Proc Natl Acad Sci USA 83:6377–6381

Rohwer RG 1984 Scrapie infectious agent is virus-like in size and susceptibility to inactivation. Nature (Lond) 308:658–662

Schnölzer M, Haas B, Ramm K, Hofmann H, Sänger HL 1985 Correlation between structure and pathogenicity of potato spindle tuber viroid (PSTV). EMBO (Eur Mol Biol Organ) J 4:2181–2190

Westaway D, Prusiner SB 1986 Conservation of the cellular gene encoding the scrapie prion protein. Nucl Acids Res 14:2035–2044

DISCUSSION

Almond: How clean is your globin mRNA preparation?

Oesch: It is made in an SP6 transcription system, so there may be some contamination with *E. coli* sequences.

Almond: If you don't cut all your template molecules with restriction endonuclease the polymerase will transcribe further round the plasmid from the globin cDNA.

Oesch: The plasmid used for SP6 transcription contains the same restriction site (EcoRI) twice at the end of the β-globin gene increasing the probability that the plasmids will be cut at least once. In addition, read-through transcripts would be longer than the correct size RNA. I therefore isolated the RNA of the correct size from a gel.

Almond: Another control would be to screen your candidate cDNA clones by hybridization to your plasmid preparation and discard those which are positive.

Manuelidis: When you treated with zinc ions and micrococcal nuclease, what was the infectivity before treatment and after treatment in terms of logs?

Oesch: Within the error of the assay there is no loss in infectivity. The amount of protein recovered after the treatment always relates to the titre, while the amount of nucleic acids present in such purified preparations is decreased at least tenfold by the treatment.

Prusiner: We start with 10^8 infectious units per ml, take 10 ml and concentrate it, and we recover 10^9 infectious units at the end of the experiment.

Manuelidis: When you cloned with random primers, how did you rule out that you weren't cloning DNA? Do you think you have a double-stranded RNA or single-stranded RNA? What do you think the source of your clones is, in terms of nucleic acid?

Oesch: Various forms of nucleic acid may have been cloned by this procedure. After the initial isolation of the nucleic acids the mixture is heated to 100°C probably leaving just single-stranded nucleic acids.

Manuelidis: Is 100°C going to destroy your RNA? (presumably not because you recover the globin RNA). Some double-stranded regions will rapidly snap back and renature after denaturization. Before you do the cDNA synthesis with random primer, what do you do to assure that your RNAs are entirely single stranded?

Oesch: When the primer is added, the mixture is boiled.

Manuelidis: So you could have DNA as the source of your material.

Oesch: By this procedure double-stranded DNA would be cloned.

Almond: But you would not have cloned closed circular double-stranded or closed circular single-stranded nucleic acids.

Oesch: That is the drawback of this method. Double-stranded, covalently closed circular nucleic acid, on denaturation, will probably result in Form IV DNA which probably cannot be cloned.

Almond: Yes; although some molecules might be nicked.

Oesch: If only a small percentage of the molecules are nicked then the scrapie-related clones may be too infrequent to be found. Another form of nucleic acid which may not be cloned is double-stranded RNA which may have a melting point above 100°C.

Almond: There are also small nucleic acid molecules, such as 2-5 A, which cannot be reverse transcribed.

Oesch: Branched RNA cannot be reverse transcribed, so a highly branched RNA will not be cloned either.

Almond: It depends how highly branched, you could prime beyond the branch point using your random primer approach.

Oesch: I have to do a size selection in order to separate the linker. I chose a cut off size of about 50 nucleotides, so everything smaller than that is not cloned.

Almond: You could use a homopolymer tail rather than a linker.

Oesch: With homopolymer tails there is the problem of sizing the insert. If you have a homopolymer tail of 20 nucleotides on each side, 40 nucleotides of the insert is useless and you would probably have to sequence in order to determine the size of the heteropolymeric sequence of a clone.

Diringer: In your experiment you started with 10^8 infectious units, how many brains did these come from?

Prusiner: In a typical preparation we start with a 1000 brains which is about 10^{12} infectious units. So 10^8 infectious units represents one-tenth of a brain, assuming 100% efficiency.

Diringer: When you said you couldn't find any nucleic acid by conventional methods, how sensitive is your test? How many milligrams of brain would you have to take to detect about 1 ng of nucleic acid?

Oesch: Using reverse transcriptase and measuring the incorporation we got down to about 100 pg, but if you calculate one nucleic acid of approximately 100000 daltons per infectious unit you get an estimate of 10 pg, therefore we did not get down to the sensitivity at which we can say that there is definitely no nucleic acid.

Diringer: But you would say that there was less than 1 ng per brain?

Oesch: In this purified preparation there is certainly less than 1 ng per 10^8 ID_{50}, which correspond to 10% of the total amount of infectivity in a brain.

Diringer: If you look at such a fraction by electron microscopy do you see anything?

Oesch: We haven't done electron microscopy in Zürich.

Merz: There is a point at which electron microscopy is very useful and it is usually between something biologically detected and a direct biochemical assay as has been observed with SAF from scrapie-infected sheep (Rubenstein et al 1987). In the visualization of nucleic acids by the Kleinschmidt procedure or the diffusion method, the diluted nucleic acids are concentrated into the protein film (cytochrome C). Thus a large sample volume with a very low concentration of nucleic acid can be concentrated on this protein film for visualization. Samples as low as 2×10^{-2} ng nucleic acid in a single drop can be micro-diffused into the protein film and detected by electron microscopy (Evenson 1977).

Oesch: In the preparations not purified by micrococcal nuclease and zinc there are lots of nucleic acids. Before treatment we found nanogram amounts in a sample of 10^8 infectious units.

Prusiner: You can visualize the nucleic acids which contaminate our purified prion preparations by decoration with gene 32 protein for RNA and rec A protein for the DNA; these nucleic acids disappear when the sample is treated with micrococcal nuclease and zinc ions.

Almond: One can normally label DNA with ^{32}P to a specific activity of about 10^9 c.p.m. per microgram. If you assume that the incorporation of say 200 c.p.m. is evidence of positive reverse transcription, then you should be able to detect less than a picogram of nucleic acid, e.g. 10^6 molecules of a sequence 100 bases in length. So even if you have only 10^6 molecules in your 10^8 infectious units (and of course there should be at least 10^8) and the reverse transcription is efficient, you would be able to detect that nucleic acid by reverse transcription alone.

Oesch: The efficiency of reverse transcription varies with the preparation of RNA, it is seldom better than 20 or 30% and using random primers, the efficiency is even lower. We are dealing with very small amounts of nucleic acid. We were afraid that we would lose it so we added a carrier nucleic acid, for example poly A, then reverse transcribed in the presence of radioactively labelled dCTP. We could never convincingly detect less than 100 pg. We then dropped this approach and said let's clone it.

Almond: You were afraid of losing it at what stage, the precipitation stage?

Oesch: 10^8 infectious units is associated with a large amount of protein. To remove that and liberate the scrapie nucleic acid you have to protease digest, phenol extract and ethanol precipitate, which is the critical step.

Almond: There are other ways of concentrating, for example, reduce the volume with butanol.

Oesch: It's difficult to eliminate salts and buffers after using methods which reduce the volume.

Merz: Did you ever monitor protein loss at the different stages of your procedure?

Gabizon: Kay Gilles used to do that, the PrP is destroyed by the procedure Bruno is using; we can show by silver staining and Western blotting that nothing is left.

Dickinson: Do you think that the array of surviving nucleic acids are different after the micrococcal nuclease and zinc ion treatments from those in the original preparation or are they representative of your starting material?

Chesebro: To find out whether there is specific protection of certain sequences you could make a library from the DNA before and after micrococcal nuclease digestion and ask whether the frequency of clones in those two libraries is different.

Oesch: It should not be necessary to make a library before nuclease treatment. I do not expect randomly surviving nucleic acids to be present more than once in the library after nuclease treatment, while scrapie-related clones should be found several times.

Almond: You can't do that because you are making a cDNA and you don't know the abundance of the messenger RNA in the brain tissue.

Oesch: The RNA should be destroyed by the zinc ion treatment. That may be reflected by the clones corresponding to repetitive sequences.

Dickinson: But that assumes that nuclease and the zinc would destroy all nucleic acids, it does not allow for some sequences being specifically protected.

Prusiner: The infectivity titres of the preparations are measured after the zinc and the nuclease treatments. We are worried about what then happens to the residual nucleic acid, some molecule of which is the putative scrapie-specific nucleic acid that we are trying to find. It seems to me that our method is satisfactory because we are using the 10^8 infectious units as a denominator throughout.

Dickinson: The logic of my question is that Bruno is looking for a needle in a haystack. If you can get a lead on what that needle is going to be like from the restrictions imposed by the prior treatment, you can focus your search. So, is the nucleic acid that survives treatment a representative sample of the starting material or is there something special about it?

Prusiner: The infectivity does not change, therefore I would argue that it is representative. We are not looking at 0.01% but at nearly 100% of the infectivity with which we start.

Dickinson: That is infectivity; the point I am making is that one could be pointed towards the type of sequences involved in the scrapie genome by the peculiarities of sequences of non-scrapie related molecules which are able to survive these treatments.

Prusiner: We are looking for molecules needed for infectivity, that's our only assay for scrapie.

Chesebro: If you take clone No.1, that you think is the putative scrapie clone, you screen these two libraries and the frequency of this clone is very low in the before-treatment-with-nuclease library but noticeably higher in the library made after treatment with micrococcal nuclease that would suggest that that sequence is being selectively protected from nuclease, which would be supporting evidence for its relevance. Whereas if the frequency is the same in the two populations then these clones are just random surviving molecules.

Almond: But you should see your sequence reasonably frequently in the first library because it's a reasonably clean preparation containing a putative 10^8 infectious molecules.

Oesch: A sequence that is randomly still present after treatment, you wouldn't expect to occur more than once in that library. I start with a random distribution of hamster genomic DNA. This nucleic acid is digested and some sequences remain. Now I make the cDNA library. If the average size of my cloned inserts is 1000 nucleotides and the genome size is 10^9 base pairs, and if every individual clone is different, you need 10^6 clones in order to have each sequence. Statistically you would need more than 10 million clones for a 99% probability that each sequence is represented once in such a library. The number of clones in the library will therefore determine whether I find a given sequence more than once. By looking at 100 non-globin clones in my library it is very unlikely that any random sequence will be present more than once. In these 100 non-globin clones I expect at least 10 scrapie-related clones as judged from the cloning efficiency of the globin RNA; that's far more frequent than any random sequence can be present unless it is specifically protected. If there were hamster sequences that were specifically protected this would be interesting.

Almond: There is also the problem of repetitive DNA.

Manuelidis: But you have negative clones that are not globin and not repetitive sequences. Those would be the presumptive clones that have the nucleic acid of scrapie.

Oesch: I wouldn't draw that conclusion. To be able to say anything definite I need a positive identification and that would be hybridization of a candidate clone either to nucleic acids isolated from the infectious preparations or to the library. If you find a frequency of one copy of the corresponding nucleic acid per infectious unit, you have identified a nucleic acid which co-purifies with infectivity. However, there are technical problems with the sensitivity of the hybridization. It is much easier to screen the library, which transforms the problem of the intensity of the signal into the question of: how frequent is a given sequence in the library. For a scrapie-related sequence, I would expect it to be present more than once.

Carlson: Assuming that Alan Dickinson is correct and there is a nucleic acid protected by a host protein, the question is whether the experiment described by Bruno Oesch is a reasonable strategy to identify a scrapie-specific nucleic acid. I think most people here agree that this is a perfectly reasonable approach to identify such a nucleic acid.

Almond: I think this is a very clever, excellent way of approaching it; our discussion is centred on the fact that it is very difficult to control.

Diringer: There must have been a nucleic acid there because you cloned it!

Oesch: No, there could be contaminating nucleic acids in the restriction enzymes.

Diringer: So you think that there was nucleic acid in your starting material.

Chesebro: There were some hamster repetitive sequences.

Almond: What is it reasonable to expect in terms of number of molecules? How many molecules of prion protein are you estimating that there are per infectious unit?

Prusiner: 10000 to ten million per infectious unit.

Almond: In polio there are 240 protein molecules per RNA molecule. The particle:infectivity ratio can often be around 1000, in which case there would be 240000 protein molecules per infectious unit, so you are in the right ball park.

Merz: We calculated the particle ratio if SAF were the infectious agent (which is open to debate), to be 10^3 SAF molecules per infectious unit, which is reasonable for viral particles.

Diringer: We tried something similar. We isolated about 10^7 infectious units per brain. By chemical measurement there is less than 1 ng of nucleic acid per brain in this fraction (we see almost no protein any more by silver staining of gels). Nevertheless, by electron microscopy we can still see nucleic acid. With tissue from normal brain the result is the same: we find less than 1 ng of nucleic acid but by electron microscopy we still find different kinds of nucleic acids. The problem is to find a virus-specific nucleic acid.

Almond: In quite a lot of virus infections there are occasional cellular sequences, often RNAs, wrapped up in virus coat proteins. For example, influenza viruses contain host ribosomal RNAs in appreciable quantities, which can be detected by hybridization to a cDNA derived from ribosomal RNA. Has anyone looked at a scrapie preparation which has been through your micrococcal nuclease treatment by hybridization to a cDNA from a well-expressed RNA, such as tubulin, or actin mRNA or ribosomal RNA?

Diringer: If you do this, you select for a certain type of nucleic acid. If you don't select at all, if you just analyse by chemical means the nucleic acid content in a preparation from, for example, ten hamster brains, from such analysis one can calculate that less than one nanogram of nucleic acid per brain is present in the preparation. By electron microscopy you still find it.

Almond: But is it in sufficient amounts to account for it being part of the infectivity?

Diringer: You can't quantitate it by electron microscopy. If you measure the size to see whether by that criterion the nucleic acid could be infectious, then you find that it could be.

Bolton: Bruno, are you planning to repeat this with 10^{10} or 10^{11} infectious units? Have you tried 10^8 ID_{50} or even 10^8 particles of poliovirus and run this through the same procedure?

Oesch: That is what I am planning–to use different forms of nucleic acid such as single-stranded RNA, double-stranded RNA, double-stranded DNA or single-stranded DNA, or circular DNA as small as we can get it. We will use 10^9 infectious units, mix in 10^8 molecules of each form of nucleic acid and then run the whole mixture through the cloning procedure. Then we can show by hybridization that in this library we have cloned these different forms of nucleic acids. If a scrapie-specific nucleic acid consisted of one of these types of nucleic acid, it should be cloned with the same efficiency and therefore be ten times more frequent in the library. If we do not find any scrapie-related sequences, we can then conclude that the 'scrapie nucleic acid' is not of the type of nucleic acid we have included in the experiment.

Almond: You would also need to put in a digestion step to open up any circles.

Oesch: I can devise various strategies for what to clone and how. The optimal strategy for cloning one type of nucleic acid may conflict with strategies for other types of nucleic acid. The strategy I described here was judged by us to be the most universal. Adding a step like S1 nuclease treatment will be unfavourable for linear single-stranded RNA or DNA. However, we have to keep in mind that we do not cover the cloning of all types of nucleic acids.

Almond: The point is, if the scrapie nucleic acid were such a thing, then you would miss it.

Oesch: I am content to say that under the conditions I used I would have found it and I didn't find it. Cloning all possible forms of nucleic acids will require a major effort and I'm not sure that I would want to do it.

Almond: But the scientific community would be very unhappy if an experiment of this elegance wasn't seen all the way through to the ultimate conclusion.

References

Evenson DP 1977 Electron microscopy of viral nucleic acids. In: Maramorosch K, Koprowski H (eds) Methods in Virology 7:219–264

Rubenstein R, Merz PA, Kascsak RJ, Carp RI, Scalici CF, Fama CL, Wisniewski HM 1987 Detection of scrapie-associated fibrils (SAF) and SAF proteins from scrapie-affected sheep. J Infect Dis 156:36–42

Pathogenesis of amyloid formation in Alzheimer's disease, Down's syndrome and scrapie

Henryk M. Wisniewski and Monika Wrzolek*

New York State Office of Mental Retardation and Developmental Disabilities, Institute for Basic Research in Developmental Disabilities, 1050 Forest Hill Road, Staten Island, NY 10314, USA

Abstract. Paired helical filaments (PHF) are abnormal fibrous structures found in human nerve cells and their processes. Ultrastructural studies of the proto-filaments that make up the PHF revealed that the individual proto-filaments have a different substructure from normal neurofilaments or any other known fibrous profiles. Studies using immunological and biochemical methods suggested that abnormally phosphorylated tau, ubiquitin and neurofilament peptides are part of the PHF.

Deposits of amyloid fibres in Alzheimer's disease and senile dementia of the Alzheimer type (AD/SDAT) are found in meningeal and brain vessels, choroid plexus and neuritic plaques. In 1984 Glenner and Wong reported the sequence of a β-protein isolated from cerebrovascular amyloid. We used the amino acid sequence of the cerebrovascular amyloid protein to synthesize oligonucleotide probes specific for the gene encoding this amyloid protein. Screening of a human brain cDNA library allowed us to isolate a clone which encodes the amyloid peptide. *In situ* hybridization studies and Southern blot analysis of a DNA sample isolated from a human-mouse hybrid cell line indicated that the corresponding genomic sequences of this cDNA clone are located on human chromosome 21. Using immunochemical and histochemical methods, we have identified the cells associated with the formation of the amyloid fibres. With immunochemical and biochemical methods we and others also showed that the protein constituting amyloid in AD/SDAT is different from amyloid in unconventional slow virus diseases.

1988 Novel infectious agents and the central nervous system. Wiley, Chichester (Ciba Foundation Symposium 135) p 224–238

Amyloidosis is a generic term encompassing a wide variety of pathological conditions in which fibrillar proteinaceous deposits called amyloid are laid down in different organs (Glenner 1980). These deposits, when stained by thioflavine-S and examined by fluorescence microscopy, show characteristic yellow-green-green fluorescence (Schwartz 1970). When stained by Congo

* Visiting Scientist from the Department of Pathology, Medical School, Gdansk, Poland

red, amyloid deposits show green birefringence under polarized light. Examination by electron microscopy shows that the amyloid deposits are made of distinct pathological fibres. There is a wide range of host proteins which can form amyloid fibres. Only some of them, for example, an immunoglobulin light chain, an acute phase serum protein, some polypeptide hormones and a prealbumin variant, have been identified. It is now well recognized that the uniform structure and tinctorial properties of amyloid fibres laid down in different tissues in many and unrelated diseases and composed of distinct proteins, result from a unique arrangement of polypeptide chains, the so-called β-pleated sheet conformation (Glenner 1981).

As data were accumulated on the primary structure of proteins in amyloid deposits, it became apparent that the peptides forming amyloid fibres are products of proteolytic cleavage of larger precursor proteins. These proteins, which can form amyloid fibres when cleaved enzymically or altered by other physicochemical means, are designated 'amyloidogenic' (Glenner 1980). In normal ageing, Alzheimer's disease/senile dementia of the Alzheimer type (AD/SDAT), Down's syndrome and unconventional slow virus diseases, there are three types of fibres exhibiting amyloid properties: (1) paired helical filaments (PHF), (2) plaque and vascular amyloid fibres, and (3) scrapie-associated fibrils (Wisniewski et al 1986).

Paired helical filaments

These are found only in pathological conditions in human nerve cells. Analysis of their distribution within the nerve cell body and the nerve processes showed that PHF occur in greater concentrations in the perikaryon area and in the axon terminals which are part of the classical or primitive plaque. PHF are more common in unmyelinated nerve cell processes than in myelinated ones. Not all human nerve cells produce PHF: they were never seen in cerebellar cortex, spinal cord or dorsal root ganglion. Recently, they were observed in superior cervical ganglion. Whether produced *in vitro* or found in animals or insects, PHF are structurally different from those described in humans (Wisniewski et al 1981).

Ultrastructural analysis of the PHF showed that the individual protofilaments of PHF have a substructure different from that of normal neurofilaments or any other published fibrous profiles. Structural and biochemical studies of PHF showed differences in their morphology (there are left-handed and right-handed PHF) and biochemistry, some PHF are readily soluble, others are difficult to dissolve (Wisniewski & Wen 1985, Wisniewski et al 1987a). Recent studies using immunological and biochemical methods showed the following proteins to be present in neurofibrillary tangles: abnormally phosphorylated tau, ubiquitin, and neurofilaments (Sternberger et al 1985, Grundke-Iqbal et al 1986, Mori et al 1987, Selkoe 1987). We also found a novel protein in PHF whose origin and peptide composition are currently being studied.

The presence of abnormally phosphorylated tau suggests that phosphorylation of tau might be a factor in the formation of PHF. Such a defect in AD/SDAT might be caused by an imbalance of the protein kinase-phosphatase system, involving either an increase of a certain protein kinase activity or a reduction in the level of phosphatase activity that would normally control phosphorylation. Protein phosphorylation is believed to be one of the major mechanisms for regulation of cellular function. Tau is a phosphoprotein (Selden & Pollard 1983). It was discovered and is best known for promoting the *in vitro* assembly of microtubules (Weingarten et al 1975). The interaction of tau with other brain proteins appears to be regulated by phosphorylation. The *in vitro* phosphorylation of tau has been reported to inhibit both the polymerization of tubulin (Lindwall & Cole 1984) and the interaction of microtubules with actin filaments (Selden & Pollard 1983). Furthermore, preliminary results suggest that there is a defect in microtubule assembly in AD/SDAT (Iqbal et al 1987). The abnormal phosphorylation of tau observed in AD/SDAT brain might depress its normal interaction with other brain proteins and could also lead to the assembly of tau, either alone or with other neuronal components, into PHF.

Earlier immunohistological studies implicated phosphorylated neurofilament epitopes as constituents of PHF (Anderton et al 1982, Perry et al 1985). However, recent studies revealed that all of the antibodies which label both phosphorylated neurofilaments and PHF cross-react with phosphorylated forms of tau protein. Thus, neurofilament antibodies that label PHF appear to recognize phosphorylation sites on tau that have conformational or sequence similarities to those of neurofilaments. In the light of the above observations, evidence for the contribution of neurofilament proteins to PHF must be re-examined (Selkoe 1987).

Recently, Mori et al (1987) identified ubiquitin as a component of PHF. Ubiquitin is a protein involved in ATP-dependent breakdown of abnormal or short-lived intracellular proteins. The target(s) of ubiquitin in PHF is unknown; however, it is possible that phosphorylated forms of tau in PHF are ubiquinated. The reason for the failure of degradation of PHF in spite of ubiquitination is not clear, although there is a good chance that a defective, possibly ATP-dependent, protease is responsible for the progressive formation and accumulation of PHF. In 1970 Johnson and Blum reported ATPase activities associated with the PHF tangles. Presumably, the cytochemical reaction for ATPases that they observed in tangles results from the ATP-dependent protease activity discussed by Mori et al (1987).

Plaques and vascular amyloid

In contrast to PHF which are formed intracellularly, the amyloid fibres in the plaques and vessels are mainly formed extracellularly. As opposed to the PHF, which are seen only in neurons and their processes, amyloid fibres in plaques and vessels are associated with a variety of brain mesodermal cells. Also in contrast to PHF, which are found in many and unrelated diseases, plaques are seen only in normal old people and animals (few), cases of AD (many), patients with Down's syndrome after the age of 40 (many), and unconventional virus infections (not in all cases and in varying numbers) both in humans and animals. Depending on the proportion of amyloid and cellular components, and the assumed temporal sequence of plaque development, the following forms of neuritic plaques are recognized (Wisniewski & Terry 1973, Wisniewski & Merz 1985): (1) a primitive, immature plaque composed of wisps of amyloid among normal, dystrophic degenerating and regenerating neuronal and fibrous astrocytic processes; (2) a classical, typical or mature plaque consisting of a central core of amyloid surrounded by a rim of neuronal and astrocytic processes as seen in primitive plaques. Since the central core of amyloid deposits varies in size depending on the thickness of the section prepared for microscopy, a plaque which appears as primitive, cut serially, may turn out to be a classical plaque. The third type of plaque, also called amyloid or 'burned out' plaque, is made up almost exclusively of amyloid deposits. AD/SDAT plaques are rich in neuritic components. The neuritic component is not prominent in plaques associated with unconventional virus infections. At this point we would like to recall that in AD/SDAT many neurites which form the corona round the central core of amyloid in the classical plaques, as well as the neurites associated with immature plaques, contain many PHF. In aged animals and unconventional virus infections, the nerve cell bodies and their processes do not make PHF; therefore, the plaque neurites do not have PHF. An exception to this rule may be old people with cortical plaques who also have Gerstmann-Sträussler syndrome or Creutzfeldt-Jakob disease.

There is an extensive literature concerning the sequence of events leading to the formation of neuritic plaques. According to one hypothesis, the first change leading to plaque formation is the deposition of amyloid fibres. A second hypothesis states that pathological changes in other brain components, blood vessels, nerve cells and/or their terminals and glial cells are responsible for the initiation of plaque formation. Studies of the pattern of degeneration of cortical terminals undergoing Wallerian degeneration due to undercutting or spindle inhibitor-induced terminal pathology, revealed that none of these changes lead to amyloid deposition or plaque formation (Wisniewski & Terry 1970, Ghetti & Wisniewski 1972). Also, in studies of infantile neuroaxonal dystrophy in humans, in which there are many dystrophic neurites in the cortex, amyloid deposits have not been observed as a response to the degeneration of neurites (Seitelberger 1971, Jellinger 1973, Wisniewski & Merz 1985). On the basis of these results we postulated that the primary aetiological and pathogenic events are associated with brain amyloidogenesis, and that the neuritic abnormalities are a secondary phenomenon. It should be stressed that in the brain cortex amyloid deposits generate an extensive reaction in the neuropil, giving rise to primitive and classical plaques. In the cerebellar cortex the reaction to amyloid deposits is poor. Therefore, the most common plaque in the cerebellum is the amyloid plaque.

By light and electron microscopy, the plaques in normal old people, people with AD and Down's syndrome look alike. However, lectin-binding studies (Szumanska et al 1987) showed a higher content of monosaccharide residues in the amyloid cores of Down's syndrome plaques than in cores of other plaques. These differences are quantitative and may be due to a gene dosage effect of the extra chromosome 21.

Biochemical and immunohistological studies showed that the amyloids in AD, Down's syndrome, normal old people and animals are similar. However, the protein making the amyloid fibres in the conditions listed above is very different from the amyloidogenic protein and amyloid fibres found in human and animal diseases caused by unconventional virus infections.

Recently, the genes encoding the amyloid proteins in unconventional virus infections and Alzheimer's disease were found (Oesch et al 1985, Robakis et al 1986, 1987a,b, Goldgaber et al 1987, Kang et al 1987). Both are host genes. In unconventional virus infections the product is a protease-resistant 33–35 kDa protein, PrP (Bolton et al 1982). In AD the product is an approximately 70 kDa protein. Its cleavage product, termed the β-peptide, Glenner protein, or A4 peptide, forms amyloid fibres. The role of PrP and the β-peptide precursor protein in normal brain function remains to be determined. Using human-rodent somatic cell hybrids it was found that the β-peptide gene is located on chromosome 21 (Robakis et al 1987a, St George-Hyslop et al 1987). This observation may partially explain why in people with Down's syndrome, aged 40 and above, the Alzheimer neuropathology is present in almost all cases (Wisniewski & Rabe 1986). Two DNA markers designated D21S1/D21S11 on the long arm of chromosome 21 showed close linkage with the β-protein gene (Tanzi et al 1987). The same DNA markers showed linkage to the gene responsible for some cases of autosomal dominant forms of AD (St George-Hyslop et al 1987). We and others (Bobin et al 1987) were unable to confirm the observations (see Masters & Beyreuther, this volume) that PHF shares a common peptide with vascular and plaque amyloid. In our recent studies on the dynamics of plaque and tangle formation in people with Down's syndrome we found that neuritic (senile) plaques in their brains occur much earlier than neurofibrillary tangles (Wisniewski et al 1987b,c). This result, and the fact that PHF may develop independently of plaques in other diseases, in our opinion supports the notion that the amyloid plaque protein and PHF proteins are different. The temporal primacy of plaques in Down's syndrome suggests the possibility of a gene dosage effect on plaque formation in these patients. There are unconfirmed reports on amyloid protein gene duplication in both familial and sporadic cases of AD (Delabar et al 1987). At this time, the cellular origin of the β-protein forming the plaque and vascular amyloid in AD, as well as the PrP protein in unconventional virus infections, is unknown. The mRNAs encoding the precursor proteins for AD and scrapie amyloids were found in neurons and non-neuronal cells in the brain, as well as in tissues of peripheral organs (Bahmanyar et al 1987). Therefore, we cannot exclude the possibility that transport of βpPP from the blood vessels contributes to the formation of plaque and vascular amyloid in AD/SDAT. However, the fact that in the areas around tumours and vascular lesions where the blood-brain barrier is changed one does not see increased deposits of amyloid, indicates that local production of amyloidogenic protein and the inability of the local processor cells to degrade this protein may be of critical importance in the pathogenesis of brain amyloid.

We have separated and quantified the core and vascular amyloid peptides. We have shown that the major peptide possesses a similar amino acid composition to that of the cerebrovascular amyloid peptide (CVAP) as determined by Glenner and Wong (1984) (Wisniewski & Miller 1986, Wisniewski et al 1987d). Furthermore, we were able to isolate and sequence a 12-residue tryptic peptide from the core amyloid protein that is identical to a peptide from CVAP, which suggests that both amyloid proteins are derived from the same precursor. Nevertheless, several observations lead us to believe that the core amyloid peptide differs in three important respects from CVAP. Firstly, the core amyloid peptide is not amenable to direct N-terminal sequencing; we conclude that its amino terminus is blocked. Secondly, it is distinctly larger than the 4000 Da reported for CVAP peptide. Thirdly, antibodies raised against synthetic CVAP react much more extensively with CVAP than with the core amyloid protein (Bobin et al 1987). We believe that these differences between CVAP and the core amyloid peptide reflect different routes of processing before the peptides are deposited.

At this point we would like to recall that, according to the current concepts based on studies of systemic amyloidosis, the formation of amyloid fibres is a two-step process involving the *production* of amyloidogenic protein, which is further *processed* either locally or at distant sites to yield amyloid fibres. This concept is supported by the observation that in a majority of amyloidoses one type of cell produces the amyloidogenic proteins, e.g., hepatocytes in secondary amyloidosis or B cells in multiple myeloma, and different cells (the reticulo-endothelial cells) process the protein. From these data a unifying concept of the amyloidosis has emerged. It was postulated that proteolytic cleavage of the precursor amyloidogenic proteins leads to the formation of peptides, which assume the β-pleated conformation and fibrillar structure characteristic of amyloid. According to this hypothesis, the actual deposition of the amyloid fibres results from an *imbalance* between the production of the precursor protein and the ability to degrade it completely. This imbalance could be a result of a gene dosage effect as in Down's syndrome, or overproduction of the amyloidogenic proteins resulting from antigenic stimulation, for example in experimental casein-induced or endotoxin-induced amyloidosis, or during chronic infections. It could also be due to gene mutation, as in some cases of familial amyloid polyneuropathy. Another possibility is that as a result of age-associated changes or gene mutation the amyloidogenic protein processor cells lose their ability to degrade correctly the amyloidogenic proteins.

In our Institute, we have identified the cells which are associated with the formation of the amyloid fibres (the amyloidogenic protein processor cells) (Wisniewski et al 1982, Merz et al 1987). These cells appear to be pericytes, microglia and as yet poorly defined cells in the walls of the large and medium size vessels. Irrespective of whether the brain reticulo-endothelial cells (pericytes, microglia) are both producer and processor cells or only processor cells, the pathogenic events in plaque and vascular amyloid formation in AD/SDAT and unconventional virus infections appear to be similar to those observed in the systemic amyloidoses.

As indicated above, the intimate structural relationship between the amyloid fibres and the microglia-like cells suggests that these cells produce the amyloid fibres. Labelling of these cell surfaces and adjacent amyloid fibres with the same lectins (Vorbrodt et al 1987) raises the possibility that glycosylation of the amyloid fibres occurs extracellularly. The major breakthrough in our understanding of the systemic amyloidoses resulted from the recognition of their chemical identity. With the availability of the Alzheimer amyloid protein gene we can expect much greater progress in understanding the sequence of events leading to brain and mind destruction in AD.

Acknowledgements

The authors wish to thank Marjorie Agoglia for editorial and secretarial assistance. Supported in part by Grant No AGO-4220 from the National Institute on Aging, NIH.

References

Anderton BH, Breinburg D, Downes MJ et al 1982 Monoclonal antibodies show that neurofibrillary tangles and neurofilaments share antigenic determinants. Nature (Lond) 298:84–86

Bahmanyar S, Higgins GA, Goldgaber D et al 1987 Localization of amyloid β protein messenger RNA in brains from patients with Alzheimer's disease. Science (Wash DC) 237:77–80

Bobin SA, Currie JR, Merz PA et al 1987 The comparative immunoreactivities of brain amyloids in Alzheimer's disease and scrapie. Acta Neuropathol 74:313–323

Bolton DC, McKinley MP, Prusiner SB 1982 Identification of a protein that purifies with the scrapie prion. Science (Wash DC) 218:1309–1311

Delabar JM, Goldgaber D, Lamour Y et al 1987 β amyloid gene duplication in Alzheimer's disease and karyotypically normal Down syndrome. Science (Wash DC) 235:1390–1392

Ghetti B, Wisniewski HM 1972 On degeneration of terminals in the cat striate cortex. Brain Res 44:630–635

Glenner GG 1981 The bases of the staining of amyloid fibers: Their physico-chemical nature and the mechanism of their dye-substrate interaction. Prog Histochem Cytochem 13:1–37

Glenner GG 1980 Amyloid deposits and amyloidosis. New Eng J Med 302:1283–1292; 1333–1343

Glenner GG, Wong CW 1984 Alzheimer's disease: initial report of the purification and characterization of a novel cerebrovascular amyloid protein. Biochem Biophys Res Commun 120:885–890

Goldgaber D, Lerman MI, McBride OW, Saffiotti U, Gajdusek DC 1987 Characterization and chromosomal localization of a cDNA encoding brain amyloid of Alzheimer's disease. Science (Wash DC) 235:877–880

Grundke-Iqbal I, Iqbal K, Tung Y-C, Quinlan M, Wisniewski HM, Binder LI 1986 Abnormal phosphorylation of the microtubule-associated protein (tau) in Alzheimer cytoskeletal pathology. Proc Natl Acad Sci (USA) 83:4913–4917

Iqbal K, Grundke-Iqbal I, Wisniewski HM 1987 Alzheimer's disease, microtubule and neurofilament proteins, and axoplasmic flow. Lancet 1:102

Jellinger K 1973 Neuroaxonal dystrophy: Its natural history and related disorders. In: Zimmerman HM (ed) Progress in Neuropathology. Grune & Stratton, New York vol 2 p 129–180

Johnson AB, Blum NR 1970 Nucleoside phosphatase activities associated with the tangles and plaques of Alzheimer's disease: a histochemical study of natural and experimental neurofibrillary tangles. J Neuropathol & Exp Neurol 29:463–478

Kang J, Lemaire H-G, Unterbeck A et al 1987 The precursor of Alzheimer's disease amyloid A4 protein resembles a cell-surface receptor. Nature (Lond) 325:733–736

Lindwall G, Cole RD 1984 Phosphorylation affects the ability of tau protein to promote microtubule assembly. J Biol Chem 259:5301–5305

Masters CL, Beyreuther K 1988 Neuropathology of unconventional virus infections: molecular pathology of spongiform change and amyloid plaque deposition. In: Novel infectious agents and the central nervous system. Wiley, Chichester (Ciba Found Symp 135) p 24–36

Merz GS, Schwenk V, Schuller-Levis G, Gruca S, Wisniewski HM 1987 Isolation and characterization of macrophages from scrapie-infected mouse brain. Acta Neuropathol 72:240–247

Mori H, Kondo J, Ihara Y 1987 Ubiquitin is a component of paired helical filaments in Alzheimer's disease. Science (Wash DC) 235:1641–1644

Oesch B, Westaway D, Wälchli et al 1985 A cellular gene encodes scrapie PrP 27–30 protein. Cell 40:735–746

Perry G, Rizzuto N, Autilio-Gambetti L, Gambetti P 1985 Paired helical filaments from Alzheimer disease patients contain cytoskeletal components. Proc Natl Acad Sci (USA) 82:3916–3920

Robakis NK, Sawh PR, Wolfe GC, Rubenstein R, Carp RI, Innis MA 1986 Isolation of a cDNA clone encoding the leader peptide of prion protein and expression of the homologous gene in various tissues. Proc Natl Acad Sci (USA) 83:6477–6381

Robakis NK, Wisniewski HM, Jenkins EC et al 1987a Chromosome 21q21 sublocalisation of gene encoding beta-amyloid peptide in cerebral vessels and neuritic (senile) plaques of people with Alzheimer disease and Down syndrome. Lancet 1:384–385

Robakis NK, Ramikrishna N, Wolfe G, Wisniewski HM 1987b Molecular cloning and characterization of a cDNA encoding the cerebrovascular and the neuritic plaque amyloid peptides. Proc Natl Acad Sci (USA) 84:4190–4194

Schwartz P 1970 Amyloidosis: cause and manifestations of senile deterioration. Thomas, Springfield, Ill

Seitelberger F 1971 Neuropathological conditions related to neuroaxonal dystrophy Acta Neuropathol (suppl V) 17–29

Selden SC, Pollard TD 1983 Phosphorylation of microtubule-associated proteins regulates their interaction with actin filaments. J Biol Chem 258:7064–7071

Selkoe, DJ 1987 Deciphering Alzheimer's disease: the pace quickens. Trends Neurosci 10:181–184

St George-Hyslop PH, Tanzi RE, Polinsky RJ et al 1987 The genetic defect causing familial Alzheimer's disease maps on chromosome 21. Science (Wash DC) 235:885–890

Sternberger NH, Sternberger LA, Ulrich J 1985 Aberrant neurofilament phosphorylation in Alzheimer disease. Proc Natl Acad Sci (USA) 82:4274–4276

Szumanska G, Vorbrodt AW, Mandybur TI, Wisniewski HM 1987 Lectin histochemistry of plaques and tangles in Alzheimer's disease. Acta Neuropathol 73:1–11

Tanzi RE, Gusella JF, Watkins PC et al 1987 Amyloid β protein gene: cDNA, mRNA distribution, and genetic linkage near the Alzheimer locus. Science (Wash DC) 235:880–884

Vorbrodt AW, Dobrogowska DH, Kim YS, Lossinsky AS, Wisniewski HM 1987 Ultrastructural studies of glycoconjugates in brain micro-blood vessels and amyloid plaques of scrapie-infected mice. Acta Neuropathol, in press

Weingarten MD, Lockwood AH, Hwo S-Y, Kirschner MW 1975 A protein factor essential for microtubule assembly. Proc Natl Acad Sci (USA) 72:1858–1862

Wisniewski HM, Merz GS 1985 Neuropathology of the aging brain and dementia of the Alzheimer type. In: Gaitz CM et al (eds) Aging 2000: our health care destiny. Springer-Verlag, New York, p 231–243

Wisniewski HM, Miller DL 1986 Morphology and biochemistry of abnormal fibrous proteins in Alzheimer's disease and senile dementia of the Alzheimer type (AD/SDAT). Neurobiol Aging 7:446–447

Wisniewski HM, Rabe A 1986 Discrepancy between Alzheimer-type neuropathology and dementia in persons with Down's syndrome. In: Wisniewski HM, Snider DA (eds) Mental Retardation: research, education, and technology. The New York Academy of Sciences, New York, Annals New York Acad Sci 477:247–260

Wisniewski HM, Terry RD 1970 An experimental approach to the morphogenesis of neurofibrillary degeneration and the argyrophilic plaque. In: Alzheimer's Disease and Related Conditions, Churchill, London (Ciba Found Symp) p 223–248

Wisniewski HM, Terry RD 1973 Reexamination of the pathogenesis of the senile plaque. Prog Neuropathol 2:1–26

Wisniewski HM, Wen GY 1985 Substructures of paired helical filaments from Alzheimer's disease neurofibrillary tangles. Acta Neuropathol 66:173–176

Wisniewski HM, Sinatra RS, Iqbal K, Grundke-Iqbal I 1981 Neurofibrillary and synaptic pathology in the aged brain. In: Johnson Jr JE (ed) Aging and Cell Structure. Plenum Publishing Corp, New York, p 105–142

Wisniewski HM, Vorbrodt AW, Moretz RC, Lossinsky AS, Grundke-Iqbal I 1982 Pathogenesis of neuritic (senile) and amyloid plaque formation. In: Hoyer S (ed) The Aging Brain — physiological and pathophysiological aspects experimental research (suppl 5) Springer-Verlag, Berlin-Heidelberg-New York, p 3–9

Wisniewski HM, Iqbal K, Grundke-Iqbal I et al 1986 Amyloid in Alzheimer's disease and unconventional viral infections. In: International Symposium on Dementia and Amyloid. The Japanese Society of Neuropathology. Neuropathology Suppl 3, p 87–94

Wisniewski HM, Iqbal K, Grundke-Iqbal I, Rubenstein R 1987a The solubility controversy of paired helical filaments: A commentary. Neurochem Res 12:93–95
Wisniewski HM, Rabe A, Wisniewski KE 1987b Neuropathology and dementia in
people with Down syndrome. In: Neurochemistry of Aging. Cold Spring Harbor
Laboratory, Banbury Report, in press
Wisniewski HM, Rabe A, Wen GY, Wisniewski KE 1987c Gene dose effect on early
formation of neuritic plaques in Down syndrome (DS). J Neuropath & Exp Neurol
46:334 (Abstr)
Wisniewski HM, Wen GY, Grundke-Iqbal I et al 1987d Pathological, biochemical, and
genetic aspects of Alzheimer's disease in aged people and Down syndrome. In:
Machleidt H (ed) Contributions of Chemistry to Health (Proc 5th Chemrawn Conf,
Heidelberg, 1986) p 297–315

DISCUSSION

Dormont: Do you have any information about the A4 mRNA in the brain of normal patients?

Masters: The mRNA for the A4 precursor protein is present in many different areas of the normal brain. The highest concentration is in the cortex and the basal nuclei; low amounts are found in the caudate, thalamus and in the cerebellum.

Almond: Have you looked by *in situ* hybridization?

Masters: Northern blot analysis shows this distribution in the human brain. *In situ* hybridizations have also been performed on rodent brain, which again shows a regional distribution within different areas of the brain. Using antibodies to the precursor, immunoreactive cells are seen as stellate interneurons located in different laminae of the cerebral cortex and in the basal forebrain nuclei. In Alzheimer's disease it seems that the amount of mRNA for the A4 precursor goes down, at least in the few cases that have been looked at. However, there are major problems in interpreting *in situ* hybridizations or Northern blots of material from terminally diseased brains.

Roberts: If the amount of A4 mRNA decreases, how do you reconcile that with your idea that amyloidogenic protein-producing cells should be turned on? According to your ideas there should be an increased level of A4 mRNA.

Wisniewski: As indicated by Colin Masters, there are major problems in interpreting *in situ* hybridization or Northern blots of material from terminally diseased brains. Moreover, the studies of A4 mRNA mentioned by Colin were carried out in patients with a 7–10 year history of Alzheimer's disease. At the end stage of AD the production of the amyloidogenic protein could be reduced as a result of a feedback phenomenon.

Roberts: There are two components of the plaques: the neuritic part which contains tau protein that is the same as the material found in tangles, and the plaque core which contains the β-pleated protein. Normally when people say there is a life cycle to a plaque, the neuritic part is formed first, so how does that fit in with your theory?

Wisniewski: The neuritic senile plaque is a complex structure made of deposits of amyloid, abnormal neurites and reactive cells and their processes. The human plaques have tau because their neurites have the paired helical filaments (PHF). In animals, neurons and their processes do not form PHF. PHF are uniquely human structures. In our opinion, PHF and amyloid deposits are composed of different proteins. That's why in animals, plaques develop without PHF. In humans there are many diseases where PHF are formed in the absence of plaques.

Roberts: According to the accepted neuropathology, there is no case of diagnosis of Alzheimer's disease when there are only plaque cores. That is regarded as an end stage.

Wisniewski: There are two hypotheses explaining formation of the plaques. According to one hypothesis, neuritic pathology occurs first and amyloid appears as a result of the neuritic pathology. A second hypothesis states that the amyloid deposits start the plaque formation. We have convincing data which show that the amyloid initiates the neuritic response and neuritic plaque formation. Therefore, amyloid seems to both start and drive plaque development.

Beyreuther: I do not agree with the localization of the message in the parts of the brain you described. Brenda Shivers (Center for Molecular Biology, Heidelberg) looked at the rat brain, because in a human post mortem brain neither the RNA nor the protein are stable. If you look at the RNA in the brain of an Alzheimer's patient, you almost never find full-length RNA. The rat is a rather good model for looking at amyloid precursor mRNA. There are rats which develop plaques; Peter Seeburg has sequenced the rat homologue of the human amyloid gene and found it to be very similar to the human gene. *In situ* hybridization with rat A4 precursor cDNA showed the rat brain displaying highest expression of A4 mRNA in, e.g. the cerebral cortex, cerebellum and thalamus (Brenda Shivers, Caroline Hilbich, Konrad Beyreuther & Peter Seeburg, unpublished work). We conclude from this study that the glial cells don't have it because non-neural brain elements show little or no A4 mRNA.

We have also shown that the A4 precursor protein is present in those cells where we see the mRNA. Brenda Shivers, using our anti-peptide antibodies against the A4 precursor protein, has found that the staining pattern is compatible with staining of receptors.

Roberts: This suggests that the cells in which the protein is made are being damaged by something and amyloid precursor is being released then processed.

Beyreuther: If you want to release amyloid you have first to destroy the cell membrane, because the amyloid precursor is a membrane protein and the A4 amyloid protein is in part derived from the transmembrane domain (see Kang et al 1987). This is relevant for therapy—retention of the membrane means protection of the molecule.

*Masters:*Henryk, did you say that all the vascular deposits of amyloid are derived from the blood?—whereas the amyloid in the neuropil is locally produced?

Wisniewski: At this time the cellular origin of the β-peptide precursor protein is unknown. However, in people with AD we do not see amyloid deposits in areas where there is no blood-brain barrier, whereas in patients with systemic amyloidosis there are deposits of amyloid in areas without the blood-brain barrier. To me these data indicate that the majority of the amyloid precursor protein in Alzheimer's disease is produced locally.

Almond: I have heard that plaques can be seen in any human brain so long as it is old enough, does that suggest that if we live long enough, we will get Alzheimer's disease?

Wisniewski: I guess more people would develop Alzheimer's disease but not all. It's very interesting, the peak of Alzheimer's is at 75–80 years and, if anything, it then declines. There are brains from people over 90 years old, which show minimal Alzheimer pathology. There is genetic selection or some other factor which determines that the disease will not affect all of us.

Dickinson: Nobody has ever seen a plaque in a senile mouse, they have been seen in other species. In those species which do show senile plaques is there any decline in amyloid protein mRNA during the course of senility?

Wisniewski: I do not know whether someone looked at the mRNA in animals where the plaques were found, such as bears, dogs, horses, monkeys and cats.

Prusiner: Why did you mention bears first?

Wisniewski: Because they are not easy to work with!

Almond: Many models of ageing involve a derepression of genes (Wareham et al 1987). Has anyone looked in a quantitative way at things like tau, PrP or this Alzheimer precursor protein, to see whether the levels of expression are higher in aged tissue than in the tissues of children?

Wisniewski: Everyone in the field is doing that right now.

Almond: What is the situation in hamsters and mice? Presumably some of the people working with scrapie have looked at PrP expression in embyros versus juveniles versus adults.

McKinley: We have looked at the levels of PrP messenger RNA expression in neonatal hamsters and we find very little PrP messenger RNA before the first week after birth. Then it rises very sharply and maintains a constant level for the rest of the life of the animal.

DeArmond: We have looked at PrP mRNA levels on a neuron by neuron basis by *in situ* hybridization over about a 100 day period of the life of the hamster. There is a constant level throughout that time, no variation and even no variation during the disease state.

Almond: That's very important because you get these cascade effects–individual cells age as well as the general ageing of the organ.

Chesebro: There is a discrepancy between not finding the mRNA of PrP in embryonic cells and yet finding it in almost all the cell lines. Most cell lines behave like embryonic cells, they are somewhat de-differentiated and rapidly dividing. There are a lot of cell lines of non-neuronal origin that produce as much PrP mRNA as the cell lines of neuronal origin.

*Wisniewski:*Maybe it has something to do with the cell lines being transformed cells.

*Manuelidis:*If, as Mike McKinley says, the neurons are really producing the majority of the PrP mRNA and protein in the brain, expression may relate to the differentiation state of specific sets of neurons at a given time. It is interesting that some of the times of PrP expression appear to coincide with synaptic development.

Gabizon: Bruce, in the cell lines where you find a lot of PrP message, you don't find any PrP protein by Western blots, whereas in the brain you have some correlations.

Chesebro: I don't put much emphasis on those Western blots because I have not looked very hard.

DeArmond: We have compared the results of *in situ* hybridization with those of immunohistochemistry in tissue sections. Using Ashley Haase's method for calculating the amount of RNA, there are approximately 50 copies of PrP mRNA in neurons. Similarly, neurons are the only cells that can be shown by immunohistochemistry to express the protein. We find very low levels of PrP mRNA in other non-neuronal cells and glial cells, less than three mRNA copies per cell, and there is no detectable expression of protein in any of those other cells. So in the case of PrP *in situ*, the cells making the highest number of mRNA copies are the ones expressing the protein.

Oesch: I have a question for Richard Kimberlin. In the different scrapie experimental systems, there are strains that form a lot of plaques and others that form few plaques. Does that correlate with the duration of the clinical course?

Kimberlin: In general terms amyloid formation occurs more frequently in the long incubation models. However, the amount of amyloid formed in brain does not correlate with clinical duration, which in rodents is fairly short, but with incubation period. Actually, from what I said in my talk, the correlation is probably with the duration of the replication phase in brain.

Wisniewski: The amyloid deposits in Alzheimer's disease are of critical importance because they destroy the brain. The amyloid deposits in unconventional virus infections do not contribute to the clinical signs and symptoms because there are not many plaques.

Kimberlin: But the simple point is that time is one of the important factors in both situations: the clinical duration in human cases and the duration of replication in the brain in i.c. injected scrapie.

Oesch: But in your talk, you said that peripheral injection leads to a short clinical course, while i.c. injection produces a relatively longer clinical course.

Kimberlin: It wasn't clinical course, it was the length of time when scrapie agent was replicating in brain and this is one contributing factor to the smaller amounts of amyloid, and indeed of vacuolation, that occur after peripheral injection compared to i.c. injection.

Fraser: If you do a sequential study of a plaque model in scrapie, at the very end of the disease in the thalamus and cerebral cortex there is a rapid increase in the number of plaques. Elsewhere plaques do occur early but only in very low numbers (Bruce 1981).

Beyreuther: The concentration of amyloid precursor protein is high in the cerebellum but there are not many plaques there. If the concentration of factors involved in amyloid generation is high in some regions and low in others, then you have to take the duration of the disease into account.

Paul Brown: It's possible that in future years, because of the growth hormone outbreak, there may be some information to bear on this problem in the human. We will know both the incubation period and the clinical duration of illness. I am sure they are both equally important. I think it is the total time rather than a clinical phase or an incubation phase.

None of the iatrogenic growth hormone cases of CJD examined so far have had significant numbers of plaques, yet some incubation periods have gone a minimum of 6–15 years, with clinical durations of between 10 and 19 months.

Dickinson: There has been a lot of enthusiasm over the discovery that the gene for the amyloid precursor protein is on chromosome 21, as is the potential gene for familial Alzheimer's disease. Of course a protein has a gene, but where is the relevant genetic variation for the condition in question? In familial Alzheimer's disease, are we expecting to find genetic variants of the gene for the A4 protein (or some other gene on chromosome 21)?

Beyreuther: The chance of the two genes—the gene for the amyloid precursor and the gene for familial Alzheimer's disease—both occurring on chromosome 21 is one in 70. Linkage analysis shows that the gene for amyloid protein is not closely linked to the gene for familial Alzheimer's disease and that these loci are genetically distinct. That both genes are *located* on chromosome 21 might reflect the possibility that the familial gene is a gene acting in *cis* (Van Broeckhoven et al 1987, Tanzi et al 1987).

Masters: As we increase the sensitivity of our techniques for detecting these amyloid plaques (Tateishi, this volume p 32) we see a dramatic increase in the numbers of plaques. We are at the moment screening Down's syndrome cases, and we see plaques in Down's syndrome cases as young as 13 years old. But they don't develop clinical symptoms until they are in their 40's and 50's. If you think in terms of time course, you have to remember that it may take many years for a plaque to develop.

References

Bruce ME 1981 Serial studies on the development of cerebral amyloidosis and vacuolar degeneration in murine scrapie. J Comp Pathol 91:589–597

Kang J, Lemaire HG, Unterbeck A et al 1987 The precursor of Alzheimer's disease amyloid A4 protein resembles a cell-surface receptor. Nature (Lond) 325:733–736

Tanzi RE, St George-Hyslop PH, Haines JL et al 1987 The genetic defect in familial Alzheimer's disease is not tightly linked to the amyloid b-protein gene. Nature (Lond) 329:156–157

Van Broeckhoven C, Genthe AM, Vandenberghe A et al 1987 Failure of familial Alzheimer's disease to segregate with the A4–amyloid gene in several European families. Nature (Lond) 329:153–155

Wareham KA, Lyon MF, Glenister PH, Williams ED 1987 Age related reactivation of an X-linked gene. Nature (Lond) 327:725–727

Novel mechanisms of degeneration of the central nervous system — prion structure and biology

Stanley B. Prusiner*†, Neil Stahl* and Stephen J. DeArmond‡

Departments of *Neurology, †Biochemistry and Biophysics, and ‡Pathology, University of California, San Francisco, California 94143, USA

Abstract. Prion is a term for the novel infectious agents which cause scrapie and Creutzfeldt-Jakob disease; these infectious pathogens are composed largely, if not entirely, of prion protein (PrP) molecules. No prion-specific polynucleotide has been identified. Considerable evidence indicates that PrP 27–30 is required for and inseparable from scrapie infectivity. PrP 27–30 is derived from a larger protein, denoted PrP^{Sc}. A cellular isoform, designated PrP^C, and PrP^{Sc} are both encoded by a single copy chromosomal gene and both proteins appear to be translated from the same 2.1 kb mRNA. Monoclonal antibodies to PrP 27–30 as well as antisera to PrP synthetic peptides, react with both PrP^C and PrP^{Sc}, establishing the relatedness of these proteins. PrP^C is completely digested by proteinase K; PrP^{Sc} is converted to PrP 27–30 under the same conditions. Detergent extraction of microsomal membranes isolated from scrapie-infected hamster brains solubilizes PrP^C but induces PrP^{Sc} to polymerize into amyloid rods. This procedure allows separation of the two prion protein isoforms and the demonstration that PrP^{Sc} accumulates during scrapie infection while the level of PrP^C does not change. The prion amyloid rods generated by detergent extraction are identical morphologically, except for length, to extracellular collections of prion amyloid filaments which form plaques in scrapie- and CJD-infected brains. The prion amyloid plaques stain with antibodies to PrP 27–30 and PrP peptides. Prion rods composed of PrP 27–30 dissociate into phospholipid vesicles with full retention of scrapie infectivity. The murine PrP gene (*Prn-p*) is linked to the *Prn-i* gene, which controls the length of the scrapie incubation period. Prolonged incubation times are a cardinal feature of scrapie and CJD. While the central role of PrP^{Sc} in scrapie pathogenesis is well established, the chemical and conformational differences between PrP^C and PrP^{Sc} are unknown but presumably arise from post-translational events.

1988 Novel infectious agents and the central nervous system. Wiley, Chichester (Ciba Foundation Symposium 135) p 239–260

Many degenerative neurological diseases are age dependent. These disorders occur at specific times in life, for example, the onset of multiple sclerosis is generally between the ages of 25 and 35 years. Patients with Gerstmann-

Sträussler syndrome (GSS) are slightly older, while patients with amyotrophic lateral sclerosis, Parkinson's disease, Creutzfeldt-Jakob disease (CJD) and Alzheimer's disease are generally between 45 and 85 years of age when their disorders become apparent. We have no understanding of what molecular mechanisms control the timing of these diseases. Perhaps biological clocks which normally operate to control physiological processes are involved in the pathogenesis of these dreaded disorders.

The study of scrapie, a model degenerative neurological disease, is beginning to uncover new mechanisms of diseases, which may be important for understanding a variety of human degenerative disorders.

Slow infections are characterized by prolonged incubation periods ranging from several months to decades followed by brief, progressive clinical courses leading to death of the host. The concept of slow infections was first introduced in 1954 by Bjorn Sigurdsson, a pathologist working in Iceland on neurological diseases in animals (Sigurdsson 1954). It appears that slow infections are caused by at least two different classes of infectious agents: viruses and prions.

Prion diseases

The unusual features of the scrapie agent have been recognized by many investigators (Alper et al 1966, 1967, Gibbons and Hunter 1967) and emphasized by such terms as 'unconventional virus' and 'virino'. The former term has been used as a synonym for the scrapie agent with its unusual characteristics in contrast to conventional viruses (Gajdusek 1977). Virino was originally defined: 'If the recent experimental results of Marsh and Malone are correct in implicating DNA as a necessary component of the infective unit of scrapie, then an appropriate name for this class of agent would be 'virinos' which (by analogy with neutrinos) are small, immunologically neutral particles with high penetration properties which need special criteria to detect their presence' (Dickinson & Outram 1979). Subsequent studies showed that the work on which this proposal was based (Marsh et al 1978, Malone et al 1979) could not be confirmed (Prusiner et al 1980d).

By 1981, convincing data for a protein component within the scrapie agent were obtained (McKinley et al 1981, Prusiner et al 1981). The next year, a new term 'prion' was suggested for this class of novel infectious agents (Prusiner 1982). Prion was defined operationally as 'small proteinaceous infectious particles which resist inactivation by procedures that modify nucleic acids'. A family of structural hypotheses were proposed for the prion: 1) proteins surrounding a nucleic acid which encodes them (a virus), 2) proteins surrounding a small non-coding polynucleotide, and 3) a proteinaceous particle devoid of nucleic acid.

While some investigators defined prions as particles consisting only of

TABLE 1 Prion diseases[a]

Disease	Natural host
Scrapie[b]	Sheep and goats
Transmissible mink encephalopathy	Mink
Chronic wasting disease	Mule deer and elk
Kuru	Humans – Fore tribe
Creutzfeldt-Jakob disease (CJD)[b]	Humans
Gerstmann-Sträussler syndrome	Humans

[a] Alternative terminologies include subacute transmissible spongiform encephalopathies and unconventional slow virus diseases (Gajdusek 1977)
[b] Prions have been shown to cause scrapie and CJD; they are presumed to cause the other diseases listed

proteins, we studiously avoided this oversimplification to exclude bias from our experimental approaches. The studies described below have limited the number of putative structures for the prion which can now be seriously considered. Results from many laboratories have made the possibility that scrapie is caused by a virus seem remote (Diener 1987, Oesch et al 1985, Gabizon et al 1987).

Six diseases, three of animals and three of humans, are probably caused by prions (Table 1). Scrapie and CJD are the best studied of these disorders. The slow infectious agents causing transmissible mink encephalopathy, chronic wasting disease, kuru and GSS are not well characterized; further knowledge about the properties of these infectious agents must be obtained before they can be firmly classified as prions. For ease of discussion, all the diseases listed in Table 1 are referred to as prion diseases even though a prion aetiology must be considered tentative until the molecular properties of each slow infectious agent are well defined (Prusiner 1984).

Prion diseases share many features. All known prion diseases are confined to the central nervous system (CNS). Prolonged incubation periods ranging from two months to more than three decades have been observed. The clinical course in these diseases is usually rather stereotyped and progresses to death. The clinical phase of prion illnesses may last for periods from a few weeks to a few years. A reactive astrocytosis is found throughout the CNS in all these diseases (Zlotnik 1962, Beck & Daniel 1964). Neuronal vacuolation is also found, but it is not a constant or obligatory feature. The infectious agents or prions causing these diseases possess unusual molecular properties which distinguish them from both viruses and viroids (Diener et al 1982, Prusiner 1982).

The three human prion diseases (kuru, CJD and GSS) are probably variants of the same disorder. By analogy with studies on experimental scrapie, it seems likely that all three of these human diseases will involve an abnormal isoform of the prion protein. The prion protein is encoded by a single copy gene in hamsters and mice (Oesch et al 1985, Basler et al 1986, Sparkes et al 1986). Both chromosomal localization (Sparkes et al 1986) and Southern analysis of human DNA (Hsiao et al 1987) suggest that the human PrP gene is single copy.

Mechanisms of degeneration of the central nervous system

The human prion diseases illustrate three mechanisms by which CNS degeneration might arise: slow infection, sporadic disease, and genetic alteration. That the three human prion diseases can be transmitted by inoculation to experimental animals is well documented (Gajdusek et al 1966, Gibbs et al 1968, Masters et al 1981a). Kuru is thought to have been spread exclusively through the slow infectious mechanism by ritual cannibalism (Gajdusek 1977, Alpers 1979).

While a few CJD cases can be traced to inoculation of material contaminated with prions, i.e. human growth hormone (Gibb et al 1985, Koch et al 1985, Tintner et al 1986, Weller et al 1986), cornea transplantation (Duffy et al 1974) and cerebral electrode implants (Bernoulli et al 1977), the vast majority appear to be sporadic, despite considerable effort to implicate scrapie-infected sheep as an exogenous source of prions. Certainly, sporadic CJD could be explained by prions being ubiquitous in our food chain with a very low efficiency of infection. We have shown that scrapie prion infection in hamsters by the oral route is 10^9 times less efficient than intracerebral inoculation in hamsters (Prusiner et al 1985). Whether or not CJD can arise endogenously without any molecules being contributed from exogenous prions remains to be established. If it is possible for prions to arise endogenously, then it will be important to identify the macromolecule or event(s) which initiate their synthesis.

GSS seems to represent the genetic form of prion disease although 10 to 15% of CJD may have a genetic basis (Masters et al 1979, 1981a). The genetic mechanism whereby patients develop GSS during their fifth decade of life is unknown. One possibility is that a genetic locus renders these individuals susceptible to infection by exogenous prions. Genetic control of the scrapie and CJD incubation periods in mice after inoculation with prions is well documented (Dickinson & Outram 1979, Kingsbury et al 1983, Carlson et al 1986). Alternatively, GSS might be due to a gene which activates the synthesis of the abnormal isoform of the prion protein as well as any other components of the prion, if they exist. Whether or not the PrP gene in GSS patients is different from that in unaffected family members is not known.

All of the considerations raised by these three forms of prion diseases are equally compatible with a prion structure which either is devoid of any nucleic acid or includes one. Much evidence has been accumulated showing that the abnormal isoform of the prion protein is a component of the infectious particle. No other components of the prion have been identified so far, yet many investigators continue to believe that a small nucleic acid is buried within the interior of the prion. Current data are insufficient to allow us to state that prions are devoid of nucleic acid; however, arguments in support of this hypothesis are growing.

Purification and molecular structure of prions

Progress in the purification of the hamster scrapie prion (Bolton et al 1982, Prusiner et al 1982a) led to the discovery of a unique protein, PrP 27–30, which was shown to be a major component of the infectious particle (McKinley et al 1983, Bolton et al 1984). PrP 27–30 is a sialoglycoprotein (Bolton et al 1985) and was found to polymerize into rods possessing the ultrastructural and histochemical characteristics of amyloid (Prusiner et al 1983). The development of a large-scale purification protocol provided sufficient immunogen for the production of antiserum to PrP 27–30 (Bendheim et al 1984). This antiserum has enabled the molecular comparison in rodents of the infectious particles causing scrapie with those causing CJD (Bendheim et al 1985). We have also used this antiserum to show that amyloid plaques in the brains of scrapie-infected hamsters are composed of paracrystalline arrays of prion proteins (Bendheim et al 1984, DeArmond et al 1985).

Development of an incubation time interval assay (Prusiner et al 1980a, 1982a) facilitated purification of the infectious particles (Prusiner et al 1981, 1982b, Diringer et al 1983). Partial purification of the scrapie agent led to experiments that provided convincing evidence for a protein within the prion which is required for scrapie infectivity (McKinley et al 1981, Prusiner et al 1981). Subsequently, a concerted effort was made to identify the protein (Bolton et al 1982, Prusiner et al 1982a). Using purification steps derived from earlier protocols (Prusiner et al 1978a,b, 1980a,b,c, 1981) and centrifugation through a discontinuous sucrose gradient formed in a reorienting vertical rotor, highly purified preparations of scrapie prions were obtained (Prusiner et al 1982a).

Seven lines of evidence indicate that the protein, PrP 27–30, is a component of the infectious particle or prion (Table 2). (1) PrP 27–30 and scrapie prions co-purify (Prusiner et al 1982a); PrP 27–30 is the most abundant macromolecule in purified preparations of prions (Prusiner et al 1983). In fact, PrP 27–30 is the only macromolecule found in sufficiently high concentration to be considered a component of the infectious particle. During co-purification of PrP 27–30 and scrapie prions, we have enriched each species 3 000- to 10 000-fold with respect to cellular proteins. This co-purification indicates that the molecular properties of PrP 27–30 and the infectious prions must be

TABLE 2   Scrapie isoform of the prion protein is a component of the infectious prion

1. PrP 27–30 is the most abundant macromolecule in purified preparations of prions
2. PrP 27–30 concentration is proportional to prion titre
3. Hydrolysis, denaturation or selective modification of PrP 27–30 results in a diminution of prion titre
4. PrP gene is linked to the *Prn-i* gene controlling scrapie incubation times
5. PrP 27–30 and prion infectivity partition together in membranes, rods, spheres, detergent-lipid-protein complexes and liposomes
6. PrP 27–30 is specific for prion diseases
7. Cultured neuroblastoma cells infected with prions produce PrP[Sc]

extremely similar. (2) PrP 27–30 concentration is proportional to prion titre (Bolton et al 1982, McKinley et al 1983). PrP 27–30 or its precursor PrP[Sc] is absent from uninfected, normal animals. The kinetics of PrP 27–30 appearance in scrapie-infected animals coincides with the increase in scrapie prion titre. (3) Procedures that denature, hydrolyse or selectively modify PrP 27–30 also diminish prion titre (McKinley et al 1983, Bolton et al 1984). The unusual kinetics of PrP 27–30 hydrolysis catalysed by proteases has been shown to correlate with the diminution of scrapie prion titre. Denaturation of PrP 27–30 by boiling in sodium dodecyl sulphate is accompanied by a reduction in scrapie prion titre and a change in the resistance of PrP 27–30 to proteases (Bolton et al 1984). (4) The PrP gene (*Prn-p*) in mice is linked to a gene controlling scrapie incubation times (*Prn-i*) (Carlson et al 1986). *Prn-p* and *Prn-i* form the prion gene complex (*Prn*). *Prn-p* has been mapped to murine chromosome 2 (Sparkes et al 1986). Prolonged incubation periods are a cardinal feature of both scrapie and CJD. These genetic studies argue strongly for a central role of PrP[Sc] or PrP 27–30 in the pathogenesis of scrapie. (5) PrP 27–30 and scrapie prion infectivity partitition together into many different forms: membranes, rods, spheres, detergent-lipid-protein complexes and liposomes. These markedly different physical forms all contain PrP 27–30 and high prion titres (Prusiner et al 1982a, 1983, McKinley & Prusiner 1986, McKinley et al 1986, Meyer et al 1986, Gabizon et al 1987). These experiments not only provide important evidence for the essential role of PrP 27–30 in the transmission of scrapie infection, but they also argue that it is unlikely that prions contain more than one type of macromolecule unless the two putative components are tightly bound to each other. (6) PrP 27–30 is disease specific. Protease-resistant prion proteins are found only in prion diseases: scrapie, CJD, kuru and GSS (Bockman et al 1985, Gibbs et al 1985, Kitamoto et al 1986, Roberts et al 1986). The scrapie PrP isoform is not found in other degenerative disorders (Bockman et al 1985, Brown et al 1986). (7) Cultured mouse neuroblastoma cells infected with prions produce PrP[Sc]. Uninfected cloned cells did not contain any detectable PrP[Sc] (D. Butler, M. Scott, J.

Bockman, K. Hsiao, D. Kingsbury and S. B. Prusiner, submitted for publication). All attempts to separate the scrapie isoform of the prion protein (PrP^{Sc}) from infectivity have been unsuccessful.

PrP 27–30 was further purified and subjected to gas phase amino acid sequencing (Prusiner et al 1983, 1984). Once the N-terminal sequence was determined, an isocoding mixture of oligonucleotides corresponding to a portion of this sequence was synthesized and used as a probe to select a clone encoding PrP 27–30 from a scrapie-infected hamster brain cDNA library (Oesch et al 1985). The identification of the PrP cDNA was confirmed by sequencing additional peptides from PrP 27–30 generated by cyanogen bromide cleavage and showing that all were found within the translated sequence of the cloned cDNA insert. Southern blotting with PrP cDNA revealed a single gene with the same restriction patterns in normal and scrapie-infected hamster brain DNA. A single PrP gene was also detected in murine (Chesebro et al 1985, Oesch et al 1985) and human DNA (Oesch et al 1985). PrP mRNA was found at similar levels in both normal and scrapie-infected hamster brain, and at lower levels in many other normal tissues. Using antisera raised against PrP 27–30, PrP proteins were detected in crude extracts of infected and normal brains (Oesch et al 1985); these isoforms were designated PrP^{Sc} and PrP^{C}, respectively (Barry et al 1986, Meyer et al 1986). Proteinase K digestion yielded PrP 27–30 from infected brain extract, but it completely degraded PrP^{C} in normal brain. No PrP-related nucleic acids were found in purified preparations of scrapie prions suggesting that PrP^{Sc} is not encoded by a nucleic acid carried within the infectious particles (Oesch et al 1985). Recent studies show that in scrapie-infected brains both the scrapie and cellular isoforms of PrP are present (Meyer et al 1986).

Considerable evidence suggests that the infectious particles or prions causing scrapie and CJD are composed largely, if not entirely, of protein. The possibility that prions contain a small nucleic acid molecule, though unlikely, cannot be excluded by current experimental data (Diener 1987, Gabizon et al 1987). How prions multiply is unknown, since they do not contain a gene encoding the prion protein — that gene is found in cellular DNA (Oesch et al 1985).

Prion protein isoforms

In healthy cells, the only product of the PrP gene is a protein designated PrP^{C} (Oesch et al 1985, Barry et al 1986, Meyer et al 1986). This protein has a M_r of 33 000 to 35 000, is sensitive to proteases and does not polymerize on exposure to detergents (Oesch et al 1985, Barry & Prusiner 1986, Barry et al 1986, Meyer et al 1986). The counterpart of PrP^{C} that is found only in scrapie-infected animals, PrP^{Sc}, is resistant to proteases and polymerizes into amyloid rods and filaments. The structure and organization of the PrP gene suggest that these differences arise from a post-translational event (Basler et al 1986).

Both PrP^C and PrP^{Sc} have several post-translational modifications. A signal sequence is removed during their biosynthesis (Basler et al 1986, Hope et al 1986, Hay et al 1987), and they are glycosylated at one, possibly both, of the two potential N-glycosylation sites (Bolton et al 1985, Oesch et al 1985, Hope et al 1986, Haraguchi et al 1987).

Both PrP^C and PrP^{Sc} contain a phosphatidylinositol glycolipid (Stahl et al 1987) that shares many features with those found on the carboxy termini of the variant surface glycoprotein (VSG) of *Trypanosoma brucei* (Ferguson et al 1985a,b), acetylcholinesterase (Futerman et al 1985, Haas et al 1986, Low & Finean 1977), alkaline phosphatase (Ikezawa et al 1976, Low & Zilversmit 1980), Thy-1 (Low & Kincade 1985, Tse et al 1985), and decay accelerating factor (Davitz et al 1986, Medof et al 1986). Components of the glycolipid, including ethanolamine, phosphate, *myo*-inositol, and stearic acid were identified by gas chromatography/mass spectrometry of acid hydrolysates of PrP 27–30 purified by SDS-PAGE. Incubation of purified PrP 27–30 with a phosphatidylinositol-specific phospholipase C (PIPLC) results in a decrease in the amount of covalently attached stearic acid, and allows PrP 27–30 to react on Western blots with an antiserum raised against the PIPLC-treated glycolipid attached to VSG. PrP^C also contains a glycolipid: incubation of cultured cells with PIPLC virtually abolished the cell-surface indirect immunofluorescence observed with PrP antisera, and PrP^C was found by Western blotting to be in the cell media instead of being associated with cell membranes.

The chemical and/or conformational differences between PrP^C and PrP^{Sc} remain to be determined. To elucidate the molecular structure which confers on PrP^{Sc} protease resistance and the ability to polymerize into amyloid rods is a central goal in scrapie research.

Neuropathology of prion diseases

CJD, GSS and kuru in humans and scrapie in animals are classified together because they are transmitted by atypical infectious agents or prions, and because they have similar histopathologies. The microscopic features that characterize this group of neurological disorders are spongiform degeneration of neurons, severe astrocytic gliosis which often appears to be out of proportion to the degree of nerve cell loss, and amyloid plaque formation.

The prion protein accumulates selectively and abnormally in CNS nerve cells during the course of scrapie. Immunohistochemistry with anti-PrP monoclonal antibodies shows that PrP accumulates within the neuropil where spongiform degeneration and astrocytic gliosis are most intense (Fig. 1) (DeArmond et al 1987a). Although most of our studies have focused on scrapie in hamsters, a similar relationship between the prion protein and neuropathology of prion diseases seems likely because the human PrP se-

PrP

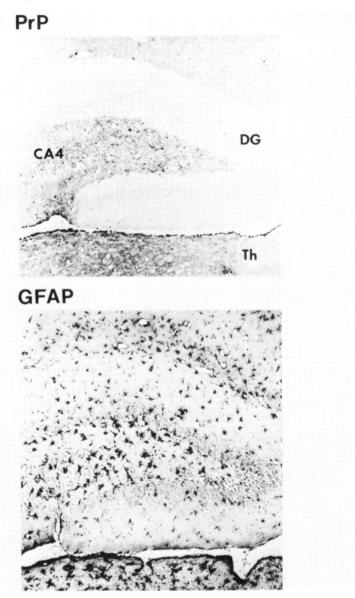

GFAP

FIG. 1.   The distribution of the scrapie prion protein (PrP) in scrapie is topographically related to the distribution of astrocytic gliosis (GFAP). Serial brain sections of hamsters terminally ill with scrapie were stained by peroxidase immunohistochemistry with monoclonal antibodies specific for PrP and GFAP. The latter was counterstained with haematoxylin. Intense neuropil staining for PrP and intense reactive astrocytic gliosis are present in CA4 region of the hippocampus and in the thalamus (Th). Little or no PrP staining is present in the dentate gyrus (DG) and, correspondingly, reactive astrocytic gliosis is significantly less intense in DG.

quence is approximately 90% homologous with hamster PrP (Kretzschmar et al 1986), and amyloid plaques in CJD, GSS, kuru and scrapie are antigenically related (see below). The human PrP gene (PRNP) is located on the short arm of chromosome 20 (Sparkes et al 1986).

The amyloid plaques of CJD, kuru, as well as natural (Beck et al 1964, Masters et al 1981a,b) and experimental scrapie are similar morphologically (Tateishi et al 1984). They consist of discrete eosinophilic glassy-appearing masses often having radiating amyloid fibrils at their periphery (Fig. 2B,C). Because this appearance of the plaques was first described in kuru, some investigators refer to these types of plaques in CJD and scrapie as 'kuru' plaques.

Only 5 to 10% of human CJD cases and 50 to 70% of human kuru cases have histochemically demonstrable plaques (Masters et al 1981a, b). All cases of GSS have plaques by definition, since the diagnosis encompasses the triad of cerebellar and/or corticospinal tract degeneration, dementia and cerebral amyloidosis (Gerstmann et al 1936). The plaques of CJD, kuru and GSS are, predictably, located in the cerebellar cortex. In GSS, amyloid plaques are numerous; they can be found throughout the cerebral cortex, thalamus and brain stem. Amyloid deposits develop in and around small blood vessels in the CNS (Fig. 2E). In the cases reported by Gerstmann and co-workers (Gerstmann et al 1936), amyloid was found in the lumen of blood vessels. Plaques in CJD are found almost exclusively in the cerebellar cortex, but they also occur in the cerebral cortex, basal ganglia and thalamus, although less frequently. The distribution of plaques in kuru is similar to that in CJD (Klatzo et al 1959).

Amyloid plaques have been found in the cerebellar cortex in natural sheep scrapie (Beck et al 1964). The plaques which developed in mice after intracerebral inoculation of scrapie prions were distributed among nerve cell bodies in the hippocampus (dentate gyrus), thalamus, hypothalamus, cerebral cortex, granular cell layer of the cerebellum, and medulla (Bruce & Fraser 1975, Wisniewski et al 1975). They were also located in the corpus callosum and along the intracerebral inoculation tract.

In our studies of the hamster scrapie model of prion diseases, every animal inoculated intracerebrally with scrapie prions and terminally ill with scrapie has been found to have cerebral amyloid plaques (Bendheim et al 1984, DeArmond et al 1985, 1987a, b). The plaques in these studies were primarily subependymal, subpial and perivascular; some were found in the cerebral neuropil and corpus callosum, but none were found in the cerebellum. Immunohistochemistry with antisera specific for the prion protein demonstrated that filaments which form the amyloid plaques contain the prion protein (DeArmond et al 1985).

In collaborative studies, we have shown that CJD amyloid plaques stain with PrP 27–30 antiserum (Fig. 2C) (Kitamoto et al 1986, Roberts et al 1986).

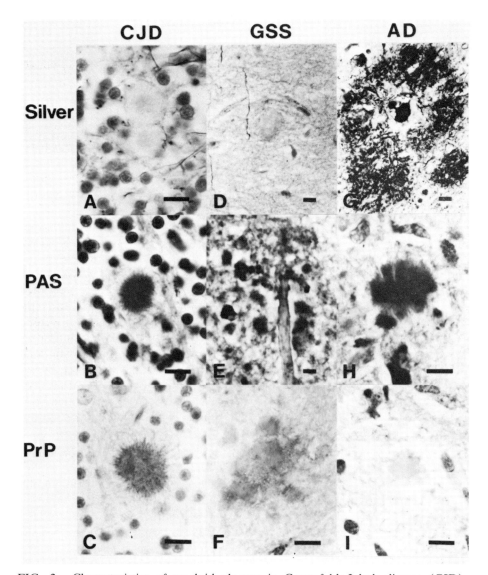

FIG. 2. Characteristics of amyloid plaques in Creutzfeldt-Jakob disease (CJD), Gerstmann-Sträussler syndrome (GSS) and Alzheimer's disease (AD). The Bielschowsky silver stain for neurites (Silver) shows that dystrophic neurites are not characteristic of amyloid plaques in CJD (A) or GSS (D), while they are the hallmark of the senile plaques of AD (G). The periodic acid Schiff (PAS) histochemical reaction stains all amyloids intensely (B, E, H). The plaques of GSS (E) are more dense than the kuru plaques of CJD (B) and similar in density to the amyloid of senile plaques (H). The plaques of GSS are typically perivascular (E). Peroxidase immunohistochemistry with an antiserum specific for the scrapie prion protein (PrP) (Bendheim et al 1984) causes strong specific staining of plaques in CJD (C) and less intense, but specific, staining of plaques in GSS (F). Amyloid in AD (I) fails to react with the PrP antiserum. (C, F and I were counterstained with haematoxylin.) Bar: 25 μm

GSS plaques were also immunoreactive (Fig. 2F). These observations were important because they link human PrP to the pathology of CJD and GSS. Other studies show that a protease-resistant form of human PrP accumulates in CJD and that this form of PrP polymerizes into amyloid rods (Bockman et al 1985, 1987).

The senile amyloid plaques of Alzheimer's disease (AD) do not react with the prion protein antisera (Fig. 2I). This agrees with amino acid sequencing studies of a protein which is thought to be a major component of amyloid plaques in AD and Down's syndrome (Glenner & Wong 1984, Masters et al 1985); the AD amyloid protein exhibits no significant sequence homology with PrP.

Prions and human degenerative neurological diseases

The approaches first developed for the investigation of experimental scrapie in rodents have proved to be directly applicable to the study of CNS degeneration in humans caused by CJD prions. Perhaps most important, the current study of prions may provide a basis for future investigations of other degenerative diseases. Many disorders may eventually be shown to be caused by prion-like macromolecules. The genetic origin of prions and the slow amplification mechanisms which account for their replication make these unique macromolecules interesting with respect to many diseases that occur later in life.

Due largely to the chemical studies described above, any clinical description of prion diseases in humans must be considered provisional and incomplete. Research on human prions is in its infancy, but the availability of both antibodies and cDNA probes should lead to an explosion of new information about their classification, aetiology, clinical course, pathogenesis and possible means of intervention during the next decade.

The above studies clearly establish that the infectious particles causing scrapie are not viruses. Using terms like 'unconventional viruses' implies that these infectious pathogens are unusual but display the basic aspects of viruses, however, they do not. Prions causing scrapie contain a protein (PrP^{Sc}) which is encoded by a cellular gene, not by a hypothetical nucleic acid hiding within the interior of the particle. The structure of the prion clearly differs from that of viruses. Viruses are infectious pathogens containing a nucleic acid genome which encodes most or all of the proteins of the virus. Progeny viruses are encoded by their genomes; progeny prion proteins are host encoded. Whether prions are devoid of nucleic acid or contain some small, as yet undetected polynucleotide is unknown presently (Diener 1987).

The study of scrapie provides a model from which to approach CNS degenerative diseases of humans for which the aetiologies remain undetermined. Of these, Alzheimer's disease, Parkinson's disease and amyotrophic lateral sclerosis are among the most common. While these degenerative diseases are not transmissible to experimental animals, it is possible that their mechanisms of pathogenesis resemble some aspects of scrapie. The accumulation of abnormal proteins causing cellular dysfunction must be considered in each of these diseases. The events leading to the conversion of normal proteins into abnormal isoforms remain undefined, but may play a central role in their pathogenesis. Also worthy of consideration is the possibility that degenerative diseases outside the CNS feature similar pathogenic mechanisms.

Acknowledgements

Important contributions from Drs R Barry, C Bellinger-Kawahara, J Bockman, R Gabizon, K Gilles, R Meyer, M McKinley, M Scott and D Westaway are gratefully acknowledged. Collaborative studies with Drs G Carlson, J Cleaver, T Diener, W Hadlow, L Hood, S Kent, D Kingsbury, B Oesch, D Riesner and C Weissmann have been important to the progress of these studies and are greatly appreciated. The authors thank K Bowman, D Groth and M Wälchli for technical assistance as well as L Gallagher for manuscript production assistance. This work was supported by research grants from the National Institutes of Health (AG02132 and NS14069), the Senator Jacob Javits Center of Excellence in Neuroscience (NS22786) and by gifts from RJR-Nabisco, Inc. and Sherman Fairchild Foundation.

References

Alper T, Haig DA, Clarke MC 1966 The exceptionally small size of the scrapie agent. Biochem Biophys Res Commun 22:278–284
Alper T, Cramp WA, Haig DA, Clarke MC 1967 Does the agent of scrapie replicate without nucleic acid? Nature (Lond) 214:764–766
Alpers MP 1979 Epidemiology and ecology of kuru. In: Prusiner SB, Hadlow WJ (eds) Slow transmissible diseases of the nervous system. Academic Press, New York, vol 1:67–92
Barry RA, Prusiner SB 1986 Monoclonal antibodies to the cellular and scrapie prion proteins. J Infect Dis 154:518–521
Barry RA, Kent SB, McKinley MP, Meyer RK, DeArmond SJ, Hood LE, Prusiner SB 1986 Scrapie and cellular prion proteins share polypeptide epitopes. J Infect Dis 153:848–854
Basler K, Oesch B, Scott M et al 1986 Scrapie and cellular PrP isoforms are encoded by the same chromosomal gene. Cell 46:417–428
Beck E, Daniel PM, Parry HB 1964 Degeneration of the cerebellar and hypothalamo-neurohypophysial systems in sheep with scrapie; and its relationship to human system degenerations. Brain 87:153–176
Bendheim PE, Barry RA, DeArmond SJ, Stites DP, Prusiner SB 1984 Antibodies to a scrapie prion protein. Nature (Lond) 310:418–421
Bendheim PE, Bockman JM, McKinley MP, Kingsbury DT, Prusiner SB 1985 Scrapie and Creutzfeldt-Jakob disease prion proteins share physical properties and antigenic determinants. Proc Natl Acad Sci USA 82:997–1001
Bernoulli C, Siegfried J, Baumgartner G et al 1977 Danger of accidental person to person transmission of Creutzfeldt-Jakob disease of surgery. Lancet 1:478–479

Bockman JM, Kingsbury DT, McKinley MP, Bendheim PE, Prusiner SB 1985 Creutzfedt-Jakob disease proteins in human brains. N Engl J Med 312:73–78

Bockman JM, Prusiner SB, Tateishi J, Kingsbury DT 1987 Immunoblotting of Creutzfeldt-Jakob disease prion proteins – host species-specific epitopes. Ann Neurol 21:589–595

Bolton DC, McKinley MP, Prusiner SB 1982 Identification of a protein that purifies with the scrapie prion. Science (Wash DC) 218:1309–1311

Bolton DC, McKinley MP, Prusiner SB 1984 Molecular characteristics of the major scrapie prion protein. Biochemistry 23:5898–5905

Bolton DC, Meyer RK, Prusiner SB 1985 Scrapie PrP 27–30 is a sialoglycoprotein. J Virol 53:596–606

Brown P, Coker-Vann M, Pomeroy K et al 1986 Diagnosis of Creutzfeldt-Jakob disease by Western blot identification of marker protein in human brain tissue. N Engl J Med 314:547–551

Bruce M, Fraser H 1975 Amyloid plaques in the brains of mice infected with scrapie: morphological variations and staining properties. Neuropathol Appl Neurobiol 1:189–202

Carlson GA, Kingsbury DT, Goodman P, Coleman S, Marshall ST, DeArmond SJ, Westaway D, Prusiner SB 1986 Prion protein and scrapie incubation time genes are linked. Cell 46:503–511

Chesebro B, Race R, Wehrly K et al 1985 Identification of scrapie prion protein-specific mRNA in scrapie-infected and uninfected brain. Nature (Lond) 315:331–333

Davitz MA, Low MG, Nussenzweig V 1986 Release of decay-accelerating factor (DAF) from the cell membrane by phosphatidylinositol-specific phospholipase C (PIPLC). J Exp Med 163:1150–1161

DeArmond SJ, McKinley MP, Barry RA, Braunfeld MB, McColloch JR, Prusiner SB 1985 Identification of prion amyloid filaments in scrapie-infected brain. Cell 41:221–235

DeArmond SJ, Mobley WC, DeMott DL, Barry RA, Beckstead JH, Prusiner SB 1987a Changes in the localization of brain prion proteins during scrapie infection. Neurology 37:1271–1280

DeArmond SJ, Kretzschmar HA, McKinley MP, Prusiner SB 1987b Molecular pathology of prion diseases. In: Prusiner SB, McKinley MP (eds) Prions – novel infectious pathogens causing scrapie and Creutzfeldt-Jakob disease. Academic Press, Orlando, in press

Dickinson AG, Outram GW 1979 The scrapie replication-site hypothesis and its implications for pathogenesis. In: Prusiner SB, Hadlow WJ (eds) Slow transmissible diseases of the nervous system. Academic Press, New York, vol 2:13–31

Diener TO 1987 PrP and the nature of the scrapie agent. Cell 49:719–721

Diener TO, McKinley MP, Prusiner SB 1982 Viroids and prions. Proc Natl Acad Sci USA 79:5220–5224

Diringer H, Gelderblom H, Hilmert H, Ozel M, Edelbluth C, Kimberlin RH 1983 Scrapie infectivity, fibrils and low molecular weight protein. Nature (Lond) 306:476–478

Duffy P, Wolf J, Collins G, Devoe A, Streeten B, Cowen D 1974 Possible person to person transmission of Creutzfeldt-Jakob disease. N Engl J Med 290:692–693

Ferguson MAJ, Hadlar K, Cross GAM 1985a *Trypanosoma brucei* variant surface glycoprotein has a sn-1,2-dimyristyl glycerol membrane anchor at its COOH terminus. J Biol Chem 260:4963–4968

Ferguson MAJ, Low MG, Cross GAM 1985b Glycosyl-sn-1,2-dimyristylphosphatidylinositol is covalently linked to *Trypanosoma brucei* variant surface glycoprotein. J Biol Chem 260:14547–14555

Futerman AH, Low MG, Michaelson DM, Silman I 1985 Solubilization of membrane-bound acetylcholinesterase by a phosphatidylinositol-specific phospholipase C. J Neurochem 45:1487–1494

Gabizon R, McKinley MP, Prusiner SB 1987 Purified prion proteins and scrapie infectivity copartition into liposomes. Proc Natl Acad Sci USA 84:4017–4021

Gajdusek DC 1977 Unconventional viruses and the origin and disappearance of kuru. Science (Wash DC) 197:943–960

Gajdusek DC, Gibbs CJ Jr, Alpers M 1966 Experimental transmission of a kuru-like syndrome to chimpanzees. Nature (Lond) 209:794–796

Gerstmann J, Sträussler E, Scheinker I 1936 Über eine eigenartige hereditär-familiäre Erkrankung des Zentralnervensystems zugleich ein beitrag zur Frage des vorzeitigen lokalen Alterns. Z Neurol 154:736–762

Gibbons RA, Hunter GD 1967 Nature of the scrapie agent. Nature (Lond) 215:1041–1043

Gibbs CJ Jr, Gajdusek DC, Asher DM et al 1968 Creutzfeldt-Jakob disease (spongiform encephalopathy): transmission to the chimpanzee. Science (Wash DC) 161:388–389

Gibbs CJ Jr, Joy A, Heffner R et al 1985 Clinical and pathological features and laboratory confirmation of Creutzfeldt-Jakob disease in a recipient of pituitary-derived human growth hormone. N Engl J Med 313:734–738

Glenner GG, Wong CW 1984 Alzheimer's disease and Down's syndrome: sharing of unique cerebrovascular amyloid fibril protein. Biochem Biophys Res Commun 122:1131–1135

Haas R, Brandt PT, Knight J, Rosenberry TL 1986 Identification of amine component in a glycolipid membrane-binding domain at the C-terminus of human erythrocyte acetylcholinesterase. Biochemistry 25:3098–3105

Haraguchi T, Groth D, Barry RA et al 1987 Deglycosylation demonstrates two forms of the scrapie prion protein. Fed Proc 46:1319 (Abstr)

Hay B, Barry RA, Lieburburg I, Prusiner SB, Lingappa VR 1987 Biogenesis and transmembrane orientation of the cellular isoform of the scrapie prion protein. Mol Cell Biol 7:914–920

Hope J, Morton LJD, Farquhar CF, Multhaup G, Beyreuther K, Kimberlin RH 1986 The major polypeptide of scrapie-associated fibrils (SAF) has the same size, charge distribution and N-terminal protein sequence as predicted for the normal brain protein (PrP). Eur Mol Biol Organ (EMBO) J 5:2591–2597

Hsiao K, DeArmond SJ, Prusiner SB 1987 Human prion protein gene. Neurology, 37 (suppl 1):342 (Abstr)

Ikezawa H, Yamanegi M, Taguchi R, Miyashita T, Ohyabu T 1976 Studies on phosphatidylinositol phosphodiesterase (phospholipase C type) of *Bacillus cereus*: I. Purification, properties, and phosphatase releasing activity. Biochim Biophys Acta 450:154–164

Kingsbury DT, Kasper KC, Stites DP, Watson JC, Hogan RN, Prusiner SB 1983 Genetic control of scrapie and Creutzfeldt-Jakob disease in mice. J Immunol 131:491–496

Kitamoto T, Tateishi J, Tashima T, Takeshita I, Barry RA, DeArmond SJ, Prusiner SB 1986 Amyloid plaques in Creutzfeldt-Jakob disease stain with prion protein antibodies. Ann Neurol 20:204–208

Klatzo I, Gajdusek DC, Zigas V 1959 Pathology of kuru. Lab Invest 8:799–847

Koch TK, Berg BO, DeArmond SJ, Gravina RF 1985 Creutzfeldt-Jakob disease in a young adult with idiopathic hypopituitarism: possible relation to the administration of cadaveric human growth hormone. N Engl J Med 313:731–733

Kretzschmar HA, Stowring LE, Westaway D, Stubblebine WH, Prusiner SB, DeArmond SJ 1986 Molecular cloning of a human prion protein cDNA. DNA 5:315–324

Low MG, Kincade PW 1985 Phosphatidylinositol is the membrane-anchoring domain of the Thy-1 glycoprotein. Nature (Lond) 318:62–64

Low MG, Zilversmit DB 1980 Role of phosphatidylinositol in attachment of alkaline phosphatase to membranes. Biochemistry 19:3913–3918

Low MG, Finean JB 1977 Non-lytic release of acetylcholinesterase from erythrocytes by a phosphatidylinositol-specific phsopholipase C. FEBS (Fed Eur Biochem Soc) Lett 82:143–146

Malone TG, Marsh RF, Hanson RP, Semancik JS 1979 Evidence for the low molecular weight nature of scrapie agent. Nature (Lond) 278:575–576

Marsh RF, Malone TG, Semancik JS, Lancaster WD, Hanson RP 1978 Evidence for an essential DNA component in the scrapie agent. Nature (Lond) 275:146–147

Masters CL, Gajdusek DC, Gibbs CJ Jr, Bernoulli C, Asher DM 1979 Familial Creutzfeldt-Jakob disease and other familial dementias: an inquiry into possible modes of virus-induced familial diseases. In: Prusiner SB, Hadlow WJ (eds) Slow transmissible diseases of the nervous system. Academic Press, New York, vol 1:143–193

Masters CL, Gajdusek DC, Gibbs CJ Jr 1981a Creutzfeldt-Jakob disease virus isolations from the Gerstmann-Sträussler syndrome. Brain 104:559–588

Masters CL, Gajdusek DC, Gibbs CJ Jr 1981b The familial occurrence of Creutzfeldt-Jakob disease and Alzheimer's disease. Brain 104:535–558

Masters CL, Simms G, Weinman NA, Multhaup G, McDonald BL, Beyreuther K 1985 Amyloid plaque core protein in Alzheimer disease and Down syndrome. Proc Natl Acad Sci USA 82:4245–4249

McKinley MP, Prusiner SB 1986 Biology and structure of scrapie prions. Int Rev Neurobiol 28:1–57

McKinley MP, Masiarz FR, Prusiner SB 1981 Reversible chemical modification of the scrapie agent. Science (Wash DC) 214:1259–1261

McKinley MP, Bolton DC, Prusiner SB 1983 A protease-resistant protein is a structural component of the scrapie prion. Cell 35:57–62

McKinley MP, Braunfeld MB, Bellinger CG, Prusiner SB 1986 Molecular characteristics of prion rods purified from scrapie-infected hamster brains. J Infect Dis 154:110–120

Medof ME, Walter EI, Roberts WI, Haas R, Rosenberry Tl 1986 Decay accelerating factor of complement is anchored to cells by a C-terminal glycolipid. Biochemistry 25:6740–6747

Meyer RK, McKinley MP, Bowman KA, Barry RA, Prusiner SB 1986 Separation and properties of cellular and scraple prion proteins. Proc Natl Acad Sci USA 83:2310–2314

Oesch B, Westaway D, Wälchli M et al 1985 A cellular gene encodes scrapie PrP 27–30 protein. Cell 40:735–746

Prusiner SB 1982 Novel proteinaceous infectious particles cause scrapie. Science (Wash DC) 216:136–144

Prusiner SB 1984 Prions – novel infectious pathogens. Adv Virus Res 29:1–56

Prusiner SB, Hadlow WJ, Eklund CM, Race RE, Cochran SP 1978a Sedimentation characteristics of the scrapie agent from murine spleen and brain. Biochemistry 17:4987–4992

Prusiner SB, Hadlow WJ, Garfin DE et al 1978b Partial purification and evidence for multiple molecular forms of the scrapie agent. Biochemistry 17:4993–4997

Prusiner SB, Groth DF, Cochran SP, Masiarz FR, McKinley MP, Martinez HM 1980a Molecular properties, partial purification and assay by incubation period measurements of the hamster scrapie agent. Biochemistry 19:4883–4891

Prusiner SB, Garfin DE, Cochran SP, McKinley MP, Groth DF 1980b Experimental scrapie in the mouse: electrophoretic and sedimentation properties of the partially purified agent. J Neurochem 35:574–582

Prusiner SB, Groth DF, Cochran SP, McKinley MP, Masiarz FR 1980c Gel electrophoresis and glass permeation chromatography of the hamster scrapie agent after enzymic digestion and detergent extraction. Biochemistry 19:4892–4898

Prusiner SB, Groth DF, Bildstein C, Masiarz FR, McKinley MP, Cochran SP 1980d Electrophoretic properties of the scrapie agent in agarose gels. Proc Natl Acad Sci USA 77:2984–2988

Prusiner SB, McKinley MP, Groth DF, Bowman KA, Mock NI, Cochran SP, Masiarz FR 1981 Scrapie agent contains a hydrophobic protein. Proc Natl Acad Sci USA 78:6675–6679.

Prusiner SB, Bolton DC, Groth DF, Bowman KA, Cochran SP, McKinley MP 1982a Further purification and characterization of scrapie prions. Biochemistry 21:6942–6950

Prusiner SB, Cochran SP, Groth DF, Downey DE, Bowman KA, Martinez HM 1982b Measurement of the scrapie agent using an incubation time interval assay. Ann Neurol 11:353–358

Prusiner SB, McKinley MP, Bowman KA, Bolton DC, Bendheim PE, Groth DF, Glenner GG 1983 Scrapie prions aggregate to form amyloid-like birefringent rods. Cell 35:349–358

Prusiner SB, Groth DF, Bolton DC, Kent SB, Hood LE 1984 Purification and structural studies of a major scrapie prion protein. Cell 38:127–134

Prusiner SB, Cochran SP, Alpers MP 1985 Transmission of scrapie in hamsters. J Infect Dis 152:971–978

Roberts GW, Lofthouse R, Brown R, Crow TJ, Barry RA, Prusiner SB 1986 Prion protein immunoreactivity in human transmissible dementias. N Engl J Med 315:1231–1233

Sigurdsson B 1954 Rida, a chronic encephalitis of sheep with general remarks on infections which develop slowly and some of their special characteristics. Br Vet J 110:341–354

Sparkes RS, Simon M, Cohn VH et al 1986 Assignment of the human and mouse prion protein genes to homologous chromosomes. Proc Natl Acad Sci USA 83:7358–7362

Stahl N, Borchelt DR, Hsiao KK, Prusiner SB 1987 Glycolipid modification of the scrapie prion protein. Cell 51:229–240

Tateishi J, Sato Y, Nagara H, Boellaard JW 1984 Experimental transmission of human subacute spongiform encephalopathy to small rodents. IV. Positive transmission from a typical case of Gerstmann-Sträussler-Scheinker's disease. Acta Neuropathol 64:85–88

Tintner R, Brown P, Hedley-Whyte ET, Rappaport EB, Piccardo CP, Gajdusek DC 1986 Neuropathologic verification of Creutzfeldt-Jakob disease in the exhumed American recipient of human pituitary growth hormone: epidemiologic and pathogenetic implications. Neurology 36:932–936

Tse AGD, Barclay AN, Watts A, Williams AF 1985 A glycophospholipid tail at the carboxy terminus of the Thy-1 glycoprotein of neurons and thymocytes. Science (Wash DC) 230:1003–1008

Weller RO, Steart PV, Powell-Jackson JD 1986 Pathology of Creutzfeldt-Jakob disease associated with pituitary-derived human growth hormone administration. Neuropathol Appl Neurobiol 12:117–129

Wisniewski HM, Bruce ME, Fraser H 1975 Infectious etiology of neuritic (senile) plaques in mice. Science (Wash DC) 190:1108–1110
Zlotnik I 1962 The pathology of scrapie: a comparative study of lesions in the brain of sheep and goats. Acta Neuropathol suppl 1:61–70

DISCUSSION

Hope: Did you say that PrP^{Sc} is not found in amyloid plaques?

Prusiner: No, PrP^{Sc} is found in amyloid plaques, although I can't say that unequivocally. The problem is that we don't have an antibody that can discriminate PrP^{C} from PrP^{Sc}. Also, these are operational definitions of these two molecules: PrP^{C} is a protein which is solubilized by detergents and sensitive to proteinase K; PrP^{Sc} forms a rod-shaped molecule when we add detergents to membranes containing it and is resistant to proteinase K degradation, except for the N-terminal 67 amino acids which are cut off. So I cannot be sure what is in the amyloid plaques; in Alzheimer's disease there is clearly no PrP^{Sc}.

Hope: Concerning the sequencing of PrP^{C}, have you noticed any modification of the arginine at residues 3 or 15?

Prusiner: The data are very preliminary: this was work done by D. Teplow in collaboration with Leroy Hood, and Eric Turk has been doing the PrP^{C} purification. At this point I don't know, but we shall certainly look having heard your findings.

Beyreuther: Neil, you mentioned that the number of ethanolamine molecules per mole of protein was 2.8. Can you comment on that?

Stahl: The glycolipid found on the variant surface glycoprotein from *Trypanosoma brucei* has one ethanolamine which links the phosphatidylinositol glycan to the carboxy terminus. Every mammalian glycolipidated protein where the ethanolamine analysis has been done has more than one ethanolamine. Thy-1 has two moles of ethanolamine. Acetylcholinesterase and decay accelerating factor, which is a regulatory protein in the complement system, contain three ethanolamines: it is thought that two are connected to the glycan through their hydroxyl groups by phosphodiester bonds. These extra ethanolamines, as well as the hexosamine residue of the anchor, all have free amino groups.

Chesebro: I was interested in your results on the tissue culture cells, what species were they from?

Stahl: One mouse, one rat and one hamster.

Prusiner: The cultured mouse cells are the same C 1300 neuroblastoma cells that you obtained from David T. Kingsbury. It is mouse scrapie. When we tried hamster scrapie at the same multiplicity of infection, no PrP^{Sc} or infectivity was found.

Chesebro: Rick Race has also done this experiment and we have fairly similar results in that we have some clones that are positive for infectivity at about the same level you describe, but we haven't yet detected PrP^{Sc} in those clones. I would like to process our cells and try to detect PrP^{Sc} using exactly your technique.

Prusiner: Briefly, what we did was to make a membrane preparation, extract that with detergent and treat it with proteinase K. Using normal whole cells you cannot detect PrP^C by Western blotting, but you can detect it by immuno-fluorescence. If you take the whole cell pellet without proteinase K treatment you can't detect PrP^{Sc} in the scrapie preparations; the proteinase K step is needed to reduce the background and to enable enough protein to be loaded onto the gel for the PrP^{Sc} to be seen.

Dormont: Did you find any difference in the cell growth of your infective clones versus the non-positive clones?

Prusiner: We have not seen any difference in cell growth. We have looked for cytopathic effects and occasionally there are some little vacuoles in the cells but these are also in normal cells.

Dormont: Did you try to infect glial cells?

Prusiner: Yes, but we were unsuccessful.

Dormont: Did you try to co-cultivate your infective clone with normal astrocytes or glial cells?

Prusiner: Those kinds of studies are in progress.

Manuelidis: In CJD we find that proteinase K decreases infectivity by about 1.5 logs even after half an hour incubation. Dave Bolton, however, in contrast to your data, mentioned that he had better yields of infectivity without pro-teinase K treatment. Could it be that proteinase K insensitivity (of the infec-tious agent) is related to scrapie rather than CJD agents?

*Dickinson:*How do you neutralize the enzyme after treatment, before injec-tion of the inoculum?

Manuelidis: We neutralize with phenylmethyl sulphonyl fluoride (PMSF) (Manuelidis et al 1985); dilution of the PMSF prior to incubation is sufficient, as judged from control experiments, not to give any neurological damage in the animals.

Gabizon: That is not enough to keep the PrP intact.

Manuelidis: I disagree, we have gels which show that the PrP is intact by all your criteria.

Gabizon: You checked that after injection it was the same?

Manuelidis: Yes. Parallel identical material was assayed on blots. Analysis several weeks later showed that it was still the same and that the PMSF was effective even in samples stored at 4°C.

Stahl: I think that different strains of scrapie probably have different sensiti-vities to proteinase K.

Manuelidis: That's why it would be interesting to know if everybody has identical infectivity results with proteinase K.

Bolton: In Staten Island we have never checked the infectivity by comparing the same procedure with and without proteinase K digestion during the purification. We have digested HaSp33-37 fractions with trypsin and have not seen a decrease in titre (Bolton et al 1987). In San Francisco we digested purified PrP27-30 fractions for 30 minutes with 100 mg/ml proteinase K and saw no decrease in infectivity. That may be due to the aggregated state of the material at that time. That was the 263K strain of scrapie.

Prusiner: Our only extensive experiments are with the golden hamster, a random-bred LVG strain from the Charles River laboratories. Using a hamster-adapted isolate that we received from Dick Marsh early on (Prusiner et al 1980), which Richard Kimberlin would say has all the properties of 263K, the animals are getting sick at about 65 days. Under the conditions of our experiments we see this extreme proteinase K resistance: only after a prolonged digestion of hours do we begin to see a decrease in the amount of protein and in the titre of scrapie infectivity. The early studies with mouse scrapie were done at Compton, England and those clearly showed that with scrapie 139A there was much more sensitivity of both the infectivity and PrP^{Sc} to proteinase K treatment.

Chesebro: Have you compared the *in vivo*-derived mouse strain and the *in vitro* propagated one in terms of their relative proteinase K sensitivities? It would be really interesting to know whether the same strain of scrapie passaged in your tissue culture cells and in mice has the same proteinase K sensitivity. You should be able to define conditions in which you see a drop of a couple of logs.

*Prusiner:*I think we can get 4.5 logs: that is a good experiment, we will try it.

*Dickinson:*Interpretation of any apparent differences in proteinase sensitivities would have to bear in mind the weaknesses of titre estimates in a system where infectivity is liable to aggregate. Let's assume that the proteinase K is doing two things—one is inactivating some of the infectious units, but the enzyme is also likely to have a disaggregating effect which would increase the estimated titre.

Furthermore, referring to an earlier point, I do not accept that this incubation assay is 'one of the agreed parameters': one needs to be very careful about using incubation period as an assay. Another point is that Stan showed a slide that said I/Ln mice have 'long incubation periods' and also referred to dominance in this respect, but until one has stated which strains of scrapie are being used one cannot make those statements.

On another point, I think use of the word genetic as opposed to the word familial for GSS is misleading. If the operational restraints that one has to accept with human studies were applied to the sheep data, then scrapie would be described as a genetic disease in sheep. Remove the operational restraints, do difficult experiments, and one finds that 'genetic' is no longer an appropriate way of describing it.

Prusiner: With respect to bioassays, we need to think about this in slightly broader terms. A bioassay is always very difficult. We have to consider what we are trying to assay and how good the assay needs to be–there are no absolutes in bioassays. These incubation time assays, when used to study the physical properties of these particles, have been very effective, especially with respect to purification. That does not mean that every aspect of the study of the particle or every aspect of the study of the influence of host genetics can be done with an incubation time assay. The results over the past five years are a testament to the use of these incubation time assays but they are not an absolute gold standard. No assay is, because each time one carries biology to another level of refinement, one needs new assays and new measurements with increased levels of precision.

F. Brown: How exactly do you do the neutralization tests?

Prusiner: These studies come from controls for experiments to optimize the conditions for immunoprecipitation of a detergent-lipid-protein complex. Previously we could never even do an immunoprecipitation experiment of anything associated with infectivity because it was in the rod form. With the detergent-lipid-protein complex we have these small, functionally soluble complexes composed of detergent, lipid, protein and possibly something else. Under these conditions, we can do immunoprecipitation experiments which show neutralization of scrapie infectivity with PrP antisera. In contrast we cannot neutralize the infectivity of the rods.

Dickinson: Is a distinction being made between aggregation and neutralization? Are the assays counting the number of aggregates?

Gabizon: This experiment is not done with aggregates but with a detergent-lipid-protein complex. The decrease in infectivity in logs is much greater than the increase by rod solubilization and clearly any aggregation caused by the antibody is smaller than the rod form.

Dickinson: Is the antibody causing aggregation so that your assay is really of the numbers of dispersed aggregates?

Gabizon: Definitely no.

F. Brown: Neutralization of viruses is a very complex subject; it could be by aggregation, it could be by blocking attachment or, having got inside the cell, it could prevent infection. There is a whole series of mechanisms of neutralization which are not understood in virology.

Bolton: The term neutralization as used in virology does not apply. You are not taking antibody-liposome complexes and inoculating the animals, but depleting the supernatant of protein-liposome complexes then measuring the reduction in infectivity in the supernatant. Is this correct?

Prusiner: Not in these studies. The numbers I showed were the controls for those kinds of experiments. We added everything together before centrifugation and inoculated it into the animal.

Bolton: So you *are* looking at antibody- antigen complexes.

Gabizon: We also looked at the supernatant and pellets after immunoprecipitation: there was less infectivity in the supernatant but we didn't precipitate any infectivity into the pellets. We didn't understand what was happening, until we saw the results from the controls, showing that there was a neutralization effect.

Chesebro: But presumably you did aggregate the PrP that is in these preparations.

Prusiner: No; immunoelectron microscopy studies show that PrP antibody reacted with PrP27-30 in liposomes. The liposomes are not pulled together; our results show where the antibody is attached.

Chesebro: The antibodies could be aggregating the proteins in the membranes of the liposome; immunogold would not show that.

Prusiner: Within a specific liposome that may be true, but the antibody is not pulling large numbers of liposomes together. For the immunoprecipitation to work we have to add a second antibody plus some large carrier, such as protein A Sepharose.

Chesebro: I think we agree that in the liposomes there could be massive aggregation of molecules by IgG antibody.

Gabizon: It is possible but it is probably much less than it was in the rods. The decrease in infectivity is greater than the increase by solubilization of the rods.

Almond: Do experiments in progress include some using Fab fragments?

Prusiner: Next week!

Carp: In your tests of dominance, have you used ME7 scrapie in your F1 mice, the NZW × I? In our hands, in the C57BL × I F1 mice the incubation period is exactly in the middle of that in the two parent strains: about 200 days versus 300 days in I mice and about 140 days in C57BL, so we don't see any dominance.

Carlson: Those preparations have been inoculated into mice; we don't have the results yet.

References

Bolton DC, Bendheim PE, Marmorstein AD, Potempska A 1987 Isolation and structural studies of the intact scrapie protein. Arch Biochem Biophys 258:579–590

Manuelidis L, Valley S, Manuelidis EE 1985 Specific proteins in Creutzfeldt-Jakob disease and scrapie share antigenic and carbohydrate determinants. Proc Natl Acad Sci USA 82:4253–4267

Prusiner SB, Groth DF, Cochran SP, Masiarz FR, McKinley MP, Martinez HM 1980 Molecular properties, partial purification, and assay by incubation period measurements of the hamster scrapie agent. Biochemistry 19:4883–4891

Final general discussion

Merz: One of the continuing enigmas in unconventional agent research is the nature of the causative agent. Evidence to date indicates that infectivity co-purifies with scrapie-associated fibrils (SAF), which are composed of a normal host protein (33-35 kDa) or its cleavage product PrP (protease resistant protein) of 25-27 kDa. At present, the SAF can be considered to be 1) a form of the transmissible agents composed either entirely of protein (prion) or of protein and a nucleic acid which does not code for the PrP, or 2) a pathological product which happens to co-purify with infectivity.

The biological evidence suggests that an agent-specific nucleic acid is required, since individual scrapie strains have been characterized. The morphology of the SAF and the Western blot profiles of the SAF PrP proteins reflect the biological diversity observed with particular scrapie strains.

In 1983, Dr Heino Diringer asked us for verification that the structures he had isolated from hamster brains infected with scrapie strain 263K were SAF. The structures were SAF and close observation of the electron micrographs indicated that a few (around 1 in 100 to 1000 SAF) had a very thin tail associated with the end of the SAF. During the course of isolating SAF and infectivity from the brains of scrapie-infected mice (scrapie strains ME7 and 139A), the thin tails were observed occasionally in preparations from ME7-infected brains and very frequently in preparations from 139A-infected brains. But the presence of the tails was inconsistent from preparation to preparation. The isolation procedure employed the proteolytic enzyme, proteinase K. The SAF and PrP proteins from 263K-infected hamsters are very resistant to this enzyme, while those from ME7 are moderately sensitive and SAF from 139A-infected brains are very sensitive to this enzyme (Kascsak et al 1985). These observations were controlled by using another type of abnormal filament, paired helical filaments (PHF), which can also be isolated under these conditions (Rubenstein et al 1986).

The presence of the tails associated with SAF suggested that the tails could be nucleic acid adventitiously bound to the SAF or released from the interior of the structure. Absence of the tails in over 100 PHF preparations observed indicated that the SAF tails may be associated with the interior of the SAF structure and not just inadvertently bound to the structure. Of course, normal animal and human brain preparations were also studied but since the abnormal fibrils are not observed in these preparations it is not surprising that the thin tails were also not observed.

Ultrastructural observations of nucleic acids extracted from normal and SAF preparations were performed but this line of experiments was discontinued for several reasons. A scrapie-specific nucleic acid has never been detected with biochemical methods, either because of the detection limits of the assay system or possibly because the nucleic acid is bonded in an unusual way which allows the nucleic acid to stay either in the phenol phase or in the protein interface. If, by chance, a distinct nucleic acid was detected in the scrapie preparations, the structure from which it originated would be unknown.

With this reasoning and the previous observations of tails associated with the SAF, experiments were designed to control the release of this tail material onto the electron microscope grid. These experiments were similar in design to those employed in the study of tobacco mosaic virus or other viruses.

The experimental design employed replicate samples placed on electron microscope grids: one was washed and negatively stained; others were exposed to various chemicals, washed and negatively stained. The experimental samples were SAF from scrapie strains 139A-, ME7- and 263K-infected animal brains. Control preparations included: similar preparations from normal animal brains: PHF from the brains of humans with Alzheimer's disease, Semliki Forest virus preparations and the bacteriophage Qβ. The samples were evaluated in the electron microscope for the presence and number of SAF, and the presence or absence of tails associated with the SAF or any other structure.

Tails associated with the SAF were not observed at a range of ionic strengths or pH levels. Low levels of sodium dodecyl sulphate (SDS) (0.1%) had no effect but tails were observed when 0.1% β-mercaptoethanol was added to the 0.1% SDS. Urea (4M) in combination with 0.8 mM dithiothreitol and 0.08 mM EDTA also revealed tails associated with SAF (Fig.1). No tails were observed with other preparations except preparations of the viruses.

Due to the difficulties of ultrastructural observation of negatively stained material, the initial tests to determine the nature of the tails employed Zn^{2+} (2-10 mM) and basic pH. The use of an enzyme could cause the deposition of a thin protein layer, obscuring the presence or absence of the tails. With this in mind, Zn^{2+}, as zinc chloride in 10 mM Tris buffer, and acid and basic pHs in 10 mM Tris buffer (adjusted with HCl or NaOH) were employed. The design of these experiments again utilized replicate samples exposed to nothing, to 4M urea, to Zn^{2+} (2-10 mM) or pH (3-13) alone, and to 4M urea plus Zn^{2+} (2-10 mM) or pH (3-13). Similar controls were employed as above.

The tails were observed with the urea treatment, and were not seen when the urea treatment was followed with Zn^{2+} or basic pH (11-13) treatment. The SAF were still present but no thin material was associated with the structures, whereas thin material had been associated with the SAF after urea treatment. To determine if the thin material was just lying along the exterior of the SAF, zinc treatment (2-10 mM) was performed before and after treatment with urea (4M). Prior treatment with the zinc ions had no effect on the release of the thin material by the urea treatment. Once the thin tails had been observed, further

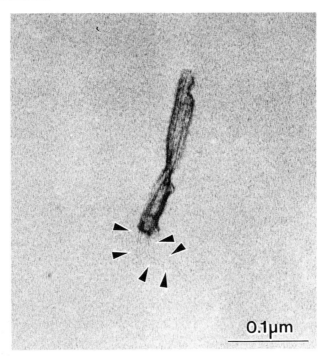

FIG. 1. (Merz) An electron micrograph illustrating the presence of tails associated with SAF isolated from mouse brains infected with scrapie strain 139A. The preparation was stained with aqueous uranyl acetate. Magnified x 198 000.

treatment with zinc ions caused the disappearance of the thin tails. Similar results were obtained with the control viral preparations.

The nature of the scrapie agent is still unsolved. The presence of the thin tails associated with the structure of SAF indicates the potential for these structures to contain additional material in the interior of the fibril. Evidence to date indicates that this material may be an RNA, since the tails are sensitive to zinc ions and basic pH. Absolute proof that this thin material is RNA is missing. Additional experiments employing nucleic acid binding proteins and hybridization studies with different nucleic acid synthetic probes are underway. If this material is related to the scrapie agent, then infectivity studies employing similar treatments may indicate its requirement for infectivity. One of the difficulties with the infectivity experiments is that they are conducted in suspension, while the above experiments were performed on biological material immobilized on the electron microscope grid. Only further experiments will reveal whether the above results reflect the nature of the scrapie agent or are tantalizing evidence of a red herring.

*Stahl:*Did you try decorating the tail with any proteins that bind nucleic acids?

Merz: I want to use an RNA binding protein and RecA. We are attempting to do nucleic acid hybridization on the grid, which has not been done. We are also attempting other mechanisms of radiolabelling on the grid and then possibly isolation–it's extremely difficult.

Hope: Have you seen any background tails without fibrils?

Merz: No, I didn't see them in the controls and I didn't see them in the background of the grid. This is 5 ml of material put on a grid from 5 ml of material.

DeArmond: One thing that all amyloids seem to have in common is that they all bind glycosaminoglycans (GAGs), in particular, heparan sulphate. We don't know whether the rods also contain GAGs, as far as I know that has not been examined. It would seem likely that there will be some GAGs associated with the SAF. Have you tried ruthenium red?

Merz: No, we have not tried ruthenium red. We have tried other reagents and the tails remained.

DeArmond: All of these amyloids are complex structures, they contain a lot of prion protein but they also probably contain glycosaminoglycans.

Almond: These are negatively stained preparations, have you shadowed?

Merz: No.

Almond: By shadowing you might be able to tell whether these tails have the thickness of a double or single strand of nucleic acid.

Prusiner: What were your conditions for the RNAse digestion and the zinc treatment?

Merz: The pre-treatment was 2 to 10 mM zinc ions, incubated at room temperature or at 37 °C. The incubation time was one hour or half an hour; the pH was neutral to acid.

Prusiner: We used a 24 hour digestion at 65 °C, pH 7 and 2 mM zinc ions; that's very different from what you have just stated.

Merz: If you go back to the original papers on zinc treatment you don't need that amount of time (Eichhorn et al 1971, Butzow & Eichhorn 1971, Butzow & Eichhorn 1975).

Prusiner: It takes about two hours at pH 7 at 65 °C to reduce RNA to mononucleotides.

Merz: Not according to the original paper. We are using labelled RNA and labelled Qβ virus for exactly that reason, to prove that an RNA is degraded under these conditions.

Prusiner: If you think that it's RNA, to hydrolyse it you should incubate your samples longer. We know that scrapie infectivity is not altered after 24 hours at 65 °C.

Merz: Are you asking about the pre-treatment, which was done to see whether or not this material was sitting alone outside the fibril and readily accessible? If that is the case, pre-treatment with zinc ions should get rid of that material and you should not then see it after opening up or disaggregating the fibril.

Prusiner: Can you see these tails without loosening up the fibril?

Merz: The initial observation was that these tails occur infrequently in 263 K isolates and very frequently in 139A isolates but I had absolutely no control over why they were there. I established conditions to try to get a good control on this observation so that I could analyse it.

Prusiner: So what do you do to open up the fibril?

Merz: Treat with 4M urea or low levels of SDS and β-mercaptoethanol.

*Prusiner:*And does that alter the infectivity?

Merz: That is being tested. I would predict that it does not alter infectivity because urea has been shown not to alter infectivity (Brown et al 1986).

Oesch: What is the frequency of these tails with respect to infectious units?

Merz: I don't know the frequency per infectious unit. The frequency of the tails per SAF, that are sitting on the grid as you open them up, is between 1 in 10 and 1 in 12. There is a 50-90% loss of SAF on the grid after treatment with urea. We have measured the number of SAF per square on grids, used that to estimate the concentration of SAF in solution, then measured the infectivity titre of the solution. The answer is 10^3 SAF per infectious unit.

Oesch: From your calculation 100 of these filamentous structures make up one infectious unit. Do these tails have a unit length?

Merz: The length varies depending on the strain of scrapie. We have used SAF isolated from 139A, ME7 and 263K scrapie. The range of tail length is 100 to 200 nm.

Beyreuther: That corresponds to about 300–600 base pairs.

Diringer: There are about 25 mg of SAF per brain in the hamster. So if you take 200 mg from 10 hamster brains, you should be able to find this nucleic acid.

Merz: There is the possibility of a small piece of nucleic acid, attached to a protein, going into the interface during protein extraction. During isolation of the nucleic acid, if you don't take this into consideration you don't know if you would even have that nucleic acid present to begin with. One reason why I gave up doing nucleic acid isolates was because there were so many assumptions built into that release.

Almond: The procedures for nucleic acid extraction use heavy protease digestion, which would chop off any terminally linked protein. If the 'nucleic acid tail' is 600 bases in length, it would be hydrophilic enough to go into the aqueous phase and not into the interface.

Paul Brown: This discussion is moving back towards the idea of a virus. With the human diseases, although it is extraordinarily difficult to conceive of sporadically occurring CJD as a contagious disease, one explanation that is still plausible is that a more or less conventional virus is being transferred at a very early age with a decades-long incubation period. It would account for the fact that the virus is not spread between people who are clinically ill. There are precedents in conventional virology, for example chicken pox, which spreads by the respiratory route during the pre-clinical stage of disease and not by the cutaneous vesicles during the clinical stage: by the time the vesicles appear infectivity is essentially finished. If you take that time period and stretch it out over decades instead of weeks, you could make a case for CJD being a contagious disease.

References

Brown P, Rohwer RG, Gajdusek DC 1986 Newer data on the inactivation of scrapie virus or Creutzfeldt-Jakob disese virus in brain tissue. J Infect Dis 153:1145–1148

Butzow JJ, Eichhorn GL 1971. Interaction of metal ions with nucleic acids and related compounds. 17. Mechanism of degradation of polyribonucleotides and oligoribonucleotides by zinc (II) ions. Biochemistry 10:2019–2027

Butzow JJ, Eichhorn GL 1975 Different susceptibility of DNA and RNA to cleavage by metal ions. Nature (Lond) 254:358–359

Eichhorn GL, Tarien E, Butzow JJ 1971 Interaction of metal ions with nucleic acids and related compounds. 16. Specific cleavage effects in depolymerization of ribonucleic acids by zinc (II) ions. Biochemistry 10:2014–2019

Kascsak RJ, Rubenstein R, Merz PA, Carp RI, Wisniewski HM, Diringer H 1985 Biochemical differences among scrapie-associated fibrils support the biological diversity of scrapie agents. J Gen Virol 66:1715–1722

Rubenstein R, Kascsak RJ, Merz PA, Wisniewski HM, Carp RI, Iqbal K 1986 Paired helical filaments associated with Alzheimer's disease are readily soluble structures. Brain Res 372:80–88

Summary

F. Brown

Wellcome Biotechnology Ltd, Langley Court, Beckenham, Kent BR3 3BS

1988 Novel infectious agents and the central nervous system. Wiley, Chichester (Ciba Foundation Symposium 135) p 267–268

The nature of the agents causing scrapie, kuru and Creutzfeld-Jakob disease has remained an enigma for more than two decades. However, the discovery in 1981 of scrapie-associated fibrils in extracts prepared from the brains of affected animals represented the starting point in an upsurge of work on this problem. With the major advances made since then on the physicochemical nature of the scrapie agent, it was inevitable that most of the discussion at the meeting should focus on this issue.

The apparent co-purification of infectivity with the fibrils and, crucially, the failure to find a scrapie-specific nucleic acid led to the controversial prion hypothesis, which postulated the existence of a self-replicating protein. The isolation of the protein in a highly purified form allowed 'reverse genetics' to be used to identify the gene coding for it. Surprisingly, it transpired that the protein is encoded by a single cellular gene which is transcribed in normal as well as scrapie-infected brains. However, the proteins from normal and infected brains differ in their susceptibility to proteinase K and it seems the differences between the two forms may be due to post-translational modification.

If the prion rods are in fact infectious, then expression of the gene in a suitable system should result in an infectious product. So far this has not been demonstrated. Whether post-translational modification of the gene product is a necessary step for infectivity to be demonstrated is a topic for urgent examination. Such a demonstration would, of course, settle the issue, but experimental evidence is required.

In the more conventional approach, the crucial issue has been the failure so far to detect a scrapie-specific nucleic acid in the purified product. If one actually exists, and the central dogma would accept no less, then precise analysis of purified brain extracts should reveal it. However, if we are dealing with low recoveries of infectivity, of the order of 1%, then the nucleic acid could easily be overlooked in the final product.

The observation made in the electron microscope by Pat Merz that the fibrils possess a fine tail-like structure, similar to that found in preparations of tobacco mosaic virus from which part of the protein shell has been removed, could be crucial to the entire problem and provide the final word. If the fractionation procedures can be refined sufficiently to allow these structures to be isolated without damaging the tails, there seems to be no reason why careful analysis should not settle the issue. Clearly, it will be vital to conduct the fractionation experiments in media which inhibit the activity of nucleases so that the tail-like structures (provided that they are in fact nucleic acid) are preserved intact. A necessary part of the experiment will be the near quantitative recovery of the infectivity of the initial extracts.

There seems to be no reason why these goals should not be achieved within the next few years. Fractionation procedures have reached a stage of refinement which should allow the tail-like structures to be isolated in reasonable yields. In addition, genetic engineering methods should allow the product obtained by expressing the prion gene to be manipulated in ways which should enable its potential infectivity to be tested. Irrespective of the route chosen and the final outcome, the nature of the scrapie agent should soon be settled.

Index of contributors

Non-participating co-authors are indicated by asterisks. Entries in bold type indicate papers; other entries refer to discussion contributions

Indexes compiled by John Rivers

Subject index